Clinics in Developmental Medicine No. 153/4
THE BIOLOGY OF THE AUTISTIC SYNDROMES
3rd Edition

© 2000 Mac Keith Press
High Holborn House, 52–54 High Holborn, London WC1V 6RL

Senior Editor: Martin C.O. Bax
Editor: Hilary M. Hart
Managing Editor: Michael Pountney
Project Editor: Sarah Pearsall

Set in Times and Avant Garde on QuarkXPress
by Keystroke, Jacaranda Lodge, Wolverhampton

First published in this edition 2000

British Library Cataloguing-in-Publication data:
A catalogue record for this book is available from the British Library

ISSN: 0069 4835
ISBN: 1 898683 22 0

Printed by The Lavenham Press Ltd, Water Street, Lavenham, Suffolk
Mac Keith Press is supported by Scope (formerly The Spastics Society)

Clinics in Developmental Medicine No. 153/4

The Biology of the Autistic Syndromes

3rd Edition

CHRISTOPHER GILLBERG
Sahlgren University Hospital
Göteborg, Sweden

MARY COLEMAN
Georgetown University School of Medicine
Washington, DC, USA

2000
Mac Keith Press

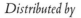 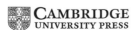

Distributed by CAMBRIDGE UNIVERSITY PRESS

AUTHORS' AFFILIATIONS

CHRISTOPHER GILLBERG, M.D., Ph.D.   Professor of Child and Adolescent
Psychiatry; Head, Child
Neuropsychiatry Clinic, University of
Göteborg, Sweden

MARY COLEMAN, M.D.   Clinical Professor Emeritus,
Department of Pediatrics,
Georgetown University School of
Medicine, Washington, DC, USA

CONTENTS

ACKNOWLEDGEMENTS

The authors wish to thank the Health Service Library of Columbia–Presbyterian Medical Center, New York and also Sasha Stallone Ash, George T. Capone, M.D., Cure Autism Now, Barbara Smith Coleman, Ira L. Cohen, Ph.D., E.H. Cook, Jr., M.D., Robert DeLong, M.D., Laura Greiner of the PARIS project, Dr. Anthony Hardan, Kathy Hunter of the International Rett Syndrome Association, Emily Kingsley, Andrea Kirshoff, Marit Korkman, M.D., Marc Lalande, Ph.D., Nancy Minshew, M.D., Tahma Metz of the Purine Research Society, Lena Nilelasson, B.A., Agneta Nydén, Ph.D., Theodore Page, Ph.D., Maria Råstam, M.D., Anna Rönneholm, John M. Shoffner, M.D., Glenn Vatter, Jan Wahlström, M.D., Lorna Wing, M.D., and Michele Zappella, M.D.

This book is dedicated to
Henri and Juliette Doucet, to Gunilla Gerland
and all the other valiant parents and
individuals affected by autism

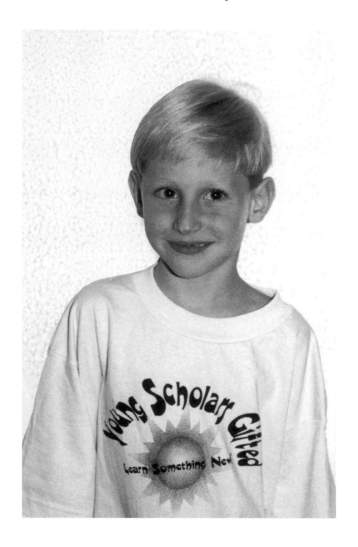

PREFACE

This book is called *The Biology of the Autistic Syndromes* because it refers to autism as a series of *syndromes*, not as a *spectrum*. There is an important distinction to be made between syndromes and spectrums; it has profound significance for diagnosis, prevention and medical therapy and needs to be fully understood.

A spectrum describes clinical variations found *within* the same disease. It is likely to be found in most diseases. For example, phenylketonuria (PKU), whose enzyme and genetic error have already been identified (see pp. 148–149), has a clinical spectrum ranging from a child with profound retardation/autism to that of a woman with such mild PKU that she is able to be married and have children (who, alas, are then damaged *in utero* by her abnormal biochemistry). PKU is an example of the wide spectrum of clinical symptoms within any one given disease entity.

In fact, when one is dealing with a single medical disease, it makes sense to talk about the often wide spectrum of clinical presentations which vary according to many factors. In psychiatry, to the extent that the underlying disease is etiologically linked to a single medical disease of the brain, the same factors influence psychiatric presentation of that disease entity. Some of the factors already known which directly affect the spectrum of clinical presentation in psychiatry in a single disease are:

- the age of the patient when the disease presents (i.e. PKU)
- different genetic alleles (*i.e.* adult metachromatic leukodystrophy – a form of schizophrenia)
- the length of the trinucleotide repeats in the newly discovered DNA triplet repeat form of genetic diseases (*i.e.* Huntington disease).

Autism, however, is not one single disease entity. It does not have one etiology. In medicine, the word "syndrome" means that a series of totally different diseases can present clinically through a final common pathway so that they resemble each other and can be confused with each other. One hundred and fifty years ago, all forms of mental retardation* were thought to be caused by the same disease, and their differences were thought to be mere clinical variations on a spectrum of mental retardation. Then Dr. John Langdon Down (1866) clinically differentiated infantile hypothyroidism (cretinism) from trisomy 21 (the chromosomal error causing Down syndrome), even though both diseases caused mental retardation and had, as a symptom, large protruding tongues in infancy. The *spectrum* of mental retardation turned into a series of different *syndromes* causing mental retardation.

---

*UK usage – learning disability.

This is the situation in autism today. Autism, like mental retardation, is a syndrome or series of syndromes caused by many different, separate individual diseases. These various diseases, some of which have specific treatments, injure that same final common pathway in the brain of a very young child which causes him or her to present with autistic symptoms. The autistic syndrome is an age-dependent behavioral disorder caused by the many diseases discussed in this textbook. Just as in mental retardation, careful differentiation of the specific cause of the autistic symptoms in each child (see Chapter 16) is already leading toward accurate genetic counseling, measures for prevention, and even specific medical therapies in some disease entities.

Is the use of the term "autistic spectrum" (Wing 1996) ever appropriate? The answer is "yes" in sorting out the exact clinical presentations (which range from infantile autism to Asperger syndrome) in an individual not yet diagnosed with a specific disease. It is a particularly useful term during the fine-tuning of educational evaluations. However, in the end, those of us who are medical doctors cannot avoid the task of diagnosing the specific underlying disease entity of each child.

Mary Coleman
Christopher Gillberg

REFERENCES

Down, J.L.H. (1866) 'Observations on an ethnic classification of idiots.' *Clinical Lectures and Reports by the Medical and Surgical Staff of the London Hospital*, **3**, 259-262.
Wing, L. (1996) *The Autistic Spectrum*. London: Constable.

1
INTRODUCTION

BE SAL U.TA-ma AMA-su I-zir
"If a woman gives birth and the infant rejects his mother"
Summa Izbu IV 42

Thousands of years ago in ancient Mesopotamia, between the Tigris and Euphrates rivers, medical information was written down on a set of durable clay tablets which have survived to the present day. The sentence above was inscribed in cuneiform signs on a tablet of medical omens. Could this be the first written description of an infant who is autistic? Sometimes an infant with autism is born so sensitive to touch at birth that the mother cannot even hold her own baby, and, in modern times, has to feed her infant by holding a bottle over the crib without touching the child (for an example, see the case history in Chapter 17, p. 271). If the medical omen above described such an infant, it is worth noting that the ancient Mesopotamians had got it right. They were clear that it was the baby, not the mother, who was doing the rejecting.

In modern times, autism was first identified by Kanner in 1943. He described 11 children who came to his office who displayed similar behavior patterns and had in common "extreme aloneness from the beginning of life and an anxiously obsessive desire for the preservation of sameness." He called them "autistic." The words "autistic/autism" have been used in different ways by different investigators causing semantic confusion. Bleuler (describing a symptom of schizophrenia) and Kanner (describing a symptom of his new disease) initially used it as an adjective; the word then became a noun (Kanner's later use and DSM-III) used to refer to a disease (Ritvo and Ritvo 1992). In 1944, Asperger described his syndrome (see Chapter 6), but it was 1981 before it obtained its status as a named syndrome (Wing 1981).

Initially, psychodynamic theories regarding the etiology of autism prevailed. These implicated parents as being the cause of the child's deviant and delayed development. As Kanner said in a popular magazine, "children with early infantile autism were the offspring of highly organized, professional parents, cold and rational, who just happened to defrost long enough to produce a child" (*Time*, July 25, 1960). Bettleheim (1967) agreed. During this period, Kanner criticized the "blindness" of colleagues (*e.g.* van Krevelen 1952, Benda and Melchior 1959) who looked for physiological causes of autism rather than focusing on parental behavior. Later Kanner (1969) said "Herewith I especially acquit you people as parents. I have been misquoted many times." He was clearly ambivalent about what was going on in these relationships. A very recent study of infants raised in Romanian orphanages has shown that autistic-like patterns of behavior have been noted in a small percentage of these truly abandoned children (Rutter *et al.* 1999).

1

There is now evidence that the right cerebral hemisphere is more developed than the left at birth in human children (Geschwind and Galaburda 1985). One theory holds that this development occurred because of the importance of right-hemisphere-mediated visual–spatial and emotional interactions with the mother as part of the bonding process. Mothers (even left-handed women) tend to cradle infants with the left arm against the left breast. This allows the infant's left visual field to see, and the left ear to hear, the mother better, since such inputs go more directly to the right hemisphere (Brumback *et al.* 1996). In babies with autism, there is a great deal of evidence of right-hemisphere dysfunction, as is documented throughout this book. Thus Kanner's initial observation of the imperfection of the mother–child relationship in autism may not have been completely wrong – simply incorrect about why it was happening and who was responsible. Professionals working in autism all know of heroic mothers of children with autism who manage to establish close bonding with their infant in spite of major obstacles in the baby's receptivity to close human relationships, but some young children with autism simply cannot tolerate such contact, no matter what is done.

Today the past controversies appear to be behind us. Almost all major psychiatric and medical centers working with autism agree that the symptoms of autism, with the possible exception of abandoned infants, are a behavioral response by young children to an organic disease of their brains. There are only a finite number of ways in which the brain can respond to injury – in the very young brain, one of those ways is what is labeled as the behavioral symptoms of autism. In fact, today it is understood that autism is a complex developmental syndrome representing a heterogeneous group of individuals with similar symptoms but multiple biological etiologies. Realizing that autism is not one disease but is a syndrome can only enhance the understanding of etiologies, prevention and treatment of this puzzling disorder. In this book, the word "autism" is used as a shorthand for "the autistic syndromes."

Throughout this textbook, autism is referred to as a behavioral syndrome, which is how it is defined. Of course, behavior is a product of many complex brain functions. Social behaviors consist of signals, generated by the motor system, processed by the perceptual systems and regulated by an elaborate cognitive system. These processes are subserved by a hard-wired, widely-distributed network that has evolved in parallel with the complex social–cultural milieu of *Homo sapiens* (Voeller 1996). The more we understand human social behavior, the more we shall understand about the failures of this system, such as autism.

One of the most encouraging developments in the field of autism is the fact that some forms of autism can now be prevented. PKU autism (see p. 148) and rubella autism (see p. 163) should become diseases of the past. In the case of PKU autism, infant-screening programs can detect this metabolic disease in the neonatal period and babies can start a therapeutic diet that will prevent the development of the disease in the first place. In the case of rubella autism, girls can be inoculated against the rubella virus prior to puberty so that there is no chance they will become infected while they are pregnant and pass the virus on to their fetuses.

Although a great deal more is known now than at the time of the writing of the second edition of this book, this third edition has few final answers. There are a series of fascinating theories about the changes in the developing brain that cause autism. The hypotheses range from the biochemical (altered serotonin modulation of the thalamo-cortical pathway (Chugani *et al.* 1999)) to the neurostructural (abnormally wired neural networks (Cohen 1994)). Many patients with an autistic syndrome do not yet have a true diagnosis of a well-defined disease entity; the majority do not have adequate medical therapies available. Important strides have been made regarding educational intervention (Chapter 18), and every child with autism needs, at a minimum, an individualized program tailored to the child's particular profile.

REFERENCES

Asperger, H. (1944) 'Die "autistischen psychopathen" im Kindesalter.' *Archiv fur Psychiatire und Nervenkrankheiten*, **117**, 76–136.

Benda, C.E., Melchior, J.C. (1959) 'Childhood schizophrenia, childhood autism and Heller's disease.' *International Record of Medicine*, **172**, 137–154.

Dettlcheim, B. (1967) *The Empty Fortress: Infantile Autism and the Birth of the Self* New York: Free Press

Bleuler, E. (1911) *Dementia Praecox or the Group of Schizophrenias*. Vienna. Translated 1952 by J. Zinkin. New York: International Universities Press.

Brumback, R.A., Harper, C.R., Weinberg, W.A. (1996) 'Nonverbal learning disabilities, Asperger's syndrome, pervasive developmental disorder – should we care?' *Journal of Child Neurology*, **11**, 427–429.

Chugani, D.C., Muzik, O., Behen, M., Rothermol, R., Janisse, J.J., Lee, J., Chugani, H.T. (1999) 'Developmental changes in brain serotonin synthesis capacity in autistic and nonautistic children.' *Annals of Neurology*, **45**, 287–295.

Cohen, I.L. (1994) 'An artificial neural network analogue of learning in autism.' *Biological Psychiatry*, **36**, 5 20.

Geschwind, N., Galaburda, A.M. (1985) 'Cerebral lateralization: biologic mechanisms, associations and pathology.' *Archives of Neurology*, **42**, 128–459.

Kanner, L. (1943) 'Autistic disturbances of affective contact.' *Nervous Child*, **2**, 217–250.

—— (1969) Keynote Address given at the Annual Meeting of the National Society of Autistic Children, Washington, DC.

Ritvo, E.R., Ritvo, R. (1992) 'Autism syndrome as a final common pathway of behavioral expression for many organic disorders. Reply.' (Letter) *American Journal of Psychiatry*, **149**, 146–147.

Rutter, M., Andersen-Wood, L., Beckett, C., Bredenkamp, D., Castle, J., Groothues, C., Kreppner, J., Keaveney, L., Lord, C., O'Conner, T.G. (1999) 'Quasi-autistic patterns following severe early global privation. English and Romanian Adoptees (ERA) Study Team.' *Journal of Child Psychology and Psychiatry*, **40**, 537–549.

van Krevelen, A.v.D. (1952) 'Early infantile autism.' *Zeitschrift fur Kinderpsychiatrie*, **19**, 91.

Voeller, K.K.S. (1996) 'Brief report: Developmental neurobiological aspects of autism.' *Journal of Autism and Developmental Disorders*, **26**, 189–193.

Wing, L. (1981) 'Asperger's syndrome: a clinical account.' *Psychological Medicine*, **11**, 115–129.

2
CLINICAL DIAGNOSIS

Autism is not a disease entity in the sense that for instance phenylketonuria is. Rather, the concept of autism (autistic disorder, childhood autism, infantile autism) represents a comprehensive diagnosis along the same lines as cerebral palsy, epilepsy or mental retardation (Gillberg 1992a). In addition, autistic disorder is but one of the variants of the many behavioral symptom constellations that occur on the so-called autism spectrum (Wing 1996). Several hundreds of papers and books have already been written under the impression that autism will one day turn out to be a disorder with a single etiology, be it psychogenic or historical. However, the behavioral syndrome of autism represents the final expression of various etiological factors (Harris 1995b). Furthermore, even within a purely behavioral phenomenological framework of autism, the complexity of the symptomatology and the difficulty of fitting all individual cases into one operational diagnostic model are striking. Hence the plural form (autistic syndromes) in the title of this book.

The term autism was coined by Bleuler (1911) to designate a category of the thought disorder that is present in schizophrenic syndromes. He saw the egocentric thinking as a core symptom of schizophrenia, and derived the word autism from the Greek word "autos" which means "self." When Kanner (1943) described infantile autism (or, rather, autistic disturbances of affective contact in young children), he used the term differently, although with special reference to schizophrenia, which he at first thought was related to infantile autism but later tried to distinguish clearly from the "Kanner syndrome." The use of the word autism in connection with this latter syndrome is somewhat misleading, implying as it does a (spurious or perhaps even non-existent) link with schizophrenia and also that "extreme aloneness" (synonymous with autism according to Kanner) is at the etiological root of the syndrome. On the other hand, there is now an emerging consensus that egocentric thinking is a central symptom in Kanner syndrome, and so autism might not be seen as a misnomer after all. In more recent years, some authors have argued for the use of terms other than autism, but so far without much success. Autism will probably be used as a descriptive term for years to come in connection with children and adults who at one time in their life show the marks of the Kanner syndrome.

Kanner's description of children with autism was accurate enough, and even though substantial progress has been made since 1943 as regards the pathogenetic mechanisms in autism, few later authors, with the possible exception of Wing (1980) and Frith (1989), have given a more vivid or clear presentation of them. Certainly, major developments in diagnostic criteria have occurred since Kanner's time, but for a classic presentation of a typical case of "narrow" autism, one is well advised to study Kanner's 1943 paper.

The diagnostic label of autism

The autistic syndromes (Coleman 1976, Coleman and Gillberg 1985) are variously referred to as *childhood autism* (Wing 1980, World Health Organization (WHO) 1993), *infantile autism* (Rutter 1978, American Psychiatric Association (APA) 1980), *autistic disorder* (APA 1987, APA 1994), *pervasive developmental disorder* (APA 1980, 1987, 1994, WHO 1993), *Kanner syndrome* (Arvidsson *et al.* 1997), *childhood psychosis* (Fish and Ritvo 1979), or just simply *autism* (Rutter and Schopler 1978). The narrow syndrome as outlined by Kanner is sometimes also referred to as *classic autism*. Of these categories, those that contain the word autism have received the most attention, and there has emerged some consensus with regard to diagnostic criteria for childhood autism and autistic disorder, which are the two concepts now most widely employed.

Autism is sometimes divided into low- and high-functioning cases, and there have also been references to middle-functioning cases in some reports. *High-functioning autism (HFA)* is the term most often used for individuals who meet diagnostic criteria for autism but whose general intellectual functioning is not in the mentally retarded range. There are considerable clinical similarities between HFA and *Asperger syndrome*. Many individuals not meeting the full criteria for HFA or Asperger syndrome (see below) fall into the category of *atypical autism*.

Several of the criteria regarded necessary for a diagnosis of autistic disorder have also been listed among the crucial features of so-called childhood psychosis/childhood schizophrenia. The label of childhood psychosis has been considered a comprehensive diagnostic term, with infantile autism constituting one of the subgroups. During the last decades of the twentieth century, leading authorities agreed to abandon the term psychosis in connection with the autistic syndromes and suggested the substitution of "developmental disorder" or "pervasive developmental disorder." The move away from the psychosis/schizophrenia branch was clearly already evident in the late 1970s when the leading scientific journal in the field changed its name from *Journal of Autism and Childhood Schizophrenia* to *Journal of Autism and Developmental Disorders*. Neither the DSM-III-R/DSM-IV (APA 1987, APA 1994), nor the ICD-10 (WHO 1993) mention the term childhood psychosis. Both diagnostic systems now refer to pervasive developmental disorders instead. The removal of the psychosis label seems to indicate a step forward in the understanding of the autistic syndromes. However, the term "pervasive developmental disorder" is not the final answer. For one thing it is unclear why severe and profound mental retardation are not included as *pervasive* developmental disorders? Also, it would seem more appropriate to regard autism as a specific rather than a pervasive disorder, particularly since it has become clear that high-functioning cases are not as rare as previously believed (Gillberg and Wing 1999).

In recent years there has been concern that Kanner's concepts have been stretched too much and that the autistic-like conditions have come to be lumped with the Kanner syndrome in an all-inclusive group of disorders or social relatedness (Rutter and Schopler 1987). Conversely, others have argued for a broadening of the concept of autism (Wing and Gould 1979, Waterhouse and Fein 1989, Wing 1989, Gillberg 1992a). Even though most authors agree that it is possible to "branch off" Kanner's form of autism from the

5

broader group now receiving diagnoses of autism and autistic-like conditions, there is no good clinical or scientific support for the notion that Kanner autism is a more "specific" kind of autism than are other forms (Gillberg 1992a, Wing 1996). For instance, the evidence of stronger validity for Kanner syndrome than for so-called Asperger syndrome (I.C. Gillberg and Gillberg 1989a, Miller and Ozonoff 1997) just is not there. Kanner, among his original criteria, included both good intellectual potential and lack of neurological dysfunction. Given today's methods of examination, these two criteria would exclude virtually all children diagnosed by Kanner himself as autistic from that category. The best-validated category appears to be a rather broader concept as advocated by Wing (1989). Her "triad of social, communication and imagination impairment" does have some better validity (Wing and Gould 1979, Steffenburg 1991, Nordin and Gillberg 1996a).

The most common term now used for the broader group of syndromes symptomatically associated with autism is *autism spectrum disorders*. However, there is some confusion over the use of this term in that it may be taken to either include or exclude autistic disorder. Thus, some authors refer to *autism spectrum disorders* (Gillberg 1990), others to *autism and autism spectrum disorders* (Szatmari 1992), and yet others to *autism and its spectrum disorders* or to *autism and related disorders*. Lorna Wing sometimes uses the term *autistic continuum* (Wing 1989). There is also synonymous use of the concept of *autism and autistic-like conditions* (Steffenburg 1991). All of these broader terms are used in roughly the same way as "pervasive developmental disorders." The authors of the present volume no longer feel confident that parents and children with autism have benefited from Kanner's original publications, implying as they did the uniqueness of a syndrome that is probably not so unique after all.

Under the broader label of autism spectrum disorders, as used by Gillberg (1990), one would find included:

1 autistic disorder
2 Asperger syndrome
3 disintegrative disorder
4 other autistic-like conditions (equivalent to *atypical autism* or *pervasive developmental disorder not otherwise specified (PDDNOS)*).

(See Fig. 2.1.)

The diagnostic criteria for autism
The criteria for autism (autistic disorder, childhood autism, autistic syndromes) currently agreed upon by most authorities are:

1 severe abnormality of reciprocal social relatedness
2 severe abnormality of communication development (including language)
3 restricted, repetitive behavior (and patterns of behavior), interests, activities and imagination
4 early onset (before age 3 to 5 years).

Umbrella term: the autism spectrum			

Synonyms:
autism spectrum disorders, autism and its spectrum disorders, autism and autistic-like conditions, autistic continuum, pervasive developmental disorders, empathy disorders

Named syndromes in the spectrum
(and the synonyms)

Kanner syndrome	*Asperger syndrome*	*Heller syndrome*	*Atypical autism*
autistic disorder	Asperger's disorder	disintegrative disorder	other autistic-like conditions
childhood autism	autistic psychopathy	dementia infantilis	PDDNOS
infantile autism	schizoid personality disorder*		
early infantile autism	high-functioning autism**		
classic autism			

Fig. 2.1 The autism spectrum.

* overlapping but not synonymous
** some authors regard this as synonymous, others as overlapping with Asperger syndrome

The first three of these criteria are usually inferred when reference is made to the *triad of social impairment* (also *triad of social, communication and imagination impairments* or, simply, *Wing's triad*) (Wing and Gould 1979).

The four criteria agree well with those set out for infantile autism by Rutter (1978) and the DSM-III (APA 1980). They are very similar to those for childhood autism in the ICD-10 (*e.g.* WHO 1993). The DSM-III-R (APA 1987) and the DSM-IV also agree that criteria 2, 3 and 4 in the above definition are essential for a diagnosis of autistic disorder to be made. However, in the DSM-III-R no specified age of onset is required (only that onset shall be in childhood and that age shall be specified) (see Table 2.1). A statistical analysis of a series of autism spectrum cases found criteria A1 and C4 of the DSM-III-R (see Table 2.1) to have the strongest discriminating capacity of the 16 criteria in differentiating autistic disorder from other conditions (Siegel *et al.* 1989). These two criteria are very similar to those considered essential by Kanner and Eisenberg (1956) – that is, autistic aloneness and elaborate repetitive routines.

Many authors (*e.g.* Coleman 1976, Ornitz 1983, Coleman and Gillberg 1985) would consider a fifth criterion important for a definite diagnosis to be made, namely abnormal responses to sensory stimuli. This criterion is supported by a number of studies on early

TABLE 2.1
Diagnostic criteria for autism according to different manuals/authors

Diagnostic criteria for infantile autism according to DSM-III (APA 1980)
1 Onset before 30 months of age.
2 Pervasive lack of responsiveness to other people (autism).
3 Gross deficits in language development.
4 If speech is present, peculiar speech patterns such as immediate and delayed echolalia, metaphorical language, pronominal reversal.
5 Bizarre responses to various aspects of the environment, *e.g.* resistance to change, peculiar interest in or attachments to animate or inanimate objects.
6 Absence of delusions, hallucinations, loosening of associations, and incoherence as in schizophrenia.

Diagnostic criteria for autistic disorder according to DSM-III-R (APA 1987)
At least eight of the following sixteen items must be present, these to include at least two items from A, one from B, and one from C.

Note: consider a criterion to be met *only* if the behavior is abnormal for the person's developmental level.

A Qualitative impairment in reciprocal social interaction as manifested by the following:

(*Note*: the examples within parentheses are arranged so that those first mentioned are more likely to apply to younger or more handicapped, and the later ones to older or less handicapped, persons with this disorder.)

1 Marked lack of awareness of the existence of feelings of others (*e.g.* treats a person as if he or she were a piece of furniture; does not notice another person's distress; apparently has no concept of the need of others for privacy).
2 No, or abnormal, seeking of comfort at times of distress (*e.g.* does not come for comfort even when ill, hurt, or tired; seeks comfort in a stereotyped way, *e.g.* says "cheese, cheese, cheese" whenever hurt).
3 No, or impaired, imitation (*e.g.* does not wave bye-bye; does not copy mother's domestic activities; mechanical imitation of others' actions out of context).
4 No, or abnormal, social play (*e.g.* does not actively participate in simple games; prefers solitary play activities; involves other children in play only as "mechanical aids").
5 Gross impairment in ability to make peer friendships (*e.g.* not interested in making peer friendships; despite interest in making friends, demonstrates lack of understanding of conventions of social interaction, *e.g.* reads phone book to uninterested peer).

B Qualitative impairment in verbal and non-verbal communications, and in imaginative activity, as manifested by the following:

(The numbered items are arranged so that those first listed are more likely to apply to younger or more handicapped, and the later ones to older or less handicapped, persons with this disorder.)

1 No mode of communication, such as communicative babbling, facial expression, gesture, mime, or spoken language.
2 Markedly abnormal non-verbal communication, as in the use of eye-to-eye gaze, facial expression, body posture, or gestures to initiate or modulate social interaction (*e.g.* does not anticipate being held, stiffens when held, does not look at the person or smile when making a social approach, does not greet parents or visitors, has a fixed stare in social situations).
3 Absence of imaginative activity, such as play-acting of adult roles, fantasy characters, or animals; lack of interest in stories about imaginary events.
4 Marked abnormalities in the production of speech, including volume, pitch, stress, rate, rhythm, and intonation (*e.g.* monotonous tone, question-like melody, or high pitch).
5 Marked abnormalities in the form of content of speech, including stereotyped and repetitive use of speech (*e.g.* immediate echolalia or mechanical repetition of television commercial); use of "you" when "I" is meant (*e.g.* using "You want cookie?" to mean "I want cookie"); idiosyncratic use of words or phrases (*e.g.* "Go on green riding" to mean "I want to go on the swing"); or frequent irrelevant remarks (*e.g.* starts talking about train schedules during a conversation about sports).

6 Marked impairment in the ability to initiate or sustain a conversation with others, despite adequate speech (*e.g.* indulging in lengthy monologues on one subject regardless of interjections from others).

C Markedly restricted repertoire of activities and interests, as manifested by the following:

1 Stereotyped body movements, *e.g.* hand-flicking or -twisting, spinning, head-banging, complex whole-body movements.
2 Persistent preoccupation with parts of objects (*e.g.* sniffing or smelling objects, repetitive feeling of texture of materials, spinning wheels of toy cars), or attachment to unusual objects (*e.g.* insists on carrying around a piece of string).
3 Marked distress over changes in trivial aspects of environment, *e.g.* when a vase is moved from its usual position.
4 Unreasonable insistence on following routine in precise detail, *e.g.* insisting that exactly the same route always be followed when shopping.
5 Markedly restricted range of interests and a preoccupation with one narrow interest, *e.g.* interested only in lining up objects, in amassing facts about meteorology, or in pretending to be a fantasy character.

D Onset during infancy or childhood
   Specify if childhood onset (after 36 months of age).

Diagnostic criteria for autistic disorder according to DSM-IV (APA 1994), similar to ICD-10 (WHO 1993)

A A total of six (or more) items from 1, 2, and 3 with at least two from 1, and one each from 2 and 3:

1 Qualitative impairment in social interaction, as manifested by at least two of the following:
   a marked impairment in the use of multiple non-verbal behaviors, such as eye-to-eye gaze, facial expression, body postures, and gestures to regulate social interaction
   b failure to develop peer relationships appropriate to developmental level
   c a lack of spontaneous seeking to share enjoyment, interests, or achievements with other people (*e.g.* by a lack of showing, bringing, or pointing out objects of interest)
   d lack of social or emotional reciprocity

2 Qualitative impairment in communication as manifested by at least one of the following:
   a delay in, or total lack of, the development of spoken language (not accompanied by an attempt to compensate through alternative modes of communication such as gesture or mime)
   b in individuals with adequate speech, marked impairment in the ability to initiate or sustain a conversation with others
   c stereotyped and repetitive use of language or idiosyncratic language
   d lack of varied, spontaneous make-believe play, or social imitative play, appropriate to developmental level

3 Restricted repetitive and stereotyped patterns of behavior, interests and activities, as manifested by at least one of the following:
   a encompassing preoccupation with one or more stereotyped and restricted patterns of interest, which is abnormal either in intensity or focus
   b apparently inflexible adherence to specific, non-functional routines or rituals
   c stereotyped and repetitive motor mannerisms (*e.g.* hand- or finger-flapping or -twisting, or complex whole-body movements)
   d persistent preoccupation with parts of objects

B Delays or abnormal functioning in at least one of the following areas, with onset prior to age 3 years:

1 Social interaction.
2 Language as used in social communication.
3 Symbolic or imaginative play.

C The disturbance is not better accounted for by Rett's disorder or childhood disintegrative disorder.

symptoms in autism (Dahlgren and Gillberg 1989, Ornitz 1989, Gillberg *et al.* 1990). However, in order to achieve consensus in the criteria, we have decided not to include it among the necessary diagnostic items, since we consider that criteria 2, 3 and 4 are necessary and sufficient and that the "purity" of autism would not be enhanced by demanding the inclusion of the abnormal sensory response criterion.

Before discussing specific criteria, we need to be aware that a majority of children with autism are also mentally retarded. We have to bear this in mind in order that distinctions between autism and mental retardation "symptoms" are kept as clear as possible. A minority of children with classic autism function in the normal or near-normal IQ range. The behavior patterns unique to autism are often most clearly evident in such children.

Also, we need to keep in mind that Kanner autism, as already mentioned, is possibly on a spectrum not only with Asperger syndrome (Wing 1981a) and other high-functioning autistic-like conditions – not uncommonly encountered in "DAMP" (deficits in attention, motor control and perception) (I.C. Gillberg and Gillberg 1989b) and "ADHD" (attention-deficit/hyperactivity disorder) (APA 1994) – but also with low-functioning conditions – often referred to as "the triad of social impairments with severe mental retardation" (Wing and Gould 1979). Any cut-off between the various subcategories on the autism spectrum appears to be relatively arbitrary. The overlap of classic autism and the afore-mentioned syndromes, plus the fact that in certain individuals with other diagnoses (obsessive-compulsive disorder, tic syndromes, anorexia nervosa, paranoid syndromes) there may be a history – or even persistent symptoms – of autism, have led some authors to speculate that underlying all the phenomenological syndromes might be a common psychological denominator. In the chapter on neuropsychology (Chapter 9) we shall see that autism spectrum disorders share a common lack (or failure of normal development) of a "theory of mind" (the ability to conceive of other people as having mental states). Having a well-developed theory of mind might be seen as synonymous with having "empathy." This, in turn, has led to the suggestion that autism might be but one of several subclasses among *"disorders of empathy"* (Gillberg 1992a). Individuals with autism and autistic-like conditions also appear to share a deficient "drive for central coherence" (the ability to piece together details so as to arrive at a comprehensive/whole picture/concept). This neuropsychological deficit could be another common denominator linking classic autism with other neuropsychiatric syndromes with autistic symptomatology.

EARLY ONSET

With regard to the age of onset, most clinicians and researchers seem to agree that the behavioral disorder – or some major indication of abnormal development – must have been apparent before age 30 to 36 months (Rutter 1978, APA 1980, Coleman and Gillberg, 1985, WHO 1993). However, some would require an even earlier age of onset, while others (Lotter 1966, Wing and Gould 1979) would allow the appearance of first symptoms to be delayed until the child's fifth birthday. Some authors have gone further still (Bohman *et al.* 1983) and have accepted cases with onset up to the age of 7 years. Certain manuals (*e.g.* the DSM-III-R) do not specify a precise age-of-onset criterion at all. Nevertheless, the age limit of 2½ to 3 years is widely accepted.

Evans-Jones and Rosenbloom (1978), while arguing that disintegrative psychosis (childhood disintegrative disorder in the ICD-10) forms a separate diagnostic category from autism, maintain that sometimes the symptoms (which are often symptoms compatible with a diagnosis of autism) may begin before 2½ years of age, and yet not qualify the child for a diagnosis of autism but rather for disintegrative disorder (see Table 2.2 on p. 25). There is a problem in the diagnostic manuals that are currently used (DSM-IV, ICD-10), in that there is confusion with regard to the age-of-onset criterion that is supposed to separate autism from disintegrative disorder: autism should be diagnosed when specific criteria apply before age 3 years, but disintegrative disorder can be diagnosed when those same criteria apply after age 2 years. Adding to this confusion is the introduction of the label "late onset autism" (Volkmar and Cohen 1989), which is intended for cases with autistic symptoms emerging after the age of about 18 to 24 months (as opposed to "early onset autism" with symptoms of autism before that age).

Even though the criterion of early onset rarely causes much dispute in controversies over diagnostic symptoms in autism, the description of typical autistic syndromes beginning in previously normal people between the ages of 4 and 31 years in connection with herpes encephalitis (DeLong *et al.* 1981, Gillberg 1986, I.C. Gillberg 1991) shows clearly that the matter cannot be regarded as settled. As has already been noted, the DSM-III-R does not include specified early onset among the diagnostic criteria.

In the great majority of cases with autistic syndromes, however, onset is quite clearly during the first years and often even in the first six months of life. Wing (1989) has suggested that "infantile autism" is congenital in approximately 80 per cent of cases. In the remaining 20 per cent there is either too scanty evidence from the medical history, or there are definite clues that the typical symptoms began at some time between the ages of 6 and 20 months. Only rarely are there cases that commence around age 30 months or later. Cases with documented set-back after a period of clearly normal development are rare, but their relative frequency within the whole group is not known. The possibility of an underlying seizure disorder should always be considered in cases with autistic regression around 18–30 months (Rapin and Katzman 1998).

Many authors have assumed that the early onset of the disorder is one of the reasons for symptoms taking on such a stereotyped and primitive appearance. While this seems reasonable in a developmental–theoretical perspective, the whole notion is contradicted by the clear documentation of Kanner-type autism with onset as late as 14 years of age.

Conversely, it should be made clear that symptom onset after, for instance, 18 months of age does not mean that the disorder may not be congenital. One possibility in such cases is that there may be a brain abnormality allowing normal development up to a specific age, but that, later, the available neural circuitries can no longer match the requirements for further development and only then will symptoms begin to appear.

SEVERE RESTRICTION OF THE ABILITY TO ENGAGE IN RECIPROCAL SOCIAL INTERACTION

The disturbance of social relatedness – as with all other symptoms – has to be out of proportion in comparison with the often concomitant mental retardation. The central

11

features of this abnormality are a markedly decreased capacity for reciprocity in social interactions, with resulting extreme egocentricity and a failure to recognize the uniqueness of other human beings (Rutter 1983, Wing 1989, Gillberg 1992a).

Frith (1989) has suggested that the basic failure in autism is the lack of early development of a "theory of mind" or the ability to "mentalize," such that a child with autism cannot conceive that other people think and feel and certainly cannot intuit *what* they think and feel (see Chapter 15). This "underdeveloped" mentalizing capacity will inevitably lead to extreme deficits in empathy, showing in all interactions with people. The empathy deficits, however, will not affect the ability to observe the world or to reason logically about visible and audible realities. Neither will basic emotions such as anger, fear or happiness necessarily be affected.

Antecedents of the restriction in mentalizing abilities can be seen in reduced capacity for "shared attention" (Sigman *et al.* 1986) and in failure to develop skills associated with attracting other people's attention, such as pointing (Baron-Cohen 1995).

Some children with autism, during the first three years of life (and to a lesser extent later also) already display, in Kanner's words (1943), an "extreme autistic aloneness." Others are described as "easy so long as they are left to themselves in their bed or in their room." Still others are difficult, "terrible," or scream at all hours and need little sleep. Imitation and imitation play is abundant in some children, but absent in others (Wing 1980).

The "typical" child with autism fails to follow the gaze direction of other people (and is therefore sometimes said to lack the so-called eye direction detector), avoids eye contact, stares into thin air or is observed to have an abnormal gaze contact, from before the end of the first year of life (Mirenda *et al.* 1983). Many children gaze out of the corner of the eye or cast fleeting glances at people or goings-on. Quite a number do not show anticipatory movements when about to be picked up, may resist being held or touched, and will not "adjust" to "fit" in a hug or something similar. However, contrary to popular belief, many children with autism enjoy body contact, which may constitute their only mode of "communication" with other people. Infants who later receive a diagnosis of autism have often seemed to lack initiative, and the interested curiosity and exploratory behavior seen in normal babies are often completely lacking.

Frequent comments include: "He was so happy if we left him all to himself, but started to scream as soon as someone picked him up"; "She was so stiff to hold"; or "I don't know what it was, but he just wasn't 'there.'" There is an impression that humans, animals and soft and hard objects are treated alike. People are often treated by the children as if they were technical tools, there only for the benefit of the children to reach certain objects (exemplified by the child who leads their mother's hand, not only by the hand but by the wrist, to their spoon, and then directs the spoon via the mother's hand/wrist to their own mouth). The child does not usually come to parents, brothers or sisters – or anybody else for that matter – for help or comfort or to share positive experiences.

However, not all children with autism show these typical features and, even in those who do, there is often a gradual decrease in the severity of symptoms after the first three to five years of life.

Typical of all in the early preschool years is a failure to develop normal relationships with age-peers. This inability persists throughout childhood, adolescence and often into adult life.

As the child grows older, the abnormalities of social relatedness become less immediately obvious, particularly if the child is seen in familiar surroundings. The resistance to being touched and held often decreases with age, even though rough-and-tumble play is sometimes preferred to gentle stroking. The delayed and abnormal gaze behaviors may decrease, particularly if concrete cues such as pointing are provided (Leekam *et al.* 1998). There is evidence (Rutter 1978, Mirenda *et al.* 1983, Willemsen-Swinkels *et al.* 1998) to suggest that it is not the amount of gaze contact that is abnormal in autism, but rather that – at least after infancy – there is qualitative difference, the gaze of people with autism being stiffer and lasting longer on an individual basis. The most striking feature in school-age children and adolescents is often that of a "wide-open, unknowing" gaze that may be interpreted as showing "confusion." The ability to use gaze contact for regulation of the ongoing social interaction is markedly reduced in a vast majority of all cases (APA 1994). However, as already noted, it is not the actual amount of gazing that is abnormal, but rather a deficit in the "checking" function of gaze, such as evidenced in the decreased returning of gaze and following the direction of gaze in others. In some instances – *e.g.* autism associated with the fragile X chromosome abnormality – there is clear gaze avoidance (Hagerman 1989), and it seems likely that, with the emergence of more and more etiological subgroups, a multifaceted view of gaze abnormalities in autism will emerge. What is already quite clear at this stage is that gaze avoidance is definitely not a necessary feature of autism at any age.

Symptoms pertaining to the avoidance of visual or physical contact are often classified in the category of social abnormalities. However, several authors, including Wing (1980) and the present authors (Coleman and Gillberg 1985, Gillberg *et al.* 1990), would argue that these abnormalities are best dealt with in the context of abnormal sensory responses. Be that as it may, as these symptoms reduce, the child becomes somewhat more cooperative and easy to relate to. Unfortunately, in most cases the inability to play reciprocally with age-peers remains sadly unchanged throughout the years, although this characteristic may not be as conspicuously apparent in the school-age child with autism as it was during the preschool years.

In some cases, and at some stages of development, the abnormality of social relatedness takes on the form of a lack of selectivity and distance. However, even in children with autism who show seemingly attention-seeking, distance-lacking behavior, the inability to reciprocate and the failure to treat humans as anything but objects are clearly evident. These hallmarks differentiate their behavior from superficially similar behavior seen in emotionally deprived children.

SEVERE RESTRICTION OF THE ABILITY TO COMMUNICATE RECIPROCALLY
The decreased capacity for communication – verbally *and* non-verbally – is difficult, if possible at all, to separate out from the reduced ability to interact socially. Some

authorities argue that the communicative problems in autism underlie the social impairments, whereas others see them as two slightly different symptoms of a common underlying abnormality; that is, the reduced capacity to understand the *meaning* of interaction. In any case, it is essential to understand that the communication deficit in autism is not to do with spoken language *per se*, but with a failure to grasp the meaning of communication (Frith 1989).

Usually from a very early age, the child with autism shows major problems in the comprehension of human mime, gesture and speech, and, accordingly, shows little social use of communication skills. Social imitation is lacking or deficient (Heimann *et al.* 1995), and common early imitation play such as waving bye-bye or playing pat-a-cake is not elicitable (Baron-Cohen *et al.* 1992). Some – though by no means all, perhaps not even the majority (Gillberg *et al.* 1990) – do not babble, and some yield strange monotonous sounds instead of the varied babble patterns heard in normal children.

Abnormal babbling is often inferred to be a crucial symptom of abnormal language development in autism. Actually there is little scientific evidence to uphold such a view, and some children with autism have seemingly normal early language development (according to parental interview data), which might be taken to contradict clear-cut abnormalities of babble (Dahlgren and Gillberg 1989, Gillberg *et al.* 1990). In fact, language and babbling may be more discrete functions and not as intrinsically interwoven as hitherto believed (Zetterström 1983).

Almost without exception, children with autism are delayed in their development of spoken language. However, it is quite common for children with autism to develop anything from a few to several dozen words before the age of 2 years, only to stop speaking for one or several years – or, indeed, for ever. The expressive language delay runs parallel with an impairment in the understanding of spoken language, which may vary from an almost total lack of understanding to more subtle deviancies leading to literal interpretation. An example of this kind of literal interpretation is provided by a 10-year-old girl with autism, with a full-scale WISC IQ of 100, who appeared panic-stricken when a nurse, about to do a simple blood test said: "Give me your hand; it won't hurt." The girl calmed down immediately when another person, who knew her well, said: "Stretch out your index finger." The girl had understood, at the first instruction, that she was required to cut off her hand and give it to the nurse. Comprehension is usually severely impaired in those high-functioning persons with autism who excel in the use of vocabulary.

Many children with autism learn to follow simple instructions if given in a particular social context, but appear to fail to grasp the meaning of these instructions when given out of that context. Quite unlike deaf children, children with autism make little, if any, use of mime or gesture. Often they seem totally to misinterpret human facial expressions and begin to laugh when somebody cries or vice versa.

Approximately one in two children with autism fails to develop useful spoken language. The vast majority of these are also mentally retarded (usually severely or profoundly so). Of those who do develop speech, all show major abnormalities of speech development, such as sustained phases of seemingly non-communicative, immediate and/or delayed echolalia (which is present only during short phases and integrated with the development of communicative speech in normal children), avoidance or confusion of personal pronouns (such as the substitution of "you," "he" or the child's first name for "I," "he" for "she" and "you" for "we," thought to be a consequence of the echolalia), confusion of prepositions, and repetitive speech which involves talking *to* rather than *with* someone. The echolalia encountered in autism is often so well developed that the casual listener/observer will have difficulty in recognizing the severity of the abnormality of language.

Some may parrot whole conversations and go on talking as if at a cocktail party or ask endless questions. Those who constantly ask questions often become very irritating for people around them. It is sometimes difficult to understand why they should want to ask all these questions when everybody knows that they know all the answers. If a theory of mind deficit underlies autism, it becomes easier to accept that people with autism can only ask questions to which they already know the answers. If you cannot conceive that other people have mental states or, as it were, "inner worlds," how can you ask them about matters unknown to you? They observe that other people ask questions and respond to them, but they do not know the true meaning of asking questions (the wish/need to acquire new knowledge, whether about basic facts or about mental states such as thoughts, beliefs and feelings). Hence, all they can do is to remain mute, or, if feeling the need to take after other people in whatever minor ways, to ask only those questions to which they already know the answers.

We have come across quite a number of people with autism who eventually develop some communicative language, but who, nevertheless, retain some of their echolalia in that they whisper in an echolalic fashion every question directed at them. This may be particularly common in autism associated with the fragile X chromosome abnormality (Gillberg 1992b). Palilalia (the repetition of your own single words or phrases) is also quite common in higher-functioning individuals – just as it is in Tourette syndrome.

A minority of people with autism not only parrot conversations in an echolalic fashion, but imitate one's every movement and gesture. This phenomenon is sometimes referred to as echopraxia.

Some talking children with autism have very good rote memory skills and can repeat whole conversations word for word. However, these same children may find it very difficult, or may not be able at all, to extract meaning from sentences based on the order and the meaning of the words (Hermelin and O'Conner 1970).

Non-speaking people with autism may be able to imitate and sing songs with baffling accuracy and some may even know the words of the song without being able to repeat them without singing.

In speaking children with autism it has been commonly noted that they can relate a series of real events if allowed to do so according to their own rigid structure of telling about the events, but cannot do so if interrupted by questions or remarks. Especially in brighter children with autism, there may be quite a lot of spontaneous speech. Rarely, if ever, do they communicate to others about their feelings and needs. They may hold lengthy and detailed disquisitions on the subject of a given, concrete experience, such as a dinner, or travelling on a bus, but will usually be unable to answer even simple questions about this same topic, in spite of having no difficulty at all "recreating" the whole journey from start to finish in their own very concrete, descriptive words.

It is important to make note of the fact that comprehension of spoken language is always seriously compromised in autism. Even in high-functioning individuals who have well-developed expressive speech there are usually severe comprehension problems. They may be able to understand most single words such as substantives and verbs (and even adjectives referring to visible or audible phenomena) and yet have enormous difficulty comprehending what these words mean if sequenced together, and particularly if set in a social context. In other words, their pragmatic comprehension skills are very limited. Some high-functioning people with autism may have better skills with regard to language comprehension if they are allowed to read a text than if they hear the same text spoken by somebody. It appears that spoken language produces few, if any, "mental states/pictures" in people suffering from the syndrome of autism.

There are often grammatical immaturities consistent with the overall developmental level of the child's speech (Bartak *et al.* 1975).

Typically there are peculiarities in respect to vocal volume and pitch, with a tendency to use staccato-like or scanning speech. Problems of pronunciation arise when using spontaneous, but not echo, phrases (Wing 1966, Howlin 1982). This can mean that when language spoken by people with autism sounds stiff or monotonous it is more likely to be communicative than when it sounds "perfect" or "just as though it had been spoken by somebody else."

Judging from the, so far limited, study of high-functioning people with autism, it appears that a flat prosody may be more characteristic than any other problems in the language domain. Also, it is important to note the abnormalities of mime and gesture which usually prevail throughout the life of people on the autism spectrum. Little facial mimicry (including stiff and stereotyped smiles on the one hand, and "depressed" appearance on the other) and an extreme poverty, or indeed absence, of gesture are typical of almost all cases.

SEVERE RESTRICTION OF IMAGINATIVE ABILITIES WITH A SMALL AND RIGID BEHAVIORAL REPERTOIRE

Children with autism often form bizarre attachments to certain objects or parts of objects, such as stones, curls of hair, pins, pieces of plastic toys or metals. They may also be fascinated by any object that glitters (glasses, earrings, necklaces, etc.). The objects are usually selected because of some particular quality (*e.g.* colour, surface texture) and are carried or followed around by the child, who becomes distressed or even frantic if anybody tries to remove them. Other children line up toys or household equipment for hours on end. Round and spinning objects, such as wheels of toy cars, coins, CDs and cassette-players often hold a distinct fascination for children with autism (see Fig. 2.2).

Many children, adolescents and adults with autism demand that certain routines be adhered to in a pathologically rigid fashion. One 6-year-old boy insisted that his mother had to put the frying pan on the stove and heat some butter in it before he would have his breakfast. This "show," as it was, had to be put on every morning or he would scream for

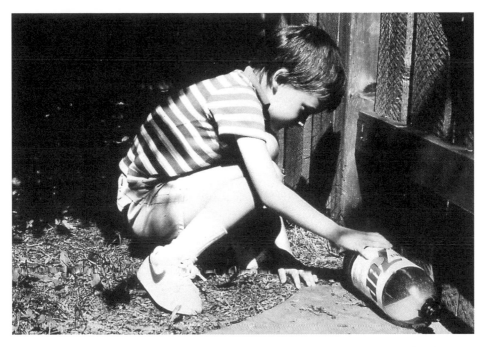

Fig. 2.2 *(Above)* Children with autism often prefer to play with shiny or mobile trash rather than toys. *(Below)* Even a flickering birthday candle can be a source of visual stimulation.

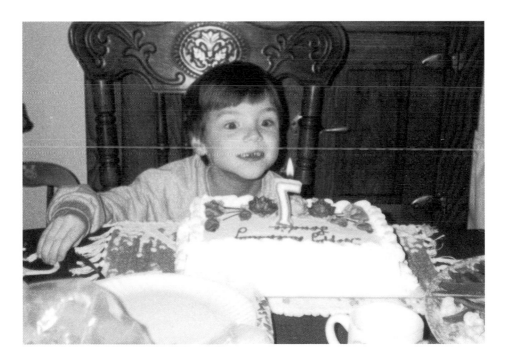

hours, refusing to eat altogether. Another boy of 7 would eat only if one of the legs of his father's chair was one inch away from one leg of the dinner table and his mother had one elbow on the table. A girl of 4 would scream in rage if her mother did not always take her twice around the block going to the right (as she had done the very first time she took her out in the pram).

It is often impossible to predict what environmental change will cause the emotional outbursts. On the whole, it appears that minor changes tend to be more upsetting and to cause more severe temper tantrums than do major changes. For instance, a 5-year-old boy cried desperately for almost an hour until his mother realized that she had removed a book from one of the shelves of the bookcase. When she put it back, he stopped crying within seconds. This boy, who was considered by his parents and professionals as unable to cope with even the smallest kind of environmental change, accepted going abroad without any outward reaction at all.

The "insistence on sameness" may also affect the verbal skills of the child, who may demand that only certain words or phrases be used or that things be talked about or repeated in exactly the same fashion. As noted above, standard questions with demands for standard answers are common.

Especially during the school years and after, some relatively brighter persons with autism show unusual preoccupations with, for example, weather reports, birthdays or train schedules.

Various other ritualistic and obsessive-compulsive phenomena are common. Some people with obsessive-compulsive disorders are very much aware that their rituals are unhelpful and limit their capacity for doing other things. People with autism are usually not as well aware of the disabling nature of their own rituals, but their obsessive-compulsive behaviors may be very similar to those of people who are diagnosed as suffering from obsessive-compulsive disorder. Also, among children with the latter diagnosis, there are many who are not aware that their rituals are "negative." It has been our experience that some children receive a diagnosis of obsessive-compulsive disorder when, in fact, they show all the hallmarks of autism. Conversely, many children with classic autism would also qualify for a diagnosis of obsessive-compulsive disorder.

Some authors include less complex stereotypic behavior – such as simple stereotypies or toe-walking – among the elaborate repetitive routines. Even though some stereotypies – especially hand-flapping with flexion of the elbows and extremely "high" tip-toeing – appear to be rather typical of autism, most authors do not include these kinds of stereotypic behaviors as *necessary* criteria for a diagnosis of autism. Nevertheless, in low-functioning individuals with autism, elaborate motor routines (stereotypies) may be the only way of "expressing" the repetitive behavior pattern considered essential for a diagnosis of autism to be made. The stereotypies are sometimes difficult to separate from simple or complex motor tics (Comings 1990), and it is possible that these different labels are sometimes applied to the same motor phenomena.

One way of looking at the "behavioral criterion" of the autism diagnosis would be to say that the restricted pattern reflects the fact that you can only do what you know how to do. People with autism, because of their inability to communicate with the "inner worlds" of other people, have to learn through copying what they see, hear or sense in other ways. This will necessarily mean a severe restriction of the behavioral repertoire even in high-functioning cases. In low-functioning individuals, repetitive motor patterns may be the only behaviors that individuals with autism may know, whereas in higher-functioning cases more elaborate patterns of behavior may be possible.

Symptoms which are almost universal but not among the diagnostic criteria

There are many symptoms commonly encountered in autism that are currently not considered part of the set of diagnostic criteria necessary and sufficient for a diagnosis to be made. Abnormal sensory responses are the most important of these, in that they are probably universally occurring and may actually underlie some of the symptoms considered primary for the diagnostic decision.

ABNORMAL RESPONSES TO SENSORY STIMULI

One of the most characteristic symptoms of autism in young children – the markedly abnormal responses to sensory stimuli – is not currently among the defining diagnostic features of the disorder. However, in our experience, all children with typical autism have shown abnormal responses to sensory stimuli when very young.

Of these symptoms, an abnormal response to sound may be thought of as the most characteristic of all. The child who "acts deaf" and does not react at all when an explosion is unexpectedly heard nearby may moments later turn at the sound of a paper being removed from a chocolate. Many children with autism cover their ears to shut out even "ordinary" noise levels. There may also be strange reactions, such as the covering of ears or eyes at a special sound. There is often an extreme variability in the reaction to sound from one second to another.

Abnormal responses to visual stimuli are probably present in a large majority of young children with autism, who often give the impression of having difficulty recognizing the things they see. People may ask the parents if the child is blind; in fact, every now and then autism is mistaken for blindness. Some children with delayed visual maturation show many or all of the symptoms of autism (Goodman and Ashby 1990). (It may need emphasizing here that some children actually suffer from both blindness and autism – see below, p. 26.) The peculiarities of gaze reported above in the section on abnormality of social relatedness could also be taken as evidence of abnormal perceptual responses, as could the extreme fascination with contrasts of light (including that produced by shadows in the sunshine).

Reduced or in other ways abnormal sensitivity to pain, heat or cold is often encountered in autism. A typical example is that of a boy who seemingly derives pleasure by biting the back of his hand. Some children withdraw or squeal if touched or stroked lightly, but enjoy being handled roughly. Other kinds of tactile stimuli may give pleasure to a child who can stand for half an hour or so just feeling and scratching differently textured surfaces.

One boy of 7 years was "helping" his mother by the stove. He put his hand down and did not remove it until the smell of burnt flesh attracted his interest. He had to undergo several operations after this, but his hand function was never totally recovered. He did not seem to experience pain or heat from the burn wound. Another Swedish boy of 9 years got up early on one extremely cold morning and went out, naked, to play in the snow for what must have been more than an hour without feeling the need for warm clothes (and, incidentally, without any untoward consequences).

Children with autism often want to smell people and objects. This is a characteristic not usually encountered in normal development or in mental retardation without major autistic features.

By and large, clinical experience suggests that perceptions relating to auditory and tactile stimuli may be more impaired in autism than are perceptions of visual and, especially, olfactory stimuli. The two latter functions make their first intracranial nerve connections at a higher level in the nervous system than do the two former. A preference for proximal stimuli has also been experimentally evidenced in autism (Hermelin and O'Conner 1970). Masterton and Biederman (1983) have argued that proprioceptive input dominates over visual input in children with autism. They see this dominance as the effect of an alternative strategy to compensate for a lack of visual control over fine motor performance. In this context, it is of some interest that certain children, who otherwise yield good gaze contact, can talk coherently only when avoiding gaze contact.

Although abnormal sensory responses in autism are regarded by many as "primary," and in their view should therefore be included among the diagnostic criteria, the most influential diagnostic manuals do not do so. Nevertheless, most authorities agree that, for instance, "undue sensitivity to sound" is an extremely common feature in autism and that it differentiates autism from, for instance, dysphasia (Rutter 1978, 1983). In a prospective study of children with autism seen before their third birthday, "abnormal responses to sensory stimuli" was the class of symptoms that most clearly distinguished autism from mental retardation (Gillberg *et al.* 1990). Ornitz (1989) reported similar findings.

ABNORMAL ACTIVITY LEVELS

Children with autism can be hyperactive or hypoactive (see also the section below on comorbidity, pp. 25–28). Only relatively few are normally active in infancy and the preschool period. There is often a characteristic trajectory of development in this respect, with hyperactivity in the preschool years followed by more normoactive behavior in the early school years and a tendency to hypoactivity from early adolescence.

Fluctuating activity levels are common throughout the life-span of some individuals with autism, and there is sometimes concern that the individual might be suffering from manic-depressive mood swings or outright bipolar disorder. In high-functioning patients with autism it has been well documented that there is an increased risk of bipolar disorder, both in the patients themselves and their close relatives (DeLong and Dwyer 1988).

Extreme degrees of hyperactivity are often encountered in individuals with autism who suffer from the fragile X syndrome. This is also true in many cases of autism combined with tuberous sclerosis. The hyperactivity is usually most pronounced in the first ten years of life, and may, particularly in cases with the combination of autism and tuberous sclerosis, be linked to severe bouts of aggression and destructive behaviors.

ABNORMAL EATING BEHAVIORS

Problems with eating – including particular food refusal, food fads, pica, hoarding, overeating and various degrees of anorectic behaviors, including complete food refusal and compulsive ordering of food on the plate – are extremely common in autism, and a major eating behavior disorder is more common than not.

Some children with autism appear to prefer only soft foods and may have difficulty chewing (or rather knowing that they are expected to chew). Others prefer only solid foods and appear nauseated when expected to eat certain minced foods. It is very common for children with autism to accept only pasta and French fries. Low-functioning individuals may "eat" anything within reach, including pieces of paper, cigarettes, flowers and even needles and pins.

Food faddism is dealt with in more detail in Chapter 7.

ABNORMAL SLEEP PATTERNS

Sleep patterns are abnormal in autism in a majority of all cases (Richdale and Prior 1995). They may be most striking in infancy and the first few years of life, when the child may keep the whole family awake by crying, but may sometimes continue right through to adulthood.

It is not uncommon for major sleep problems to be the first obvious outward sign that something is seriously at fault in an infant who does not receive a diagnosis of autism until years later.

AGGRESSION

Aggressive behaviors are common in autism at all ages, but perhaps particularly in the adolescent and young adult groups. The aggressive acts can take on frightening proportions and can lead to the requirement for heavy medication or treatment in high-security wards.

Nevertheless, it is important to note that the majority of individuals with autism are not aggressive and that it is rare for really dangerous situations to develop, even in the group which does exhibit severely aggressive behaviors.

SELF-INJURY

Self-injurious behaviors (SIBs) are said to abound particularly in children with the combination of autism and mental retardation. However, SIB is also common in individuals with high-functioning autism. Some of the most common manifestations of SIB are head-banging, wrist- or knuckle-biting, chin-knocking, cheek-smacking, eye-poking, hair-tearing, and clawing.

SIB is dealt with in more detail in Chapter 7.

TICS

It is only recently that it has become widely accepted that tics are very common in autism (see also the section below on comorbidity, p. 25). Typical simple motor and vocal tics are common, as are more elaborate and complex motor movements that appear to have a compulsive quality. As has already been noted, it is often difficult to separate tics from motor stereotypies, and it is possible that the distinction is sometimes artificial.

Several reports (*e.g.* Ehlers and Gillberg 1993, Kerbeshian and Burd 1996, Nass and Gutman 1997) have documented the co-occurrence of Tourette syndrome and Asperger syndrome. Some authors have taken this type of comorbidity as a predictor of better outcome in autism, but the evidence is not yet sufficient to warrant such a conclusion.

Cognitive profile

Many children with autism are mentally retarded. However, it appears that there are certain characteristics in the cognitive patterns of a majority that differentiate them from children without autism regardless of whether they are mentally retarded or not.

First, it is well established (Shah and Frith 1983) that some, though not all, show "islets" of special abilities, particularly in the fields of rote memory (*e.g.* numerical skills), music, art and visuospatial skills (such as is sometimes demonstrated in a particular aptitude with jigsaw puzzles).

Second, many seem to have an impaired memory for recent events (Boucher 1981). Specifically, their memory difficulties impair their ability to recall past activities in response to "open" or "uninformative" questions (Boucher and Lewis 1989). Such problems would be compatible with underlying theory of mind problems. The memory difficulties might therefore not be "true" memory deficits but depend on the way in which the "memory imprint" is approached.

Third, children with autism perform better than mental-age-matched retarded and normal children in respect to "concrete" discrimination. However, tasks requiring "formal" discrimination are more difficult for the child with autism (Maltz 1981). Their concrete way of interpreting and solving problems is often evident throughout life, even in those few with relatively high intellectual functioning.

Fourth, on the Wechsler scales, there is a particular test profile with peaks and troughs (Dartak *et al.* 1975, Ohta 1987, Rumsey and Hamburger 1988, Happé 1994, Ehlers *et al.* 1997) in certain areas. A recent study has shown a particular profile also on the Griffiths test (Dahlgren-Sandberg *et al.* 1993). Visuospatial skills show superior results, whereas language-associated and "intuition/empathy"-associated tests yield extremely low results. In high-functioning individuals – particularly those receiving diagnoses of Asperger syndrome – some of the language subtests reflecting learned or "crystallized" abilities (as opposed to more basic "fluid" abilities) may instead yield superior results.

It is the unusual cognitive profile of children with autism that has given rise to the widespread speculation that they are indeed of superior intelligence, and are just hiding their phenomenal capacity behind a shell of autism. Unfortunately, a large body of research is agreed that this view of autism is mistaken and that most children with autism, even those showing almost unbelievable splinter skills, are clearly mentally retarded. All have cognitive problems (Rutter 1983, Frith 1989, Happé 1996).

The cognitive profiles of individuals on the autism spectrum will be discussed in more depth in Chapter 9 on neuropsychology.

Gender differences in symptomatology

It has long been known that among individuals *diagnosed* with autism females have lower IQs than males (Wing 1981b, Lord *et al.* 1982). There is indirect evidence that girls with autism are more severely brain-damaged than boys. The hypothesis has been put forward that, because social and communicative behavior patterns in the general population are (a little) more towards the high-functioning end of the autism spectrum in males than in females, the insult to the brain required to push an individual over the edge "into autism" would have to be greater for females (Wing 1981b, Gillberg 1992a). This, in turn, has led to the suspicion that the behavioral phenotype of autism may be different in girls and that autistic disorder may sometimes remain undiagnosed in girls (Kopp and Gillberg 1992). To date, the few autism studies that have been performed in order to analyze this issue (*e.g.* Pilowsky *et al.* 1998) have not supported this hypothesis.

However, the documentation of previously undiagnosed autism and autism spectrum disorders in female cases with selective mutism (Wolff and McGuire 1995, Kopp and Gillberg 1997) and anorexia nervosa (Wentz-Nilsson *et al.* 1999) distinctly raises the possibility that our current clinical prototype for autism may have to be revised. In an ongoing study of females with severe social interaction problems, preliminary findings suggest that girls in the higher-functioning portion of the autism spectrum (whether diagnosed as having autistic disorder, Asperger syndrome or atypical autism) tend to be referred later, and may have fewer special interests, slightly better superficial social skills, a greater tendency to avoid demands, and (at least in the group with a diagnosis of autism or atypical autism) better expressive language skills. They also tend to be somewhat less hyperactive and considerably less aggressive, which may, in part, explain why they have not attracted enough attention to warrant consultation with child psychiatric services at an earlier age. These preliminary findings should be interpreted with caution and need to be replicated by other groups before conclusions can be drawn.

Summary of diagnostic criteria

AUTISM SPECTRUM (THE TRIAD OF SOCIAL IMPAIRMENTS)

At the present stage we would argue for an umbrella definition, such as the "autistic syndromes," "autism spectrum" or "autism and autistic-like conditions," to cover the whole group of severe disorders on the autism spectrum. In DSM-IV language, the most appropriate synonym would be "pervasive developmental disorders," but we consider this term to be conceptually more confusing. Based on the foregoing discussion, all disorders in the autism spectrum, according to our view, share the following characteristic triad of symptoms:

1   Severe restriction of the ability to interact reciprocally with other people in a social context.
2   Severe restriction of the ability to communicate reciprocally, often prominently noted in abnormalities of the production and, perhaps particularly, comprehension of spoken language as a means of communication, and in many other aspects of non-verbal communication.

3   Rigid and restricted behavioral repertoire and imaginative skills, as manifested in elaborate routines, insistence on sameness, restricted play patterns or interests, and motor stereotypies.

All symptoms have to be out of phase with the overall intellectual level of the child.

AUTISTIC DISORDER AND KANNER SYNDROME

For a diagnosis of the "complete autistic syndrome," "childhood autism," "autistic disorder" or just "autism," all three symptoms have to be present in severe and typical form.

It is possible that a fourth criterion should be added – that is, that the clinical picture does not better fit that of disintegrative disorder (see below). The vast majority of individuals meeting the full triad criteria will have had onset of symptoms long before their third birthday, and, in those few who have not, a criterion relating to set-back after normal early development would allow the diagnosing of disintegrative disorder even in cases meeting symptomatic criteria for autism.

Within the category of childhood autism/autistic disorder, a nucleus subgroup showing elaborate repetitive routines and autistic aloneness would be diagnosed as having Kanner syndrome.

ASPERGER SYNDROME

The diagnosis of Asperger syndrome would be made in cases who meet the criteria – without showing severe language problems – plus additional criteria as outlined in Chapter 3 (which is entirely devoted to Asperger's disorder).

DISINTEGRATIVE DISORDER

There are instances of disintegrative disorder commencing around the age of 3 to 4 years and usually characterized by restlessness and hyperactivity during the first three to nine months of illness before the child becomes very much like a child with autism. Such cases (see Table 2.2) were often referred to as Heller dementia (Heller 1930) in older literature, as disintegrative psychosis in the 1970s (Evans-Jones and Rosenbloom 1978), and as childhood disintegrative disorders in later writings (*e.g.* WHO 1993). Outcome appears to be at least as poor as in classic autism, and in a number of instances it is slowly realized that underlying the condition is a progressive neurological disorder.

ATYPICAL AUTISM

In cases with all three symptoms represented in atypical form, or with two of the symptoms in typical form, we suggest that "partial autistic syndrome," "autistic-like condition" or "atypical autism" be diagnosed. This ICD-10 category of atypical autism would equate with "pervasive developmental disorder not otherwise specified" in the DSM-III-R and DSM-IV.

TABLE 2.2
Diagnostic criteria for childhood disintegrative disorder

A Apparently normal development for at least the first 2 years after birth as manifested by the presence of age-appropriate verbal and non-verbal communication, social relationships, play, and adaptive behavior.

B Clinically significant loss of previously acquired skills (before age 10 years) in at least two of the following areas:

1 expressive or receptive language
2 social skills or adaptive behavior
3 bowel or bladder control
4 play
5 motor skills

C Abnormalities of functioning in at least two of the following areas:

1 qualitative impairment in social interaction (*e.g.* impairment in non-verbal behaviors, failure to develop peer relationships, lack of social or emotional reciprocity
2 qualitative impairment in communication (*e.g.* delay or lack of spoken language, inability to initiate or sustain a conversation, stereotyped and repetitive use of language, lack of varied make-believe play)
3 restricted, repetitive, and stereotyped patterns of behavior, interests, and activities, including motor stereotypies and mannerisms

D The disturbance is not better accounted for by another specific pervasive developmental disorder or by schizophrenia.

AUTISTIC FEATURES

In cases not meeting criteria for any of the above groups but showing some autistic features, we suggest that "autistic features" be diagnosed.

It is possible that in the future the triad criteria will have to be modified to take into account differences in behavioral phenotype that may exist as a consequence of sex/ gender.

Complicating disorders and comorbidity

Autism is only very rarely the sole syndrome warranting a correct diagnosis in the individual patient. The typical individual suffering from autism is one with a multitude of problems.

MENTAL RETARDATION

A majority of children with classic autism (approximately 67 to 88 per cent) are definitely mentally retarded, that is they test reliably under IQ 70 (Lotter 1966, Rutter 1978, Wing 1980, Bohman *et al.* 1983, Gillberg 1984a, Steffenburg and Gillberg 1986, Gillberg *et al.* 1991). This retardation was previously thought to be a secondary consequence of the affective disturbance, and Kanner (1943, 1949) believed that these were children with potentially superior intelligence. Now, several different lines of research have been followed and the results are in total agreement that many children with autism are indeed mentally retarded (Rutter 1983, Gillberg 1990). This intellectual retardation is not caused by motivational factors in the child and remains relatively stable over the years, with or without improvement with regard to the autistic behavior problems.

It goes without saying that the clinical picture of autism varies somewhat with the intellectual level. Severely mentally retarded children with autism (IQ <50), who constitute about 40 per cent of all children with classic autism, behave differently from mildly retarded or normally intelligent children with autism. Outcome varies with IQ and level of speech development. The speech-language competence is, of course, on the whole, closely correlated with the IQ level. Severely retarded children are less likely to have any speech at all, whereas more intelligent children with autism are the ones most likely to demonstrate a wide variety of elaborate repetitive routines and to exhibit islets of special giftedness in circumscribed areas – a symptom once mentioned as central by Kanner, but which, obviously, cannot be as conspicuous in the severely mentally retarded group. The islet abilities are sometimes referred to as "savant qualities." This area is covered in more detail in Chapter 7.

Epilepsy

Some children with autism have early onset seizures. Indeed, infantile spasms are often followed by the development of an autistic syndrome, even in infancy (Taft and Cohen 1971, Riikonen and Amnell 1981, Riikonen and Simell 1990). Equally common, however, is the development of any type of epilepsy at or near the time of puberty. One third of all children with autism (Rutter 1970, Gillberg 1984b, 1991, Olsson *et al.* 1988) develop seizures. It is a more common phenomenon among those who are also mentally retarded, but it can occur at all levels of intelligence (Gillberg *et al.* 1987). Most children who develop epilepsy in adolescence have not previously shown any outward signs of major neurological abnormality. (For more details on epilepsy in autism, see Chapter 12.)

Vision and Hearing Impairments

In a study by Steffenburg (1991), at least half of a population based group of children with classic autism had problems in the field of visual acuity (hypermetropia in most cases, myopia in a few and gradually developing blindness in one case).

It has long been suggested that blindness (especially by way of sensory deprivation) may cause autism and that blindness and autism often coexist (Keeler 1958, Rapin 1979). If autism and blindness are indeed associated, then the association might well stem from some kind of underlying central neurological deficit. Several studies have shown an increase of autism symptoms in various forms of congenital blindness (Rogers and Newhart-Larson 1989, Goodman and Minne 1995, Ek *et al.* 1998), but it appears that the association is not with blindness *per se* but rather with other associated pathologies. In one study, two groups of congenitally blind children were compared with regard to autistic symptomatology. The rate of autistic disorder was increased only in the group with retinopathy of prematurity in which additional severe brain damage was usually present (Ek *et al.* 1998).

Deafness has also been purported to be associated with autism. There is some evidence from population studies for an increased incidence of hearing problems associated with autism (Steffenburg 1991). A large-scale clinical study of comprehensively examined children with autism showed moderate hearing impairment to be relatively common, occurring at rates of 10–20 per cent, depending on the level of impairment required for a diagnosis of hearing deficit (Rosenhall *et al*. 1999).

It is rather surprising that the possible interrelationships between autism and visual/hearing impairments have attracted so little attention. Many interesting hypotheses might be tested in connection with studies undertaken in order to elucidate this association. For instance, the relative importance of periodic sensory privation versus central brain damage could be evaluated in such studies.

Based on clinical experience, it would seem that hearing impairment and deafness would be more likely than blindness to show a primary connection with autism. Throughout childhood, most children with autism show deviant reactions to sound, whereas deviant reactions to light appear to be less conspicuous. Furthermore, among individuals with autism, there are more clinically-proven cases of deafness than of blindness.

In summary, it seems that hearing and visual problems may quite often be overlooked in autism. There is a need to be aware of the relatively high rate of problems in these areas and to systematically work up all individuals with a diagnosis of autism with a view to revealing possible eye and ear problems.

ASSOCIATED MEDICAL DISORDERS

The autistic syndromes are but behaviorally-defined sets of collections of symptoms, and it is therefore quite possible to diagnose any kind of disorder in connection with autism. However, cerebral palsy (Schain and Yannet 1960) is only rarely seen in concurrence with autism and related disorders (Gillberg 1984a). The fragile X syndrome (Steffenburg and Gillberg 1986), tuberous sclerosis (Lotter 1974), neurofibromatosis (Gillberg and Forsell 1984, Gaffney *et al*. 1989), hypomelanosis of Ito (Åkefeldt and Gillberg 1991), Rett syndrome (Witt-Engerström and Gillberg 1987), achondroplasia (personal case), Moebius syndrome (Ornitz *et al*. 1977, Gillberg and Winnergard 1984), Laurence-Moon-Biedl syndrome (Steffenburg 1991), Williams syndrome (Steffenburg 1991), Angelman syndrome (Steffenburg *et al*. 1996a) and Coffin-Lowry syndrome (Bryson *et al*. 1988) have all been reported to co-occur with autism. Later in the book, we will return to a consideration of the possible implications of these connections.

DEPRESSION

Depression occurs in autism spectrum disorders at all levels of ability, and is probably underdiagnosed (Ghaziuddin and Greden 1998). A positive family history for affective disorder, a change in behavior and apathy, tearfulness, sleep problems or aggression/self-injury are markers that should alert the clinician to the possibility of comorbid depression in autism.

ATTENTION-DEFICIT/HYPERACTIVITY DISORDER

In the past, individuals with autism were only rarely diagnosed as having comorbid attention-deficit/hyperactivity disorder (ADHD). This was often due to a hierarchical system of classification in which autism was seen as the "main" diagnosis with which other problems could not "compete." Also the DSM and ICD systems precluded the possibility of making a diagnosis of ADHD in cases with an autism spectrum disorder.

Recently, it has become accepted that many individuals with autism actually meet symptom criteria for ADHD. The rate of comorbid ADHD is extremely high in Asperger syndrome (Ehlers and Gillberg 1993). Contrary to previous views, central stimulant treatment for the attention deficits may be equally as potent in this group – at least if IQ is above about 50 – as in cases with ADHD not showing autistic symptoms (Gillberg *et al.* 1997). This has led to a re-evaluation of the utility of exempting the possibility of assigning ADHD diagnoses in patients with autism. Thus, if there are clinically severe problems in the fields of attention, activity level and impulse control, an additional diagnosis of ADHD should be considered in all autism spectrum cases.

TOURETTE SYNDROME

Tics are common in autism (see above). A diagnosis of comorbid Tourette syndrome (the combination of several motor and one or more vocal tics) should be made if full DSM-IV symptom criteria for this disorder are met.

Differential diagnosis

Here we need only be concerned with those neurological, developmental and psychiatric syndromes that may cause diagnostic confusion. In the literature, often a whole list of conditions, such as rubella embryopathy, tuberous sclerosis, infantile spasms, Rett syndrome, fragile X syndrome and so on, is presented in the section on differential diagnosis. Since we consider autism to be a set of purely behavioral syndromes, regardless of underlying pathology, we will not enter into such a discussion at this stage.

DEAFNESS

Deaf children may occasionally show some autistic features, though rarely all. In the latter case they should in our view be diagnosed as suffering from deafness and autism.

BLINDNESS

Several authors (*e.g.* Wing 1980) have attested that certain patients who had been diagnosed as blind for several years were in fact seeing but suffering from autism. Interestingly, there may, in certain cases, be a connection between so-called delayed visual maturation and autistic symptoms (Goodman and Ashby 1990). As with deaf children, children with documented blindness and autism should be diagnosed as blind and as suffering from autism (Ek *et al.* 1998).

MENTAL RETARDATION

Some children with mental retardation have a number of autistic features without meeting all the necessary criteria for a diagnosis of autism (Haracopos and Kelstrup 1978, Wing and Gould 1979, Gillberg 1983, Gillberg *et al.* 1986). Conversely, children with autism, more often than not, are themselves mentally retarded. Sometimes the dividing line is indeed obscure and the allocation to diagnostic category haphazard. The studies by Wing (*e.g.* 1981c) are essential reading for anyone interested in this dichotomy.

EPILEPSY

Many individuals with the combination of epilepsy and mental retardation show autistic symptoms. The autistic behavior problems may be overlooked by specialists treating seizure disorders. In a total population study of 96 patients with the combination of epilepsy and mental retardation, 25 per cent met full criteria for autistic disorder, but only a small proportion of these had received this diagnosis prior to the study (Steffenburg *et al.* 1996b).

EMOTIONAL DEPRIVATION

Retarded children reared in institutions (especially if looked after by a large number of different carers) display, like children with autism, abnormalities of social relationships, language and behavior. However, close inspection and assessment usually make differential diagnosis easy, since such children are indiscriminate rather than aloof, language-delayed rather than deviant, and show different kinds of behavioral problems. Also, positive environmental stimulation usually leads to quick and continuing development in these cases, quite unlike the relatively minor changes seen in autism in connection with such stimulation.

INFANT DEPRESSION

Children who have developed normally in the first few years of life and who are then separated from their primary carer for an extended period sometimes develop major signs of depression (Spitz 1946). They first protest, then show sadness and withdrawal, but finally slowly adjust to the new situation. Among such children there is possibly an increased risk of depression in adulthood (von Knorring 1983).

RETT SYNDROME

Rett syndrome is also sometimes seen as an "either/or" diagnosis in relation to autism. The ICD-10 and DSM-IV have included Rett syndrome as one particular variant of the autism spectrum disorder. We consider this an absurd position. We argue that Rett syndrome and autism can co-exist and that in such cases both diagnoses should be made. However, there are cases with a mixture of Rett syndrome and autistic disorder symptoms, in which it may be difficult to determine whether or not a diagnosis of one or both disorders should be made. Rett syndrome is considered further in Chapter 11.

CHILDHOOD SCHIZOPHRENIA

There are also occasional instances of childhood schizophrenia (shown in hallucinating, thought-disordered children, who differ markedly from most children with autism). These cases probably, unlike autism, represent the early onset form of schizophrenia, and rarely commence (at least with typical symptoms) before the age of 7 or 8 years. Some US authors (*e.g.* Asarnow and Ben-Meir 1988) have argued that there are cases with early signs of autism who later develop schizophrenia. This is likely to be very rare.

SEMANTIC-PRAGMATIC DISORDER

Speech therapists often refer to "semantic-pragmatic disorder," and it is obvious that many individuals in the autism spectrum meet criteria for such a diagnosis (Bishop 1985). This will be dealt with in more detail in Chapter 3 on Asperger syndrome.

NON-VERBAL LEARNING DISABILITY

Some children with adequate language skills have great difficulty solving task problems traditionally considered to reflect "perception" and "performance." They sometimes meet criteria for a neuropsychological diagnosis termed "non-verbal learning disability" (Rourke 1988). This entity shows considerable overlap both with so-called right-hemisphere dysfunction syndromes and with Asperger syndrome, and will be considered again in Chapter 3, dealing specifically with Asperger's disorder.

ADHD/DAMP

There are quite a number of children with various combinations of deficits in attention (ADHD), motor control and perception (DAMP), who show several (usually mild) features of autism (Gillberg 1983). If the autistic features are pronounced in such cases with diagnoses of ADHD or DAMP, it is appropriate to make an additional diagnosis in the autism spectrum.

OTHER PSYCHIATRIC DISORDERS

Children with obsessive-compulsive disorders often have severe problems in the field of social relationships. Quite often they show many autistic-like features.

Children and adolescents with Tourette syndrome often have some traits – particularly empathy problems and ritualistic phenomena – reminiscent of Asperger syndrome.

School-age children and adolescents with selective mutism (the refusal to speak in certain social situations in spite of formally adequate speech–language skills) quite often have underlying autism spectrum problems which may be missed because of the alarming nature of the symptom of mutism.

Only rarely does one come across the kind of children described by Mahler and Gostiner (1955) who show a "clinging" attachment to the mother and in other respects too exhibit an overall arrest of development at the so-called symbiotic stage. These cases are extremely rare, constituting less than 1 per cent of all autism and autistic-like cases seen by us in clinical and population-based studies. It is highly doubtful as to whether they should be grouped as a separate diagnostic category. Most cases of this kind can readily be classified in other categories with the added feature of the conspicuously clinging behavior.

Comprehensive differential diagnosis

The comprehensive differential diagnosis in respect to autistic disorder, Asperger syndrome, atypical autism, disintegrative disorder, Rett syndrome, emotional deprivation and infant depression is shown in Table 2.3.

We hope that the difficulty of diagnosing autistic syndromes has not been understated in the foregoing pages. There are still many unresolved problems. In an era when operational criteria and inter-rater reliability of judgement have come into focus and taken the step from research methodology to clinical necessity, it may seem obsolete to speak of such a thing as experience. Even child psychiatrists only infrequently encounter Kanner syndrome cases. The cases fulfilling Wing's criteria for autistic disorder occur more frequently, but only those working among the mentally retarded are likely to be aware of the actual number. Clinical experience is a prerequisite seldom mentioned in writings on the diagnosis of autism, and yet this fundamental element is of utmost importance. There is a "gestalt measure" inherent in the whole concept of autism. The experienced clinician will have no difficulty in selecting the group of children in whom autistic syndromes will be found. He or she may have some trouble deciding whether to diagnose "autistic disorder," "Asperger syndrome" or "atypical autism," but the Wing category will be easier to discern. The clinically inexperienced researcher, on the other hand, may have no major difficulty in deciding that a mildly mentally retarded 4-year-old with autistic behavior does meet DSM-IV criteria for autistic disorder, but will altogether miss the possibility that a normally intelligent 8-year-old with much communicative speech belongs in that same diagnostic category. Diagnostic studies concerned with autism and autistic-like conditions require the "gestalt acumen" of the experienced clinician just as much as everyday clinical work with the people who suffer from autism does.

There will eventually be a need for new concepts and words in the field of autism diagnosis. The discovery of theory of mind deficits in autism might lead to formulations of new broad-band labels such as "disorders of empathy" (Gillberg 1992a). Nevertheless, autism and the various derivatives of that word will remain with us for many years to come. We believe that the term "pervasive developmental disorder" will die out because of its conceptual unsoundness. Diagnostic difficulties/confusions have been elegantly discussed by Waterhouse and colleagues (Waterhouse *et al.* 1984, Waterhouse and Fein 1989).

The terms "autism spectrum" and "autistic syndromes" may, by some, be taken as further evidence of the diagnostic problems relating to the area. However, at present it is our contention that these labels accord best with the current state of knowledge in so far as comprehensive categories are needed. This wording makes clear that, on balance, there is as yet no hard evidence that there exists a qualitatively unique behavioral or etiological syndrome of autism. Kanner autism does not have more validity than any of the other named syndromes on the autism spectrum (Waterhouse and Fein 1989, Wing 1989, Gillberg 1992a).

In the future it may be possible to make a definite distinction between "inborn" and "later acquired" forms of autism on some more rational criterion than the rather arbitrary 30 to 36 months onset limit proposed by influential authorities.

As time goes by, we will also be able to distinguish between etiological and behavioral subsyndromes, and in all probability the autistic syndromes will eventually be replaced by a number of different syndromes (Gillberg 1992b).

31

TABLE 2.3 Differential diagnosis for Kanner syndrome, Asperger syndrome, disintegrative disorder, Rett complex, deprivation syndrome and infant depression

Syndrome	Social relationships	Communication	Behavior	Other	Age of onset and course
Kanner syndrome	Period of autistic aloneness; lack of reciprocity	Concrete interpretation of language; comprehension of human mime and gesture impaired; muteness; echolalia	Obsessive insistence on elaborate routines; special stereotypies of hands and arms; toe-walking; lack of interests; failure to meet demands; resistance to change; overactivity alternating with apathy	Abnormal auditory perception; subgroup with large head, other with small head	From birth (minority during first 3 years); chronic; usually life-long disability
Asperger syndrome	Gradual realization that child is uninterested in peers; formal contact; odd, naive approach devoid of empathy; inability to understand perspective of others; either naive and helpless or cold, stern and "egoistic"; sometimes "regression" to autistic state	Concrete interpretation of language in spite of superficially well-developed skills; may use "old-fashioned" metaphorical language; poor pragmatics; flat prosody	Much like autism though circumscribed interests (astrology, etc.) often more conspicuous; perhaps more strikingly fixated on ideas, routines	A variant of high-functioning autism? motor clumsiness; gaucheness; personality traits? subgroup with large head	Often not obvious until the age of 3–7 years; chronic; fair (though restricted) outcome; much increased risk for psychiatric problems (depression, suicide attempts, paranoia, alcoholism, eating disorders) and bizarre criminality
Disintegrative disorder (Heller syndrome)	Regression to autistic state	Regression to level of echolalia or muteness	Partly same as autism; often extreme degrees of overactivity and motor restlessness	Confusion; variable abnormality of auditory perception	30–48 mths (small minority in the 4–10 yr age range); chronic; usually life-long disability
Rett complex	Isolation and social apraxia in stages II and III; better contact later	No language in most instances; preserved speech variant may show limited language skills	Midline hand stereotypies and loss of purposeful hand movements	Epilepsy; scoliosis; small head; motor impairment	Seemingly normal 5–18 mths, followed by regression

TABLE 2.3 (continued)

Syndrome	Social relationships	Communication	Behavior	Other	Age of onset and course
Deprivation syndrome	Lack of reticence and distance; always in pursuit of contact; understands human mime and gesture; people not objects	Delayed (not deviant) language development	Extreme overactivity; eats garbage, drinks toilet-water	Quick amelioration if early stimulation	6–30 mths; sensitive to environmental change; fair prognosis if early stimulation
Infant depression	Initial autistic-like features followed by accepting relationship with new caregiver; ambivalence upon return to primary caregiver	Initial regression	Apathy followed by adjustment to new demands	Amelioration on return to normal milieu; auditory perception normal	8–30 mths; highly age-dependent; promptly treated; risk for depression in adult life

Summary

It is now clear that autistic disorder/childhood autism is but one of several autistic syndromes belonging to the same spectrum of conditions involving a triad of social, communication and behavioral/imagination restriction. The autism spectrum comprises the syndrome described by Kanner, as well as that delineated by Asperger, plus a number of other disorders, currently less well identified. As with other developmental disorders, symptoms change over the individual's life-span. At least three different subtypes have been described: the aloof; the active but odd; and the passive and friendly. In some cases with autistic syndromes, associated problems – not the core diagnostic symptoms – can be those that cause the most suffering.

REFERENCES

Åkefeldt, A., Gillberg, C. (1991) 'Hypomelanosis of Ito in three cases with autism and autistic-like conditions.' *Developmental Medicine and Child Neurology*, **33**, 737–743.

American Psychiatric Association (1980) *Diagnostic and Statistical Manual of Mental Disorders*. Washington, DC: APA.

—— (1987) *Diagnostic and Statistical Manual of Mental Disorders. 3rd Edn (Revised)*. Washington, DC: APA.

—— (1994) *Diagnostic and Statistical Manual of Mental Disorders. 4th Edn*. Washington, DC: APA.

Arvidsson, T., Danielsson, B., Forsberg, P., Gillberg, C., Johansson, M., Källgren, G. (1997) 'Autism in 3-6-year-old children in a suburb of Göteborg, Sweden.' *Autism*, **1**, 163–173.

Asarnow, J.R., Ben-Meir, S. (1988) 'Children with schizophrenia spectrum and depressive disorders: a comparative study of premorbid adjustment, onset pattern and severity of impairment.' *Journal of Child Psychology and Psychiatry*, **29**, 477–488.

Baron-Cohen, S. (1995) *Mind Blindness. An Essay on Autism and Theory of Mind*. Cambridge: MIT Press.

Baron-Cohen, S., Allen, J., Gillberg, C. (1992) 'Can autism be detected at 18 months? The needle, the haystack and the CHAT.' *British Journal of Psychiatry*, **161**, 839–843.

Bartak, L., Rutter, M., Cox, A. (1975) 'A comparative study of infantile autism and specific developmental receptive language disorder. I. The children.' *British Journal of Psychiatry*, **126**, 127–145.

Bishop, D.V.M. (1985) 'Age of onset and outcome in "acquired aphasia with convulsive disorder" (Landau-Kleffner syndrome).' *Developmental Medicine and Child Neurology*, **27**, 705–712.

Bleuler, E. (1911) *Dementia Praecox or the Group of Schizophrenias*. Vienna. Translated 1952 by J. Zinkin. New York: International Universities Press.

Bohman, M., Bohman, I.L., Björk, P., Sjöholm, E. (1983) 'Childhood psychosis in a northern Swedish county: some preliminary findings from an epidemiological survey.' *In:* Schmidt, M.H., Remschmith, H. (Eds) *Epidemiological Approaches in Child Psychiatry*. Stuttgart: Georg Thieme, pp. 164–173.

Boucher, J. (1981) 'Memory of recent events in autistic children.' *Journal of Autism and Developmental Disorders*, **11**, 293–302.

Boucher, J., Lewis, V. (1989) 'Memory impairments and communication in relatively able autistic children.'*Journal of Child Psychology and Psychiatry*, **29**, 433–445.

Bryson, S.E., Clark, B.S., Smith, I.M. (1988) 'First report of a Canadian epidemiological study of autistic syndromes.' *Journal of Child Psychology and Psychiatry*, **29**, 433–445.

Coleman, M. (1976) *The Autistic Syndromes*. Amsterdam: North-Holland.

Coleman, M., Gillberg, C. (1985) *The Biology of the Autistic Syndromes*. New York: Praeger.

Comings, D.E. (1990) *Tourette Syndrome and Human Behaviour*. Duarte, California: Hope Press.

Dahlgren, S.O., Gillberg, C. (1989) 'Symptoms in the first two years of life. A preliminary population study of infantile autism.' *European Archives of Psychiatry and Neurological Sciences*, **238**, 169–174.

Dahlgren-Sandberg, A., Nydén, A., Gillberg, C., Hjelmquist, E. (1993) 'The cognitive profile in infantile autism – a study of 70 children and adolescents using the Griffiths Mental Development Scale.' *British Journal of Psychology*, **84**, 365–373.

DeLong, G.R., Dwyer, J.T. (1988) 'Correlation of family history with specific autistic subgroups: Asperger's syndrome and bipolar affective disease.' *Journal of Autism and Developmental Disorders*, **18**, 593–600.

DeLong, G.R., Beau, S.C., Brown, F.R. (1981) 'Acquired reversible autistic syndrome in acute encephalopathic illness in children.' *Archives of Neurology*, **38**, 191–194.

Ehlers, S., Gillberg, C. (1993) 'The epidemiology of Asperger syndrome. A total population study.' *Journal of Child Psychology and Psychiatry*, **34**, 1327–1350.

Ehlers, S., Nydén, A., Gillberg, C., Dahlgren-Sandberg, A., Dahlgren, S.-O., Hjelmquist, E., Odén, A. (1997) 'Asperger syndrome, autism and attention disorders: a comparative study of the cognitive profile of 120 children.' *Journal of Child Psychology and Psychiatry*, **38**, 207-217.

Ek, U., Fernell, E., Jacobsson, L., Gillberg, C. (1998) 'Relation between blindness due to retinopathy of prematurity and autistic spectrum disorders: a population-based study.' *Developmental Medicine and Child Neurology*, **40**, 297–301.

Evans-Jones, L.G., Rosenbloom, L. (1978) 'Disintegrative psychoses in childhood.' *Developmental Medicine and Child Neurology*, **20**, 462–470.

Fish, B., Ritvo, E. (1979) 'Psychoses of childhood.' *In:* Noshpitz, V. (Ed.) *Basic Handbook of Child Psychiatry*. New York: Basic Books, pp. 249–303.

Frith, U. (1989) 'Autism and "theory of mind."' *In:* Gillberg, C. (Ed.) *Diagnosis and Treatment of Autism*. New York: Plenum Press, pp. 33–52.

Gaffney, G.R., Kuperman, S., Tsai, L.Y., Minchin, S. (1989) 'Forebrain structure in infantile autism.' *Journal of the American Academy of Child and Adolescent Psychiatry*, **28**, 534–537.

Ghaziuddin, M., Greden, J. (1998) 'Depression in children with autism/pervasive developmental disorders: a case-control family history study.' *Journal of Autism and Developmental Disorders*, **28**, 111–115.

Gillberg, C. (1983) 'Psychotic behaviour in children and young adults in a mental handicap hostel.' *Acta Psychiatrica Scandinavica*, **68**, 351–358.

—— (1984a) 'Infantile autism and other childhood psychoses in a Swedish urban region. Epidemiological aspects.' *Journal of Child Psychology and Psychiatry*, **25**, 35–43.

—— (1984b) 'Autistic children growing up: problems during puberty and adolescence.' *Developmental Medicine and Child Neurology*, **26**, 125–129.

—— (1986) 'Brief report: Onset at age 14 of a typical autistic syndrome. A case report of a girl with herpes simplex encephalitis.' *Journal of Autism and Developmental Disorders*, **16**, 369–375.

—— (1990) 'Autism and pervasive developmental disorders.' *Journal of Child Psychology and Psychiatry*, **31**, 99–119 (published erratum appears in *Journal of Child Psychology and Psychiatry*, **32(1)**, 213).

—— (1991) 'The treatment of epilepsy in autism.' *Journal of Autism and Developmental Disorders*, **21**, 61–77.

—— (1992a) 'The Emanuel Miller Memorial Lecture 1991: Autism and autistic-like conditions: subclasses among disorders of empathy.' *Journal of Child Psychology and Psychiatry*, **33**, 813–842.

—— (1992b) 'Subgroups in autism: are there behavioural phenotypes typical of underlying medical conditions?' *Journal of Intellectual Disability Research*, **36**, 201–214.

Gillberg, C., Forsell, C. (1984) 'Childhood psychosis and neurofibromatosis – more than a coincidence?' *Journal of Autism and Developmental Disorders*, **14**, 1–8.

Gillberg, C., Wing, L. (1999) 'Autism: not an extremely rare disorder.' *Acta Psychiatrica Scandinavica*. Accepted.

Gillberg, C., Winnergard, I. (1984) 'Childhood psychosis in a case of Moebius syndrome.' *Neuropediatrics*, **15**, 147–149.

Gillberg, C., Persson, E., Grufman, M., Themnér, U. (1986) 'Psychiatric disorders in mildly and severely mentally retarded urban children and adolescents: epidemiological aspects.' *British Journal of Psychiatry*, **149**, 68–74.

Gillberg, C., Steffenburg, S., Jakobsson, G. (1987) 'Neurobiological findings in 20 relatively gifted children with Kanner-type autism or Asperger syndrome.' *Developmental Medicine and Child Neurology*, **29**, 641–649.

Gillberg, C., Ehlers, S., Schaumann, H., Jakobsson, G., Dahlgren, S.O., Lindblom, R., Bågenholm, A., Tjuus, T., Blidner, E. (1990) 'Autism under age 3 years: a clinical study of 28 cases referred for autistic symptoms in infancy.' *Journal of Child Psychology and Psychiatry*, **31**, 921–934.

Gillberg, C., Steffenburg, S., Wahlström, J., Gillberg, I.C., Sjöstedt, A., Martinsson, T., Liedgren, S., Eeg-Olofsson, O. (1991) 'Autism associated with marker chromosome.' *Journal of the American Academy of Child and Adolescent Psychiatry*, **30**, 489–494.

35

Gillberg, C., Melander, H., von Knorring, A.-L., Janols, L.-O., Thernlund, G., Hägglöf, B., Eidevall-Wallin, L., Gustafsson, P., Kopp, S. (1997) 'Long-term stimulant treatment of children with attention-deficit hyperactivity disorder symptoms. A randomized, double-blind, placebo-controlled trial.' *Archives of General Psychiatry*, **54**, 857–864.

Gillberg, I.C. (1991) 'Autistic syndrome with onset at age 31 years. Herpes encephalitis as one possible model for childhood autism.' *Developmental Medicine and Child Neurology*, **33**, 920–924.

Gillberg, I.C., Gillberg, C. (1989a) 'Asperger syndrome – some epidemiological considerations: a research note.' *Journal of Child Psychology and Psychiatry*, **30**, 631–638.

—— (1989b) 'Children with preschool minor neurodevelopmental disorders. IV: Behaviour and school achievement at age 13.' *Developmental Medicine and Child Neurology*, **31**, 3–13.

Goodman, R., Ashby, L. (1990) 'Delayed visual maturation and autism.' *Developmental Medicine and Child Neurology*, **32**, 814–819.

Goodman, R., Minne, C. (1995) 'Questionnaire screening for comorbid pervasive developmental disorders in congenitally blind children: a pilot study.' *Journal of Autism and Developmental Disorders*, **25**, 195–203.

Hagerman, R.J. (1989) 'Chromosomes, genes and autism.' *In:* Gillberg, C. (Ed.) *Diagnosis and Treatment of Autism.* New York: Plenum Press, pp. 105–132.

Happé, F. (1994) 'Wechsler IQ profile and theory of mind in autism: a research note.' *Journal of Child Psychology and Psychiatry*, **35**, 1461–1471.

—— (1996) 'The neuropsychology of autism.' *Brain*, **119**, 1377–1400.

Haracopos, D., Kelstrup, A. (1978) 'Psychotic behaviour in children under the institutions for the mentally retarded in Denmark.' *Journal of Autism and Childhood Schizophrenia*, **8**, 1–12.

Harris, J.C. (1995a) *Developmental Neuropsychiatry. I: The Fundamentals.* New York and Oxford: Oxford University Press.

—— (1995b) *Developmental Neuropsychiatry. II: Assessment, Diagnosis and Treatment of Developmental Disorders.* New York and Oxford: Oxford University Press.

Heimann, M., Nelson, K.E., Tjus, T., Gillberg, C. (1995) 'Increasing reading and communication skills in children with autism through an interactive multimedia computer program.' *Journal of Autism and Developmental Disorders*, **25**, 459–480.

Heller, T. (1930) 'Über Dementia infantilis.' *Zeitschrift für Kinderforschung*, **37**, 661–667.

Hermelin, B., O'Conner, N. (1970) *Psychological Experiments with Autistic Children.* Oxford: Pergamon Press.

Howlin, P. (1982) 'Echolalic and spontaneous phrase speech in autistic children.' *Journal of Child Psychology and Psychiatry*, **23**, 281–293.

Kanner, L. (1943) 'Autistic disturbances of affective contact.' *Nervous Child*, **2**, 217–250.

—— (1949) 'Problems of nosology and psychodynamics of early infantile autism.' *American Journal of Orthopsychiatry*, **19**, 416–426.

Kanner, L., Eisenberg, L. (1956) 'Early infantile autism: 1943–1955.' *American Journal of Orthopsychiatry*, **26**, 55–65.

Keeler, W.R. (1958) 'Autistic patterns and defective communication in blind children with retrolental fibroblasia.' *In:* Hoch, P.H., Zubin, J. (Eds) *Psychopathology of Communication.* New York: Grune & Stratton, pp. 64–83.

Kerbeshian, J., Burd, L. (1996) 'Case study: Comorbidity among Tourette's syndrome, autistic disorder, and bipolar disorder.' *Journal of the American Academy of Child and Adolescent Psychiatry*, **35**, 681–685.

Kopp, S., Gillberg, C. (1992) 'Girls with social deficits and learning problems: autism, atypical Asperger syndrome or a variant of these conditions.' *European Child and Adolescent Psychiatry*, **1**, 89–99.

—— (1997) 'Selective mutism: a population-based study: research note.' *Journal of Child Psychology and Psychiatry*, **38**, 257–262.

Leekam, S.R., Hunnisett, E., Moore, C. (1998) 'Targets and cues: gaze-following in children with autism.' *Journal of Child Psychology and Psychiatry*, **39**, 951–962.

Lord, C., Schopler, E., Revicki, D. (1982) 'Sex differences in autism.' *Journal of Autism and Developmental Disorders*, **12**, 317–330.

Lotter, V. (1966) 'Epidemiology of autistic conditions in young children.' *Social Psychiatry*, **1**, 124–137.

—— (1974) 'Factors related to outcome in autistic children.' *Journal of Autism and Childhood Schizophrenia*, **4**, 263–277.

36

Mahler, M.S., Gosliner, B.J. (1955) 'On symbiotic child psychosis: genetic, dynamic and restitutive aspects.' *Psychoanalytic Study of the Child*, **19**, 195–212.

Maltz, A. (1981) 'Comparison of cognitive deficits among autistic and retarded children on the Arthur Adaption of the Leiter International Performance Scale.' *Journal of Autism and Developmental Disorders*, **11**, 413–426.

Masterton, B.A., Biederman, G.B. (1983) 'Proprioceptive versus visual control in autistic children.' *Journal of Autism and Developmental Disorders*, **13**, 141–152.

Miller, J.N., Ozonoff, S. (1997) 'Did Asperger's cases have Asperger Disorders? A research note.' *Journal of Child Psychology and Psychiatry*, **38**, 247–251.

Miranda, P.L., Donnellan, A.M., Yoder, D.E. (1983) 'Gaze behaviour: a new look at an old problem.' *Journal of Autism and Developmental Disorders*, **13**, 397–409.

Nass, R., Gutman, R. (1997) 'Boys with Asperger's disorder, exceptional verbal intelligence, tics, and clumsiness.' *Developmental Medicine and Child Neurology*, **39**, 691–695.

Nordin, V., Gillberg, C. (1996a) 'Autism spectrum disorders in children with physical or mental disability or both. Part I: Clinical and epidemiological aspects.' *Developmental Medicine and Child Neurology*, **38**, 297–313.

—— (1996b) 'Autism spectrum disorders in children with physical or mental disability or both. Part II: Screening aspects.' *Developmental Medicine and Child Neurology*, **38**, 314–324.

Ohta, M. (1987) 'Cognitive disorders of infantile autism: a study employing the WISC, spatial relationship conceptualization, and gesture imitation.' *Journal of Autism and Developmental Disorders*, **17**, 45–62.

Olsson, I., Steffenburg, S., Gillberg, C. (1988) 'Epilepsy in autism and autistic-like conditions: a population-based study.' *Archives of Neurology*, **45**, 666–668.

Ornitz, E. (1983) 'The functional neuroanatomy of infantile autism.' *International Journal of Neuroscience*, **19**, 85–124.

—— (1989) 'Early symptoms of autism.' Paper presented at Congress of the Federation of Societies of Biological Psychiatry, Jerusalem, April.

Ornitz, E., Guthrie, D., Farley, A.J. (1977) 'The early development of autistic children.' *Journal of Autism and Childhood Schizophrenia*, **7**, 207–229.

Pilowsky, T., Yirmiya, N., Shulman, C., Dover, R. (1998) 'The Autism Diagnostic Interview-Revised and the Childhood Autism Rating Scale: differences between diagnostic systems and comparison between genders.' *Journal of Autism and Developmental Disorders*, **28**, 143–151.

Rapin, I. (1979) 'Effect of early blindness and deafness on cognition.' *In:* Katzman, R. (Ed.) *Congenital and Acquired Cognitive Disorders*. New York: Raven, pp. 189–245.

Rapin, I., Katzman, R. (1998) 'Neurobiology of autism.' *Annals of Neurology*, **43**, 7–14.

Richdale, A.L., Prior, M.R. (1995) 'The sleep/wake rhythm in children with autism.' *European Child and Adolescent Psychiatry*, **4**, 175–186.

Riikonen, R., Amnell, G. (1981) 'Psychiatric disorders in children with earlier infantile spasms.' *Developmental Medicine and Child Neurology*, **23**, 747–760.

Riikonen, R., Simell, O. (1990) 'Tuberous sclerosis and infantile spasms.' *Developmental Medicine and Child Neurology*, **32**, 203–209.

Rogers, S.J., Newhart-Larson, S. (1989) 'Characteristics of infantile autism in five children with Leber's congenital amaurosis.' *Developmental Medicine and Child Neurology*, **31**, 598–608.

Rosenhall, U., Sandström, M., Nordin, V., Gillberg, C. (1999) 'Autism and hearing loss.' Submitted.

Rourke, B.P. (1988) 'The syndrome of non-verbal learning disabled children: developmental manifestations of neurological disease.' *The Clinical Neuropsychologist*, **2**, 293–330.

Rumsey, J.M., Hamburger, S.D. (1988) 'Neuropsychological findings in high-functioning men with infantile autism, residual state.' *Journal of Clinical and Experimental Neuropsychology*, **10**, 201–221.

Rutter, M. (1970) 'Autistic children: infancy to adulthood.' *Seminars in Psychiatry*, **2**, 435–450.

—— (1978) 'Diagnosis and definition.' *In:* Rutter, M., Schopler, E. (Eds) *Autism. A Reappraisal of Concepts and Treatment*. New York: Plenum Press, pp. 1–25.

—— (1983) 'Cognitive deficits in the pathogenesis of autism.' *Journal of Child Psychology and Psychiatry*, **24**, 513–531.

Rutter, M., Schopler, E. (1978) *Autism: A Reappraisal of Concepts and Treatment*. New York: Plenum.

—— (1987) 'Autism and pervasive developmental disorders: concepts and diagnostic issues.' *Journal of Autism and Developmental Disorders*, **17**, 159–186.

Schain, R., Yannet, H. (1960) 'Infantile autism: an analysis of 50 cases and a consideration of certain relevant neuropsychological concepts.' *Journal of Pediatrics*, **57**, 560-567.

Shah, A., Frith, U. (1983) 'An islet of ability in autistic children: a research note.' *Journal of Child Psychology and Psychiatry*, **24**, 613-620.

Siegel, B., Vukicevic, J., Elliott, G.R., Kraemer, H.C. (1989) 'The use of signal detection theory to assess DSM-III-R criteria for autistic disorder.' *Journal of the American Academy of Child and Adolescent Psychiatry*, **28**, 542–548.

Sigman, M., Mundy, P., Sherman, T., Ungerer, J. (1986) 'Social interactions of autistic, mentally retarded and normal children and their caregivers.' *Journal of Child Psychology and Psychiatry*, **27**, 647–656.

Spitz, R.A. (1946) 'Anaclictic depression – an inquiry into the genesis of psychiatric conditions in early childhood.' *Psychoanalytic Study of the Child*, **2**, 313–342.

Steffenburg, S. (1991) 'Neuropsychiatric assessment of children with autism: a population-based study.' *Developmental Medicine and Child Neurology*, **33**, 495–511.

Steffenburg, S., Gillberg, C. (1986) 'Autism and autistic-like conditions in Swedish rural and urban areas: a population study.' *British Journal of Psychiatry*, **149**, 81–87.

Steffenburg, S., Gillberg, C., Steffenburg, U., Kyllerman, M. (1996a) 'Autism in Angelman syndrome. A population-based study.' *Pediatric Neurology*, **14**, 131–136.

Steffenburg, S., Gillberg, C., Steffenburg, U. (1996b) 'Psychiatric disorders in children and adolescents with active epilepsy and mental retardation.' *Archives of Neurology*, **53**, 904–912.

Szatmari, P. (1992) 'The validity of autistic spectrum disorders: a literature review.' *Journal of Autism and Developmental Disorders*, **22**, 583–600.

Taft, L.T., Cohen, H.J. (1971) 'Hypsarrhythmia and childhood autism: a clinical report.' *Journal of Autism and Developmental Disorders*, **1**, 327–336.

Volkmar, F.R., Cohen, D.J. (1989) 'Disintegrative disorder or "late onset" autism?' *Journal of Child Psychology and Psychiatry*, **30**, 717–724.

von Knorring, A.-L. (1983) 'Adoption studies on psychiatric illness. Epidemiological, environmental and genetic aspects.' Umeå University: MD thesis.

Waterhouse, L., Fein, D. (1989) 'Social or cognitive or both?' *In:* Gillberg, C. (Ed.) *Diagnosis and Treatment of Autism*. New York: Plenum Press, pp. 53–62.

Waterhouse, L., Fein, D., Nath, J., Snyder, D. (1984) *Pervasive Schizophrenia Occurring in Childhood: A Review of Critical Commentary*. Washington, DC: American Psychiatric Association.

Wentz-Nilsson, E., Gillberg, C., Gillberg, I.C., Råstam, M. (1999) 'Anorexia nervosa 10 years after onset. Personality disorders.' Submitted.

WHO (World Health Organization) (1993) *The ICD-10 Classification of Mental and Behavioural Disorders. Diagnostic Criteria for Research*. Geneva: WHO.

Willemsen-Swinkels, S.H., Buitelaar, J.K., Weijnen, F.G., van Engeland, H. (1998) 'Timing of social gaze behavior in children with a pervasive developmental disorder.' *Journal of Autism and Developmental Disorders*, **28**, 199–210.

Wing, J.K. (1966) 'Diagnosis, epidemiology, aetiology.' *In:* Wing, J.K. (Ed.) *Early Child Autism*. Oxford: Pergamon Press, pp. 3–50.

Wing, L. (1980) *Early Childhood Autism*. Oxford: Pergamon Press.

—— (1981a) 'Asperger's syndrome: a clinical account.' *Psychological Medicine*, **11**, 115–129.

—— (1981b) 'Sex ratios in early childhood autism and related conditions.' *Psychiatry Research*, **5**, 129–137.

—— (1981c) 'Language, social and cognitive impairments in autism and severe mental retardation.' *Journal of Autism and Developmental Disorders*, **11**, 31–44.

—— (1989) 'The diagnosis of autism.' *In:* Gillberg, C. (Ed.) *Diagnosis and Treatment of Autism*. New York: Plenum Press, pp. 5–22.

—— (1996) *The Autism Spectrum*. London: Constable.

Wing, L., Gould, J. (1979) 'Severe impairments of social interaction and associated abnormalities in children: epidemiology and classification.' *Journal of Autism and Developmental Disorders*, **9**, 11–29.

Witt-Engerström, I., Gillberg, C. (1987) 'Rett syndrome in Sweden.' *Journal of Autism and Developmental Disorders*, **17**, 149–150.

Wolff, S., McGuire, R.J. (1995) 'Schizoid personality in girls: a follow-up study – what are the links with Asperger's syndrome?' *Journal of Child Psychology and Psychiatry*, **36**, 793–817.

Zetterström, R. (1983) 'Infantile autism – neuropsychological correlates.' Paper read at Sävstaholm Conference on Autism, Uppsala, Sweden.

3
ASPERGER SYNDROME

The syndrome described by Asperger (1944) has now attracted widespread attention in child and adult psychiatry (Gillberg 1985, 1989, Tantam 1988, Szatmari *et al.* 1989a, WHO 1993, APA 1994), but it was not until 1981 that it received its status as a named syndrome (Wing 1981). What is currently known as Asperger syndrome had actually already been described in the 1920s by a Russian neurologist, who referred to the disorder as "schizoid personality disorder" (Ssucharewa 1926). There is an on-going debate as to whether "Kanner autism" and "childhood autistic psychopathy/personality disorder" (the original syndrome name suggested by Asperger) represent overlapping or distinct conditions (Schopler *et al.* 1998, Gillberg 1998). It is often assumed that they exist on a spectrum, with Kanner autism occupying the lower end and Asperger syndrome the upper end (Frith 1991). Some have argued that the differential diagnosis of Asperger syndrome depends only on IQ, which tends to be low or very low in Kanner autism, but normal or high (occasionally very high) in Asperger syndrome. Others regard differences in verbal ability to be the crucial differentiator, with Asperger cases generally being much more high-functioning in this respect than are those with Kanner's variant of autism. Some appear to believe that the two syndromes exist on a social deficit continuum with Kanner autism again on the lowermost portion and Asperger syndrome in the higher range. Even though all of these continuum approaches have considerable clinical credibility, Kanner autism is sometimes, albeit very rarely, diagnosed in cases with high IQ, and Asperger syndrome in cases with low (including low verbal) IQ. Also, the social deficits encountered in so-called Asperger syndrome are quite often exceptionally severe, especially if the IQ level is taken into account.

We are aware that distinguishing Asperger syndrome from autism may be an artificial venture and that the two conditions may, in the long run, be treated as one. Nevertheless, so far, the evidence is not unequivocally in favor of such an association. Clinically there is still something to be said for the use of the Asperger label for certain relatively high-functioning individuals with autistic-type empathy deficits and superficially excellent language skills. The diagnostic criteria outlined in Table 3.1 should not be thought of as an excuse either for separating out Asperger syndrome as a discrete entity, different in key aspects from all other syndromes in child psychiatry (including "autism"), or for extending the autism concept infinitely but inexplicitly to encompass all empathy deficits encountered in psychiatry. Rather, they should be regarded as a tool for distinguishing a group of children and adults with a particular conglomeration of social, communication and behavioral repertoire deficits, who either do not readily meet the clinical criteria for childhood autism or autistic disorder, or who, even if they do meet such criteria, for some reason give the impression of being "too normal" for an autism diagnosis to be

TABLE 3.1
Diagnostic criteria for Asperger syndrome/Asperger's disorder according to different manuals/authors

Gillberg and Gillberg's (1989) diagnostic criteria elaborated (Gillberg 1991)

1 Social impairment (extreme egocentricity)
  (at least two of the following):

  (a) Inability to interact with peers
  (b) Lack of desire to interact with peers
  (c) Lack of appreciation of social cues
  (d) Socially and emotionally inappropriate behavior

2 Narrow interest
  (at least one of the following):

  (a) Exclusion of other activities
  (b) Repetitive adherence
  (c) More rote than meaning

3 Repetitive routines
  (at least one of the following):

  (a) on self, in aspects of life
  (b) on others

4 Speech and language peculiarities
  (at least three of the following):

  (a) Delayed development
  (b) Superficially perfect expressive language
  (c) Formal pedantic language
  (d) Odd prosody, peculiar voice characteristics
  (e) Impairment of comprehension including misinterpretations of literal/implied meanings

5 Non-verbal communication problems
  (at least one of the following):

  (a) Limited use of gestures
  (b) Clumsy/gauche body language
  (c) Limited facial expression
  (d) Inappropriate expression
  (e) Peculiar, stiff gaze

6 Motor clumsiness
  Poor performance on neuro-developmental examination

Szatmari *et al.*'s (1989) diagnostic criteria

1 Solitary
  (two of):

  No close friends
  Avoids others
  No interest in making friends
  A loner

2 Impaired social interaction
(one of):

Approaches others only to have own needs met
A clumsy social approach
One-sided responses to peers
Difficulty sensing feelings of others
Detached from feelings of others

3 Impaired non-verbal communication
(one of):

Limited facial expression
Unable to read emotion from facial expressions of child
Unable to give message with eyes
Does not look at others
Does not use hands to express oneself
Gestures are large and clumsy
Comes too close to others

4 Odd speech
(two of):

Abnormalities in inflection
Talks too much
Talks too little
Lack of cohesion to conversation
Idiosyncratic use of words
Repetitive patterns of speech

5 Does not meet DSM-III-R criteria for:
Autistic disorder

ICD-10 (1993) research criteria (World Health Organization)

A There is no clinically significant general delay in spoken or receptive language or cognitive development. Diagnosis requires that single words should have developed by 2 years of age or earlier and that communicative phrases be used by 3 years of age or earlier. Self-help skills, adaptive behavior, and curiosity about the environment during the first three years should be at a level consistent with normal intellectual development. However, motor milestones may be somewhat delayed and motor clumsiness is usual (although not a necessary diagnostic feature). Isolated special skills, often related to abnormal preoccupations, are common, but are not required for diagnosis.

B There are qualitative abnormalities in reciprocal social interaction in at least two of the following areas (criteria as for autism):
(a) failure adequately to use eye-to-eye gaze, facial expression, body posture, and gesture to regulate social interaction
(b) failure to develop (in a manner appropriate to mental age, and despite ample opportunities) peer relationships that involve a mutual sharing of interest, activities, and emotions
(c) lack of social-emotional reciprocity as shown by an impaired or deviant response to other people's emotions, or lack of modulation of behavior according to social context; or a weak integration of social, emotional, and communicative behaviors
(d) lack of spontaneous seeking to share enjoyment, interests, or achievements with other people (*e.g.* a lack of showing, bringing, or pointing out to other people objects of interests to the individual)

C The individual exhibits an unusually intense, circumscribed interest or restricted, repetitive, and stereotyped patterns of behavior, interests, and activities in at least one of the following areas (criteria as for autism; however it would be less usual for these to include either motor mannerisms or preoccupations with part-objects or non-functional elements of play materials):

41

continued

TABLE 3.1 (continued)

    (a) an encompassing preoccupation with one or more stereotyped and restricted patterns of interest that are abnormal in their intensity and circumscribed nature though not in their content of focus

    (b) apparently compulsive adherence to specific, non-functional routines or rituals

    (c) stereotyped and repetitive motor mannerisms that involve either hand- or finger-flapping or -twisting, or complex whole-body movements

    (d) preoccupations with part-objects or non-functional elements of play materials (such as their odour, the feel of their surface, or the noise or vibration that they generate)

D The disorder is not attributable to the other varieties of pervasive developmental disorder: simple schizophrenia (F20.6); schizotypal disorder (F21); obsessive-compulsive disorder (F42); anankastic personality disorder (F60.5); reactive and disinhibited attachment disorders of childhood (F94.1 and F94.2, respectively).

DSM-IV (1994) criteria (American Psychiatric Association)

A Qualitative impairment in social interaction, as manifested by at least two of the following:

1 marked impairment in the use of multiple non-verbal behaviors such as eye-to-eye gaze, facial expression, body postures, and gesture to regulate social interaction

2 failure to develop peer relationships appropriate to developmental level

3 a lack of spontaneous seeking to share enjoyment, interests, or achievements with other people (*e.g.* by a lack of showing, bringing, or pointing out objects of interest to other people)

4 lack of social or emotional reciprocity

B Restricted repetitive and stereotyped patterns of behavior, interests, and activities, as manifested by at least one of the following:

1 encompassing preoccupation with one or more stereotyped and restricted patterns of interest that is abnormal either in intensity or focus

2 apparently inflexible adherence to specific, non-functional routines or rituals

3 stereotyped and repetitive motor mannerisms (*e.g.* hand- or finger-flapping or -twisting, or complex whole-body movements)

4 persistent preoccupation with part of objects

C The disturbance causes clinically significant impairment in social, occupational, or other important areas of functioning.

D There is no clinically significant general delay in language (*e.g.* single words used by age 2 years, communicative phrases used by age 3 years).

E There is no clinically significant delay in cognitive development or in the development of age-appropriate self-help skills, adaptive behavior (other than in social interaction), and curiosity about the environment in childhood.

F Criteria are not met for another specific pervasive developmental disorder or schizophrenia.

appropriate. Superficially, such persons may not seem to be severely disabled, but a more thorough analysis will reveal that they have extensive empathy problems that warrant further empirical study.

It needs emphasizing that the communication problems included as a diagnostic criterion might seem to differentiate Asperger syndrome as conceptualized in this chapter from that depicted in the ICD-10 (WHO 1993) and the DSM-IV (APA 1994). In these two manuals, normal language development is included as a criterion. Often, however, we are faced with "clear-cut" Asperger syndrome cases (as described by Asperger himself) *reported* to have normal or even early language development, but who, in actual fact, have not been completely normal in this respect. In our experience, on closer analysis, all such individuals have been shown to have deviant language development, at least in the context of a group of family members with superior intelligence and/or early language development. There is often a history of "relatively" late development of language followed by the emergence of perfect language skills, appropriate for an adult rather than for a young child. To be sure, such language development, taken out of its familial context, may be perceived as "normal" (and may indeed be normal as compared with the average population). However, it is definitely abnormal if analyzed in the particular family/social context. Even more commonly, we come across individuals who were late to start talking, but who, once they did, quickly seemed to develop superior expressive language skills, almost on a par with adult levels. When worked-up at the age of 6 to 8 years, they fit the clinical picture that Asperger described beautifully and do not come across as so strikingly impaired as the majority of individuals receiving a diagnosis of autism. Such cases would be diagnosed as having Asperger syndrome according to the criteria set out by Gillberg and Gillberg (1989), and fit Wing's descriptions (Wing 1981), but would be classified under childhood autism in the ICD-10, and under autistic disorder in the DSM-IV.

It is of considerable interest that none of Hans Asperger's original cases would meet the criteria for Asperger's disorder outlined in the DSM-IV (Miller and Ozonoff 1997). That they meet the Gillberg (1991) criteria is only to be expected, given that these were specifically developed on the basis of just those cases described by Hans Asperger. With the Gillberg criteria (similar to the outline provided by Wing in 1981), quite a number of individuals with severe social interaction problems would receive a diagnosis of Asperger syndrome. Using the ICD-10/DSM-IV, virtually nobody would qualify for this diagnosis, but would instead be diagnosed as having autism (Leekam *et al.* 2000).

We believe that the ICD-10/DSM-IV criteria for Asperger syndrome are inappropriate and cannot be used in clinical practice. The Asperger concept of these manuals is a theoretical artifact published in an attempt to draw a clear line between autism and Asperger syndrome. This was a legitimate effort stemming from the need to provide clear diagnostic algorithms for research, but it was not well grounded in clinical practice. Asperger individuals are not – as required by the ICD-10/DSM-IV – normal with regard to social and communicative development in the first three years of life. Furthermore, they are usually much more socially and behaviorally deviant than considered necessary for a diagnosis to be made according to these manuals.

Controversial issues in the diagnosis of Asperger syndrome

A number of issues relating to the diagnostic classification of Asperger syndrome and its distinction from high-functioning autism are unresolved. The most important of these seem to be: whether or not there may be speech and language impairment; whether clumsiness may be a specific marker; whether IQ can be in the retarded range; and whether development in the first three years of life can be abnormal.

It seems clear that the DSM-IV and ICD-10 were mistaken in suggesting that there are no speech and language problems in Asperger's disorder. The flat prosody, pedantic speech, semantic-pragmatic problems and conversational comprehension impairments are all in the speech-language domain and highly characteristic of the syndrome.

Clumsiness may not be as specific to Asperger syndrome as once believed by Asperger himself. Clumsiness is common in classic autism and in ADHD (Kadesjö *et al.* 1999). Even though motor clumsiness is included as one of the diagnostic criteria in the set outlined by Gillberg and Gillberg (1989), it should no longer be seen as a symptom that might be used to discriminate Asperger syndrome from high-functioning autism.

IQ is occasionally in the retarded range in Asperger syndrome, even though the vast majority (probably 95 per cent or more) score above IQ 70 on standardized IQ tests. In the few cases with IQs in the 60–70 range, it is usually the performance IQ that determines the classification in the retarded group.

Development in the first three years of life has to be normal for a diagnosis of Asperger syndrome according to the ICD-10 and DSM-IV. This is not in agreement with Asperger (1944), Wing (1981) or Gillberg (1991). It is extremely rare for an individual later fitting Asperger's behavioral phenotype to have had completely normal social and communication development in the early years of life. Individuals with this symptom profile and developmental background would usually be diagnosed within the category of autistic disorder in the DSM-IV, but as having Asperger syndrome according to Gillberg (1991).

Prevalence

There have been four epidemiological studies providing data on the prevalence of Asperger syndrome in the general population. Three of these are Swedish, and one originated in Iceland. This means that it is too early to draw firm conclusions regarding the rate of Asperger syndrome in the population, and whether or not prevalence is stable across cultures. Nevertheless, the four studies are in relatively good agreement with each other, meaning that, at least in the Nordic countries, there appears to be a relatively firm basis for a good estimate of the prevalence of the disorder.

The first study was one originally designed to locate those children, in the general population of 7-year-olds, with the combination of attention deficits and motor control problems. The estimated rate of Asperger syndrome in that study was 26 in 10,000 (Gillberg and Gillberg 1989). Ehlers and Gillberg (1993) screened a whole Gothenburg borough cohort of 7- to 16-year-olds and arrived at an estimate of 36 in 10,000 meeting full criteria for the disorder, according to the Gillberg (1991) definition, with another 36 in 10,000 showing many but not all of the symptoms of Asperger syndrome. The Icelandic survey (Petrusdóttir *et al.* 1994) reported finding a rate of 35 in 10,000 in Reykjavik. The most recent Swedish study, from the middle-sized town of Karlstad, found a rate of 48 in 10,000 in 7- to 11-year-olds (Kadesjö and Gillberg 1999). Thus, the range of reported rates is from 26 to 48 in 10,000, or about 0.3 to 0.5 per cent.

The male:female ratios in the studies have varied slightly, but the most common finding is about four boys to every girl. In some recent writings (*e.g.* Gillberg 1992a, Kopp and Gillberg 1992) it has been suggested that the female phenotype may be slightly different and is perhaps more prevalent than hitherto believed. For instance, one study indicated an increased frequency of Asperger syndrome and similar high-functioning autistic-like conditions in the premorbid history of some girls who developed anorexia nervosa in adolescence (Gillberg and Råstam 1992).

Familial/hereditary factors in Asperger syndrome

No major family, twin or adoption study of Asperger syndrome has been published yet. However, quite a number of clinical studies (*e.g.* Wing 1981, Gillberg 1989, Szatmari *et al.* 1989b, Volkmar *et al.* 1998) implicate a strong genetic component, with 30 to 60 per cent of affected cases having a close relative with Asperger syndrome or something very similar (such as major social difficulties or communication problems or both). Asperger himself reported that, of the approximately 200 cases that he had personally followed for many years, almost all had at least one parent with similar traits. (Asperger also drew attention to possible brain damage in his cases – see below.) Burgoine and Wing (1983) reported on monozygotic male triplets with Asperger syndrome.

A number of family case studies (*e.g.* Bowman 1988, Gillberg 1991) have shown that in certain families there is overlap of autism and Asperger syndrome. For instance, in the family described by Bowman (1988), there was a spectrum of problems in the male first-degree relatives, ranging from severe Kanner autism, through Asperger syndrome, to mild autistic traits. In the Gillberg (1991) family, the mother (highly intelligent) had Asperger traits, the eldest son had Kanner autism and mild mental retardation, the middle son had mild autistic traits (and his son in turn had Kanner autism), and the youngest son had classical Asperger syndrome with superior intelligence. The eldest son had been affected by an intrauterine rubella infection. The findings suggest that Asperger syndrome might be inherited in some fashion with variable penetrance. The added effects of certain forms of brain damage might produce full-blown autism in such families. Whether the mode of inheritance should be viewed as dominant or not is open to speculation. It appears that at least some cases (like those in the families described by Bowman and Gillberg) may be inherited in a dominant fashion. In other cases, in which both parents show some mild autistic-type traits and the child is quite severely affected, an atypical recessive mode of inheritance might be postulated. The type of oligogenic inheritance pattern now believed to account for a majority of cases with classic autism is likely to be in operation in many cases of Asperger syndrome also.

A controlled population-based study of siblings and parents of children with autism indicated a slight but significant increase in the rate of Asperger syndrome in the first-degree relatives as compared with relatives of normal children and children with learning disorders other than autism (Gillberg *et al.* 1992).

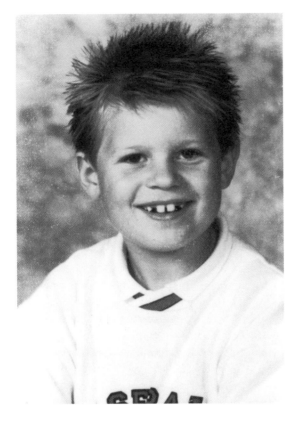

Fig. 3.1 8-year-old boy with Asperger syndrome with possible semi-dominant semi-recessive mode of inheritance.

There is a clinical impression that Asperger syndrome cases in some families segregate with obsessive-compulsive personality disorders, Tourette syndrome and simple tics. Except for one study by Comings (1990) supporting this impression, the empirical evidence in this field is lacking. A genetic link with attentional problems, elective autism and anorexia nervosa has been suggested by a few studies (Gillberg 1989, Gillberg and Gillberg 1989, Råstam 1992, Wolff 1995, Hebebrand *et al.* 1997), but there is no conclusive evidence.

Even though empirical systematic evidence from representative groups is largely lacking, the clinical evidence is such that it seems reasonable to conclude that, at least in certain cases, there is a hereditary trait common to autism and Asperger syndrome. Whether this applies to only a few, many, or even most cases with Asperger syndrome remains to be established in population studies making use of modern methodology of twin, family and adoption studies. Asperger syndrome is more common and less severe than autism. In certain instances, the cognitive style and obsessional interests may contribute to a "survival trait" which could even include "superficially normal family life" in adulthood. A hereditary link between Asperger and Kanner syndromes might account for the persistence of genetic forms of autism in the population. Kanner autism is such a severe disorder that the genetic form would be quickly extinguished if it were inherited

46

only in "pure" form, unless the genetic variants were all inherited as autosomal recessives. The bulk of the evidence is not in favor of autosomal recessive inheritance in autism/ Asperger syndrome (Bolton and Rutter 1990, Rutter *et al.* 1999b), even though some authors have argued for its importance, at least in a subgroup of patients.

Associated disorders and comorbidities in Asperger syndrome

Only occasionally is Asperger syndrome diagnosed in people with mild mental retardation (Gillberg *et al.* 1986). Asperger himself would probably have been reluctant to do this, but it is clear that there are cases with mild mental retardation who better fit the clinical picture described by him than that outlined by Kanner (Wing 1981, Gillberg 1985, Littlejohns *et al.* 1990).

Epilepsy may be marginally more common in Asperger syndrome than in the general population, but it is definitely much less common than in Kanner autism, probably affecting no more than a few per cent of the whole group (Gillberg 1989).

Occasionally, Asperger syndrome – just like autism, but less often – may be associated with specific medical conditions, such as fragile X syndrome (Hagerman 1989), tuberous sclerosis (Gillberg 1989), neurofibromatosis (Gaffney *et al.* 1988), hypothyroidism (I.C. Gillberg *et al.* 1992), Steinert's myotonic dystrophy (Blondis *et al.* 1996, Paul and Allington-Smith 1997), Marfan syndrome (Tantam *et al.* 1990), fetal alcohol syndrome (Aronson *et al.* 1997), and colobomas of the eye (Gillberg 1989).

Tics and Tourette syndrome are common in Asperger syndrome (*e.g.* Ehlers and Gillberg 1993). Symptoms or the full syndrome of ADHD are also common comorbidities. These associated neuropsychiatric problems may warrant separate symptomatic treatment.

It also appears that severe perinatal problems may be over-represented (and perhaps causative or contributory in the pathogenetic chain of events) in a subgroup (Asperger 1944, Wing 1981, Gillberg 1989, Ghaziuddin *et al.* 1995).

Unilateral brain damage has been proposed to account for the development of some cases of Asperger syndrome on theoretical grounds (Goodman 1989), and on the basis of findings obtained in individual patients (Littlejohns *et al.* 1990). Such damage would probably be most likely to affect parts of the temporal and prefrontal areas. Goodman (1989) has suggested that, whereas autism would be likely to result from bilateral brain dysfunction, Asperger syndrome could arise on the basis of unilateral dysfunction of the same brain areas. This could be either right- or left-sided if, as hypothesized, social competence and language areas are located, respectively, in these parts of the brain. During early development, these parts, by being interconnected "mirror images" of each other, could compensate to some extent for damage to the contralateral area (with a subsequent reduction of both functions).

No particular EEG, auditory brainstem response or CSF monoamine or endorphin pattern has yet been reported in Asperger syndrome (Gillberg 1989).

Medical work-up in Asperger syndrome

A medical and developmental history must be taken in all cases. Medical records from the pre-, peri- and neonatal periods should be analyzed. There should be a low threshold for

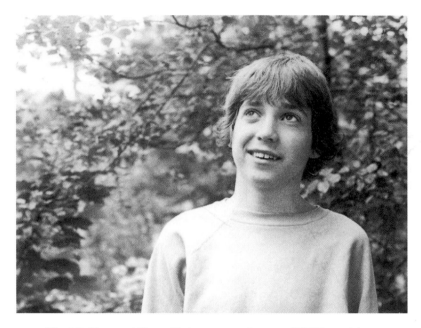

Fig. 3.2 13-year-old boy with Asperger syndrome and XYY mosaicism.

performing chromosomal analysis, particularly with a view to disclosing the fragile Xq27.3 abnormality and other sex chromosome anomalies (see Fig. 3.2). Thyroid function should be monitored. Other neurobiological examinations (such as MRI of the cortex) should be considered whenever clinical assessment and examination do not reveal a plausible cause.

Treatment/intervention

There are no specific medical treatments currently available for Asperger syndrome. Principles applied to education in autism adhere in Asperger syndrome as well, even though they have to be modified to comply with higher IQ and superficially better social functioning.

Of particular importance is the way in which bizarre interests may have to be dealt with. Many obsessive interests can be turned into something useful. However, extreme interests in areas such as gunpowder, poison, knives or violent sports should not be encouraged, and parents and teachers should be encouraged to seek alternatives in other areas. This is quite often a successful venture, but one which has to be dealt with in thoughtful ways, taking account of all sorts of factors such as family setting and child's IQ, personality and past interest patterns.

Perhaps the most important intervention of all is to make a diagnosis and inform the parents and sometimes the child. Together they will then be able to tell those people, including teachers, who would benefit from knowing that the child's social demeanor is likely to remain relatively stable over many years, regardless of treatment and other interventions. Some might consider this a nihilistic approach, but it is not. On the contrary, it means accepting somebody with a unique personality and a rather unusual set of behavioral traits without feeling the need to change him/her to achieve "normality" at any cost.

In some cases, comorbid depression or obsessive-compulsive symptoms may warrant a clinical trial of one of the selective serotonin reuptake inhibitors. These drugs are often well-tolerated and quite effective for depressive and obsessive symptoms. It is also our experience that they may be beneficial for social-withdrawal symptoms, which may sometimes be the most problematic impairment in the individual Asperger patient. Unfortunately, at the time of going to press with this volume, no randomized controlled studies have yet been published to support this clinical notion, and so no straightforward clinical recommendations can be offered.

Course and outcome in Asperger syndrome

Outcome in Asperger syndrome is very variable, ranging from excellent to poor (Asperger 1944, Wing 1981, Tantam 1988, Gillberg 1998).

It should be clear that many people with Asperger syndrome never come to the attention of psychiatrists or psychologists. They may be regarded as odd – and even aloof – but they are not perceived as psychiatrically abnormal.

Of those who do attend psychiatric services, it is possible that only a fraction apply for help in childhood. These cases have received a variety of diagnostic labels and it is only during the last decade that they have come to be diagnosed as having Asperger syndrome. "Old" labels in the field include "borderline," "borderline psychosis," "autistic traits," "minimal brain dysfunction" and occasionally even "conduct disorder." "Atypical," "schizoid" and "schizotypal" are other labels that have been employed by certain groups.

Even among those who do attend child psychiatric services, quite a number have a fair prognosis and lead independent adult lives. They will still be regarded by some as "highly original," "eccentric" or "odd," but such perceived qualities have at least as many positive as negative connotations and therefore can lead to admiration rather than rejection, and so may contribute to a good outcome. Their basic style of interaction, their concrete and formalistic treatment of spoken and written language, and their narrow interests and routines usually continue relatively unchanged throughout life. A case has been made for Asperger syndrome being associated in rare cases with artistic achievements and even philosophical writings, as exemplified by Béla Bartók and Ludwig Wittgenstein (Gillberg 1992b, Wolff 1995, Fitzgerald 1999).

Nevertheless, a proportion of young patients diagnosed with Asperger syndrome will grow up to be psychiatric patients or criminal offenders (Siponmaa *et al.* 1999). Many people with Asperger syndrome probably seek psychiatric help for the first time only in adult life. In our experience, "paranoia," "depression," "obsessive-compulsive personality disorder" and "borderline" are the most common diagnoses given by adult psychiatrists to this group. Alcohol abuse is probably much over-represented (Hellgren 1994). Some are labeled "pseudoneurotic schizophrenics." According to Wing's follow-up, suicide attempts may be relatively common (Wing 1981). Clear-cut classic schizophrenia appears to be very rare, and, so far, there is no evidence for a continuity from childhood Asperger syndrome to adult-life schizophrenia. Some of the other diagnoses given may occasionally be correct at the phenomenological level. However, the best help can be provided if the basic "Asperger traits" are recognized and many of the psychopharmacological treatments of adult psychiatry are avoided. The type of criminal offence sometimes encountered in adolescents and adults with Asperger syndrome is usually connected with extreme obsession. It could be anything from poisoning – and other variants of "experimental killing" – and arson, to bizarre violence (Baron-Cohen 1988, Tantam 1991, Siponmaa *et al.* 1999).

Summary

Even though it is far from settled where the line *vis-à-vis* autistic disorder should be drawn, it now seems clear that the diagnostic category of Asperger syndrome has become firmly rooted in clinical practice. It is conceptualized by most authorities as the highest-functioning variant of autism, but it is unclear whether or not superior functioning pertains more to language than to global cognitive skills. Outcome is much more variable than in classic autism, but psychiatric complications appear to be very common, and many individuals diagnosed with Asperger syndrome in childhood will become adult psychiatric patients. There is a need for increased awareness of Asperger syndrome in a wide variety of medical disciplines and in the education system.

REFERENCES

APA (American Psychiatric Association) (1994) *Diagnostic and Statistical Manual of Mental Disorders. 4th Edn.* Washington, DC: APA.

Aronson, M., Hagberg, B., Gillberg, C. (1997) 'Attention deficits and autistic spectrum problems in children exposed to alcohol during gestation: a follow-up study.' *Developmental Medicine and Child Neurology*, **39**, 583–587.

Asperger, H. (1944) 'Die autistischen Psychopathen im Kindesalter.' *Archiv für Psychiatrie und Nervenkrankheiten*, **117**, 76–136.

Baron-Cohen, S. (1988) 'An assessment of violence in a young man with Asperger's syndrome.' *Journal of Child Psychology and Psychiatry*, **29**, 351–360.

Blondis, T.A., Cook, E.J., Koza-Taylor, P., Finn, T. (1996) 'Asperger syndrome associated with Steinert's myotonic dystrophy.' *Developmental Medicine and Child Neurology*, **38**, 840–847.

Bolton, P., Rutter, M. (1990) 'Genetic influences in autism.' *International Review of Psychiatry*, **2**, 67–80.

Bowman, E.P. (1988) 'Asperger's syndrome and autism: the case for a connection.' *British Journal of Psychiatry*, **152**, 377–382.

Burgoine, E., Wing, L. (1983) 'Identical triplets with Asperger's syndrome.' *British Journal of Psychiatry*, **143**, 261–265.

Comings, D.E. (1990) *Tourette Syndrome and Human Behavior.* Duarte, California: Hope Press.

Ehlers, S., Gillberg, C. (1993) 'The epidemiology of Asperger syndrome. A total population study.' *Journal of Child Psychology and Psychiatry*, **34**, 1327–1350.

Fitzgerald, M. (1999) 'Did Ludwig Wittgenstein have Asperger's syndrome?' *European Child and Adolescent Psychiatry*, **8**. In press.

Frith, U. (1991) *Autism and Asperger Syndrome.* Cambridge: Cambridge University Press.

Gaffney, G.R., Kuperman, S., Tsai, L.Y., Minchin, S. (1988) 'Morphological evidence for brainstem involvement in infantile autism.' *Biological Psychiatry*, **24**, 578–586.

Ghaziuddin, M., Shakal, J., Tsai, L. (1995) 'Obstetric factors in Asperger syndrome: comparison with high-functioning autism.' *Journal of Intellectual Disability Research*, **39**, 538–543.

Gillberg, C. (1985) 'Asperger's syndrome and recurrent psychosis – a case study.' *Journal of Autism and Developmental Disorders*, **15**, 389–397.

—— (1989) 'Asperger syndrome in 23 Swedish children.' *Developmental Medicine and Child Neurology*, **31**, 520–531.

—— (1991) 'Clinical and neurobiological aspects of Asperger syndrome in six family studies.' *In:* Frith, U. (Ed.) *Autism and Asperger Syndrome*. Cambridge: Cambridge University Press, pp. 122–146.

—— (1992a) 'The Emanuel Miller Memorial Lecture 1991: Autism and autistic-like conditions: subclasses among disorders of empathy.' *Journal of Child Psychology and Psychiatry*, **33**, 813–842.

—— (1992b) 'Savant-syndrome.' *In:* Vejlsgaard, R. (Ed.) *Medicinsk årsbok*. Köpenhamn: Munksgaard, pp. 127–131.

—— (1998) 'Asperger syndrome and high-functioning autism.' *British Journal of Psychiatry*, **172**, 200–209.

Gillberg, C., Råstam, M. (1992) 'Do some cases of anorexia nervosa reflect underlying autistic-like conditions?' *Behavioural Neurology*, **5**, 27–32.

Gillberg, C., Persson, E., Grufman, M., Themnér, U. (1986) 'Psychiatric disorders in mildly and severely mentally retarded urban children and adolescents: epidemiological aspects.' *British Journal of Psychiatry*, **149**, 68–74.

Gillberg, C., Gillberg, I.C., Steffenburg, S. (1992) 'Siblings and parents of children with autism. A controlled population based study.' *Developmental Medicine and Child Neurology*, **34**, 389–398.

Gillberg, I.C., Gillberg, C. (1989) 'Asperger syndrome – some epidemiological considerations: a research note.' *Journal of Child Psychology and Psychiatry*, **30**, 631–638.

Gillberg, I.C., Gillberg, C., Kopp, S. (1992) 'Hypothyroidism and autism spectrum disorders.' *Journal of Child Psychology and Psychiatry*, **33**, 531–542.

Goodman, R. (1989) 'Infantile autism: a syndrome of multiple primary deficits?' *Journal of Autism and Developmental Disorders*, **19**, 409–424.

Hagerman, R.J. (1989) 'Chromosomes, genes and autism.' *In:* Gillberg, C. (Ed.) *Diagnosis and Treatment of Autism*. New York: Plenum Press, pp. 105–132.

Hebebrand, J., Henninghausen, K., Nau, S., Himmelmann, G.W., Schulz, E., Schafer, H. and Remschmidt, H. (1997) 'Low body weight in male children and adolescents with schizoid personality disorder or Asperger's disorder.' *Acta Psychiatrica Scandinavica*, **96(1)**, 64–67.

Hellgren, L. (1994) 'Psychiatric disorders in adolescence. Longitudinal follow-up studies of adolescent onset psychoses and childhood onset deficits in attention motor control and perception.' Göteborg University: MD thesis.

Kadesjö, B., Gillberg, C., Hagberg, B. (1999) 'Brief report: Autism and Asperger syndrome in seven-year-old children. A total population prevalence study.' *Journal of Autism and Developmental Disorders*. Accepted.

Kopp, S., Gillberg, C. (1992) 'Girls with social deficits and learning problems: autism, atypical Asperger syndrome or a variant of these conditions.' *European Child and Adolescent Psychiatry*, **1**, 89–99.

Leekam, S., Libby, S., Wing, L., Gould, J., Gillberg, C. (2000) 'Comparison of ICD-10 and Gillberg's criteria for Asperger syndrome.' *Autism*. (In press).

Littlejohns, C.S., Clarke, D.J., Corbett, J.A. (1990) 'Tourette-like disorder in Asperger's syndrome.' *British Journal of Psychiatry*, **156**, 430–433.

Miller, J.N., Ozonoff, S. (1997) 'Did Asperger's cases have Asperger disorders? A research note.' *Journal of Child Psychology and Psychiatry*, **38**, 247–251.

Paul, M., Allington-Smith, P. (1997) 'Asperger syndrome associated with Steinert's myotonic dystrophy.' *Developmental Medicine and Child Neurology*, **39**, 280–281.

Petrusdóttir, G., Sigurdsson, S., Karlsson, M.M., Axelsson, J. (1994) 'The epidemiology of autism and Asperger syndrome in Iceland: a summary of a pilot study.' Proceedings of the 9th International Congress on Circumpolar Health, June 20–25, 1993, Reykjavik, Iceland. *Arctic Medical Research*, **53**(Suppl. 2), 464–466.

Råstam, M. (1992) 'Anorexia nervosa in 51 Swedish children and adolescents. Premorbid problems and comorbidity.' *Journal of the American Academy of Child and Adolescent Psychiatry*, **31**, 819–829.

Rutter, M., Silberg, J., O'Connor, T., Simonoff, E. (1999a) 'Genetics and child psychiatry: I Advances in quantitative and molecular genetics.' *Journal of Child Psychology and Psychiatry*, **40**, 3–18.

—— (1999b) 'Genetics and child psychiatry: II Empirical research findings.' *Journal of Child Psychology and Psychiatry*, **40**, 19–55.

51

Schopler, E., Mesibov, G., Kunce, L. (Eds) (1998) *Asperger Syndrome or High Functioning Autism? Special Issue of Journal of Autism and Developmental Disorders.* New York: Plenum Press.

Siponmaa, L., Kristiansson, M., Nydén, A., Jonson, C., Gillberg, C. (1999) 'Young forensic psychiatric patients: the role of child neuropsychiatric disorders.' (In progress)

Sobanski, E., Marcus, A., Henninghausen, K., Hebebrand, J., Schmidt, M.H. (1999) 'Further evidence for a low body weight in male children and adolescents with Asperger's disorder or schizoid personality disorder.' *European Child and Adolescent Psychiatry*, **8**. In press.

Ssucharewa, G.E. (1926) 'Die schizoiden Psychopathien im Kindesalter.' *Monatsschrift für Psychiatrie und Neurologie*, **60**, 235–261.

Szatmari, P., Bartolucci, G., Brenner, R. (1989a) 'Asperger's syndrome and autism: comparisons on early history and outcome.' *Developmental Medicine and Child Neurology*, **31**, 709–720.

Szatmari, P., Brenner, R., Nagy, J. (1989b) 'Asperger's syndrome: a review of clinical features.' *Canadian Journal of Psychiatry*, **34**, 554–560.

Tantam, D. (1988) Asperger's syndrome. *Journal of Child Psychology and Psychiatry*, **29**, 245–255.

—— (1991) 'Asperger syndrome in adulthood.' *In:* Frith, U. (Ed.) *Autism and Asperger Syndrome.* Cambridge: Cambridge University Press, pp. 147–183.

Tantam, D., Evered, C., Hersov, L. (1990) 'Asperger's syndrome and ligamentous laxity.' *Journal of the American Academy of Child and Adolescent Psychiatry*, **29**, 892–896.

Volkmar, F.R., Klin, A., Pauls, D. (1998) 'Nosological and genetic aspects of Asperger syndrome.' *Journal of Autism and Developmental Disorders*, **28**, 457–463.

WHO (World Health Organization) (1993) *The ICD-10 Classification of Mental and Behavioural Disorders. Diagnostic Criteria for Research.* Geneva: WHO.

Wing, L. (1981) 'Asperger's syndrome: a clinical account.' *Psychological Medicine*, **11**, 115–129.

Wolff, S. (1995) *Loners. The Life Path of Unusual Children.* London: Routledge.

Wolff, S., McGuire, R.J. (1995) 'Schizoid personality in girls: a follow-up study – what are the links with Asperger's syndrome?' *Journal of Child Psychology and Psychiatry*, **36**, 793–817.

4
DIAGNOSIS IN INFANCY

Autism is usually diagnosed after the child's second birthday, and sometimes much later, including in adult age. Subtle symptoms of core impairments and unspecific behavior changes occur before 18 months of age in a majority of all cases of autistic disorder. In Asperger syndrome and other non-classic cases in the autism spectrum, symptoms warranting work-up and diagnosis may not appear until after the child's third birthday, and it is not uncommon for a more definitive diagnosis not to be made until the child is well into the school years.

The age of obvious clinical onset in autism can, in rare instances, be as early as the first hour of life. An infant with autism may be born with such severe haptic defensiveness (sensitivity of the tactile system) that the child screams when held, and the mother ends up feeding the infant by holding the bottle over the crib (or even tying it with ribbons to the walls of the crib) without actually touching the infant (Coleman 1989). Such infants have great difficulty tolerating breast-feeding because of the tactile interaction involved. Instead of being soothed by the mother's touch, it appears to cause the child discomfort or even pain. However, such failure to settle in the mother's arms, or lack of "cuddliness," if not in such an extreme degree, can sometimes be seen in perfectly normal children (Schaffer and Emerson 1964), so this symptom, by itself, cannot be used for screening purposes in detecting infants with autism.

Thus the question arises: are there specific or very high-risk symptoms that can alert the clinical observer to the possibility of an autistic syndrome in a very young infant? In view of the developing understanding of medical etiologies, and the specific therapies that are sometimes available, this question is no longer limited to an academic exercise. It may be quite helpful to the child if educational intervention, now possibly combined with medical treatment in some cases, can be started very early.

Since autism is a syndrome with multiple etiologies, it is not anticipated that particular specific signs and symptoms will be present in a high percentage of cases. However, when a combination of signs and symptoms is present in a neonate or a very young child, it may alert the physician and the family. In the experience of the present authors, and that of other observers in the field of autism, many parents realize that something is seriously wrong with their child from the start, or almost from the start (Gillberg 1984). Although it is quite a difficult task in many cases, it is important for physicians to use what medical knowledge exists to decide if a child is at risk for autism, while avoiding undue worry in parents of unusual but normal babies.

Early signs that may signal the risk of developing autism
Most children with autism have no obvious physical stigmata. However, a sophisticated examination of an infant could reveal signs that, in three studies, have differentiated

children with and without autism (Walker 1976, Campbell *et al.* 1978, Links *et al.* 1980). Ear anomalies were a common finding in these studies, including malformations, asymmetrical, soft or pliable ears, adherent lobes and, especially, low-set ears. (Incidentally, these ear anomalies might well account for some of the association of autism with conductive hearing loss (Smith *et al.* 1988).)

Other signs which have been shown to be statistically associated with autism, and which might alert the examiner of the infant, include hypertelorism, partial syndactyly of the second and third toes, and mouth anomalies (high palate, tongue furrows and smooth/rough spots). Although none of these signs are specific to autism and they can all be seen in other syndromes, they can be helpful when combined with the clinical symptoms in the very young patient.

Muscular hypotonia in the newborn period may signal a variety of developmental disorders including autism. For instance, in the fragile X syndrome, hypotonia is a fairly common feature, and in 20 per cent of newborns with this syndrome attention was alerted by clinically manifest hypotonia.

A systematic study of home videos of 17 infants who later developed the full syndrome of autism revealed that, without exception, there were marked abnormalities of motor performance/motor style, and/or an abnormal facial expression, including a "Moebius" mouth (Teitelbaum *et al.* 1998).

Early symptoms that may alert the clinician to the possibility of autism

There are very few studies of early symptoms (Arrieta *et al.* 1990, Wolman *et al.* 1990) and even fewer observational records available on people with autism during the first years of life. Such evidence as there is suggests that non-specific symptoms, such as lack of initiative, hyperactivity, sleep problems and feeding difficulties, are often the first to be recognized.

A series of studies is available from Göteborg, Sweden, in which early symptoms have been delineated by both retrospective and current and prospective study (Dahlgren and Gillberg 1989, Gillberg *et al.* 1990). In the Dahlgren and Gillberg study, a 130-item questionnaire was filled out by mothers of sex-, age- and IQ-matched mentally retarded and population-representative normal children, as well as by the parents of children with autism. The study was retrospective, and the subjects were 7 to 22 years old at the time the parents completed the questionnaire. In the Gillberg *et al.* study, the same questionnaire was used in a study of children with autism who were seen before age 3 years, the mothers completing the questionnaire before the child's third birthday. The children were followed up prospectively, and a diagnosis of autism established after 3 years of age. The results were contrasted with findings obtained in an age-, sex- and IQ-matched comparison group without autistic symptoms. Table 4.1 lists the 28 items which characterized the autism group in either the prospective study only (10 items) or the retrospective study only (8 items) or in both studies (10 items). Two further items pertaining to overall developmental backwardness ("late development" and "late speech development") also distinguished the autism from the non-autism retarded group in the prospective study. It is of some interest that a number of items thought to be typical of autism ("loves to spin objects," "walks on

TABLE 4.1
Items discriminating autism from mental retardation and normality under age 3 years

Area/item	Prospective study (Gillberg et al. 1990)	Retrospective study (Dahlgren and Gillberg 1989)
Social		
Appears to be isolated from surroundings	✓*	✓
Doesn't smile when expected to	✓	✓
Difficulties getting eye contact	✓	✓
Doesn't matter much whether Mum or Dad is close by or not	✓	
Doesn't like to be disturbed in own world		✓
Contented if left alone		✓
Communication		
Doesn't try to attract adult's attention to own activity	✓	✓**
Difficulties imitating movements	✓	✓
Late speech development	✓	
Doesn't point to objects	✓	
Doesn't understand what people say	✓	
Can't indicate own wishes	✓	
Play behavior		
Doesn't play like other children	✓*	✓
Occupies self only when alone	✓	✓
Plays only with hard objects	✓	✓
Odd attachments to odd objects		✓
Perception		
There is (or has been) a suspicion of deafness	✓*	✓
Empty gaze	✓	✓**
Overexcited when tickled	✓	✓
There is something strange about her/his gaze	✓	
Interested only in certain parts of objects	✓	
Exceptionally interested in things that move	✓	
Doesn't listen when spoken to	✓	
Strange reactions to sound		✓**
Doesn't seem to react to cold		✓
Engages in bizarre looking at objects, pattern and movements		✓
Rhythmicity		
There are days/periods when s/he seems much worse than usual		✓
Severe problems over sleep		✓

* 3 items with strongest discriminatory power in prospective study
** 3 items with strongest discriminatory power in retrospective study

tiptoe," "turns light on and off," "does not like to sit on somebody else's knee," "dislikes change of routine," "fascinated by sight of running water") did not discriminate between groups either in the pro- or retrospective study.

The latter study demonstrated that, in quite a number of cases of children referred in infancy with a suspicion of autism, it is possible to arrive at a correct diagnosis very early, particularly if the child is also mentally retarded. Also, at least a quarter of children believed to suffer from autism during the first few years of life will later be shown to have other developmental problems, or, in rare instances, to be perfectly normal at follow-up.

Non-specific early problems

Even though overall late development is typical both of children with autism and of children with mental retardation, there were clear trends in the Swedish studies for "abnormalities of any kind" to have been observed earlier in autism than in mental retardation. This held even if autism cases were compared with non-autism cases with severe mental retardation, provided that comparison across cases was performed at corresponding IQ levels. These findings corroborated those of Short and Schopler (1988).

Sleep problems and a strong tendency for periodicity were noted in the retrospective but not in the prospective study, implying that caution may be warranted as regards generalizability.

There is, quite naturally, considerable overlap in respect of early symptoms in autism and mental retardation. According to a study of schizophrenia with childhood onset (Watkins *et al.* 1988), there may also, in certain cases, be considerable similarity between the early histories of children with school-age onset schizophrenia and infancy onset autism.

In the Gillberg *et al.* (1990) study, mothers were asked to describe in their own words what they had first noted as possibly abnormal in the child. "Abnormalities of eye contact" was the single most common type of abnormality reported and had been noted around age 1 to 8 months. A few had worried about "strange reactions to sound" around age 1 year. Otherwise, no specific symptoms emerged as characteristic of autism. Rather, diffuse concern about something "not touchable," or "not graspable," tended to prevail.

However, it is again necessary to point out that in high-functioning children with autism there may be no characteristic (specific or non-specific) signs in infancy.

Early symptoms that may be specific to autism in infancy

Abnormal responses to sensory stimuli tend to represent the most characteristic group of symptoms in autism cases referred in infancy (Ornitz *et al.* 1978, Ornitz 1988, Gillberg 1989). In recent studies by Dahlgren and Gillberg (1989) and Gillberg *et al.* (1990), 10 out of 28 possibly specific symptoms of autism belonged in this group (see Table 4.1); this was not an effect of there being more questionnaire items in this category than in the four others (social, communication, play behavior and rhythmicity).

Except for abnormal perceptual responses, symptoms associated with "autistic aloneness," motor performance dysfunction, and abnormalities of play tend to be those most clearly evident in infants with autistic symptoms.

In a study by Sauvage *et al.* (1987), a relative lack of mimicry and an expressionless face were found to be the most common first signs of autism, at least as judged from home movies. Whether to group such symptoms with social or communication deficits is not yet obvious.

Abnormal babble, widely believed to be an early symptom of autism, has not shown up in recent studies.

In a collaborative study between the Department of Psychology at the University of London and the Child Neuropsychiatry Clinic in Göteborg, siblings of children with autism were examined at age 18 months with a view to finding symptoms of autism (and, in particular, symptoms of empathy/theory of mind deficits). A Checklist for Autism in Toddlers (CHAT) was used. Four out of 41 examined siblings were diagnosed as suffering from autism; all four could be predicted on the basis of reported deficits in two or more of imaginative play behaviors, shared attention, protodeclarative pointing, social interest and social play, at age 18 months (Baron-Cohen *et al.* 1992). In a later study, three items – protodeclarative pointing, gaze-monitoring and pretend play – on the CHAT were found to have relatively good screening ability, at least for classic autism cases (Baron-Cohen *et al.* 1996).

The clinical picture of autism developing in infancy

It appears that about three-quarters of children with autism show symptoms and signs of the disorder already in the first 18 to 30 months of life (Gillberg 1989). However, when discussing infancy in autism, it is important to keep in mind the multiple etiologies and different ages of onset. There are patients in whom one can look in vain for symptoms during early infancy (Fig. 4.1). In such cases, often a clear month of onset can be determined in the second or third year of the child's life (Wing 1980). While not disputing the existence of such forms of autism, it is clear that, even in the group with an apparent setback, careful, detailed, retrospective history-taking with the parents will often reveal that there have been early developmental delays and abnormalities (Wing 1971). Also, there are the high-functioning cases in which it may only become gradually obvious that the child is deviant. The abnormality in the brain which causes autism may well, in certain cases, have been there from before birth, but, before a certain age, the nervous system is able to deal with the demands posed by development. Gradually, the brain can no longer fully cope with these demands and the autistic symptoms appear clearly for the first time. In such cases, "autism," even if congenital, will appear to have its onset after infancy.

Many infants with autism show "no response" or "no smile." They may lack the normal anticipatory reactions typical of healthy children about to be picked up by their parents. The abnormal response to sound is often obvious in the second half of the first year, and many children with autism have been thought deaf by persons outside the immediate family (who know they cannot be). There may be major sleep problems or the child may be perceived as "too good to be true," never demanding attention. "Feeding problems," in both breast- and bottle-fed babies, are very common, the child either displaying sucking difficulties, or holding the head in stiff and strange postures, or, more rarely, actively turning away.

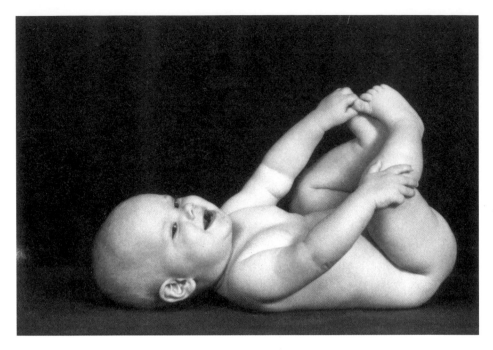

Fig. 4.1 14-month-old boy with idiopathic autism.

Many children with autism are extremely behaviorally deviant even during this first year of life. They may engage in stereotyped hand movements and be completely passive, not interested in exploring their environment – indeed, showing no initiative whatsoever, and perhaps already fiercely protesting when demands are made or routines changed. A few reject body contact. Many prefer to be left alone.

Toward the end of the first year, the child's lack of initiative and interest in exploring the environment comes into focus. The child will not look for things which disappear out of vision as normal children of that age will do. They do not show shared attention behaviors as early as other children do, and one-finger pointing is rarely achieved until several years later. They also fail to develop signs of the emergence of a theory of mind (Frith 1989). In other words, they seem to be unable to understand that other people may have minds of their own (see also Chapters 2 and 9).

Instruments developed with a view to diagnosing autism at under 3 years of age
The SAB (Symptoms of Autism in Babies) is a questionnaire which was developed by Dahlgren and Gillberg (1989). It has been used in prospective and retrospective studies (see above). On the basis of the limited empirical study and clinical experience with this instrument, a screening model for autism in infancy has been suggested (Gillberg 1989). This model (Table 4.2) should not be regarded as an "exact" device, but rather as a check-list to be used if the child has anything to suggest autism or an autistic-like condition, or if the parent is concerned about the child's behavior or development.

TABLE 4.2
Screening for autism at ages 10 and 18 months

1 The following questions to the mother provide a tentative framework for a checklist to be used whenever there is (even mild) suspicion of autistic-like behavior or autism:

Do you consider your child's eye-to-eye-contact to be normal?
Do you think that s/he listens to you or has normal hearing, or does s/he react only to particular sounds?
If there are, or have been, any feeding problems or abnormal behaviors in connection with feeding, what were they?
Is s/he comforted by proximity or body contact?
Does s/he show any interest in his/her surroundings?
Does s/he often smile or laugh quite unexpectedly?
Does s/he prefer to be left alone?
Is your child, on the whole, like other children?

2 Examine the following features systematically:

Hand stereotypies (including strange looking at or posturing of hands)
Avoidance of gaze contact
Stiff, staring gaze
Rejection of body contact
No, or very variable, reaction to strong, unexpected noise
Obvious lack of interest (e.g. does not show interest in peek-a-boo games)

The Checklist for Autism in Toddlers (CHAT) was developed by a British group in collaboration with one of the authors of the present volume (Baron-Cohen *et al.* 1992). It aims to identify children suspected of suffering from autism at around age 18 months. The checklist has now been used in several studies of very young children with autism and in general population samples, and has been shown to have relatively good validity even though it tends to under-identify a group with relatively later onset of severe/clinically important symptomatology. The CHAT is outlined in Table 4.3.

Another early autism screening checklist was developed by Uta Frith and collaborators (Johnson *et al.* 1992). These authors examined infant hearing and vision screening tests for a group of children subsequently diagnosed as autistic, and compared them with a group of children suffering from non-specific developmental delay, as well as with a random sample of records. Four categories (motor, vision, hearing and language, social) were investigated at three ages: 6, 12 and 18 months. The random sample group had a low incidence of reported problems at all ages. The learning-disabled group had a sharp increase in reported abnormalities in all categories at 12 months. The autistic group had a selective increase in the social category alone at 18 months.

The DSM-IV autistic disorder checklist has been tested for reliability, validity and stability over time in children with autism spectrum disorders under 3 years of age (Stone *et al.* 1999a). Certain items, referring specifically to peers, and language and conversational skills, are not useful in identifying these very young children with autism. This should come as no surprise, given that such skills are not well developed at a very young age in normal children either.

TABLE 4.3
Checklist for Autism in Toddlers (the CHAT)

Section A
Ask parent:

1	Does your child enjoy being swung, bounced on your knee, etc.?	Yes	No
2	Does your child take an interest in other children?	Yes	No
3	Does your child like climbing on things, such as up stairs?	Yes	No
4	Does your child enjoy playing peek-a-boo/hide-and-seek?	Yes	No
5	Does your child ever pretend, for example, to make a cup of tea using a toy cup and teapot, or pretend other things?	Yes	No
6	Does your child ever use his/her index finger to point, to ask for something?	Yes	No
7	Does your child ever use his/her index finger to point, to indicate interest in something?	Yes	No
8	Can your child play properly with small toys (*e.g.* cars or bricks) without just mouthing, fiddling, or dropping them?	Yes	No
9	Does your child ever bring objects over to you (parent), to show you something?	Yes	No

Section B
GP's or health visitor's observation:

i	During the appointment, has the child made eye contact with you?	Yes	No
ii	Get child's attention, then point across the room at an interesting object and say "Oh look! There's a (name a toy)!" Watch child's face.	Yes	No
iii	Get the child's attention, then give child a miniature toy cup and teapot, and say "Can you make a cup of tea?" Does the child pretend to pour tea, drink it, etc.?	Yes	No
iv	Say to the child "Where's the light?" or "Show me the light." Does the child point his/her index finger at the light?	Yes	No
v	Can the child build a tower of bricks? (If so, how many?) (Number of bricks …)	Yes	No

The Infant Behaviour Summarized Evaluation (ISBE) scale was developed by a French group (Barthélémy *et al.* 1990) on the basis of their Behaviour Summarized Evaluation (BSE) scale which had previously been tested for reliability and validity in several studies.

Very young children with autism show clearly different patterns of correspondence between mental age and adaptive behavior levels, as reflected in results on the Vineland scale, than do children with non-autistic developmental delay (Stone *et al.* 1999b). It appears that the Vineland scale may be one of the best tools for identifying the broader autism spectrum group in children around 3 years of age or younger.

The Autism Diagnostic Observation Schedule (ADOS) (Lord *et al.* 1989) was originally developed as a research instrument to be used in conjunction with the Autism Diagnostic Interview (ADI) (Le Couteur *et al.* 1989) for the establishment of a firm diagnosis of autism in slightly older children. There is now a prelinguistic version (Pl-ADOS) containing systematic structured observation measures which can be used in the work-up of very young children. However, it is not a screening device and should only be used by staff who have received special instruction in its use.

Summary

On the basis of the limited empirical study and clinical experience with the SAB, a screening model for autism in infancy has been suggested. This model should not be regarded as an "exact" device, but rather as a checklist to be used if the child has anything to suggest autism or an autistic-like condition, or if the parent is concerned about the child's behavior or development. The CHAT can be used as a complement or in cases where autism is suspected according to the screening model. In the future, it will be essential to try to distinguish early symptoms in autism according to the diagnosed underlying medical condition. Finding unifying features in autism will remain important for screening purposes, but differentiation of early symptoms in accordance with underlying etiology will become crucial if we are to understand brain behavior developmental relationships better.

REFERENCES

Arrieta, M.I., Martinez, B., Criado B., Simón, A., Salazar, I., Lostao, C.M. (1990) 'Dermatoglyphic analysis of autistic Basque children.' *American Journal of Medical Genetics*, **35**, 1–9.

Baron-Cohen, S., Allen, J., Gillberg, C. (1992) 'Can autism be detected at 18 months? The needle, the haystack and the CHAT.' *British Journal of Psychiatry*, **161**, 839–843.

Baron-Cohen, S., Cox, A., Baird, G., Swettenham, J., Nightingale, N., Morgan, K., Drew, A., Charman, A. (1996) 'Psychological markers in the detection of autism in infancy in a large population.' *British Journal of Psychiatry*, **168(2)**, 158–163.

Barthélémy, C., Adrien, J.L., Tanguay, P., Garreau, B., Fermanian, J., Roux, S., Sauvage, D., Lelord, G. (1990) 'The Behavioral Summarized Evaluation. Validity and reliability of a scale for the assessment of autistic behaviors.' *Journal of Autism and Developmental Disorders*, **20**, 189–204.

Campbell, M., Geller, B., Small, A.M., Petti, T.A., Ferris, S.H. (1978) 'Minor physical anomalies in young psychotic children.' *American Journal of Psychiatry*, **135**, 573–575.

Coleman, M. (1989) 'Autism: non-drug biological treatments.' *In:* Gillberg, C. *Diagnosis and Treatment of Autism.* New York: Plenum Press, pp. 219–235.

Dahlgren, S.O., Gillberg, C. (1989) 'Symptoms in the first two years of life. A preliminary population study of infantile autism.' *European Archives of Psychiatry and Neurological Sciences*, **238**, 169–174.

Frith, U. (1989) 'Autism and "theory of mind."' *In:* Gillberg, C. *Diagnosis and Treatment of Autism.* New York: Plenum Press, pp. 33–52.

Gillberg, C. (1984) 'Infantile autism and other childhood psychoses in a Swedish urban region. Epidemiological aspects.' *Journal of Child Psychology and Psychiatry*, **25**, 35–43.

—— (1989) 'Early symptoms of autism.' *In:* Gillberg, C. *Diagnosis and Treatment of Autism.* New York: Plenum Press, pp. 23–32.

Gillberg, C., Ehlers, S., Schaumann, H., Jakobsson, G., Dahlgren, S.O., Lindblom, R., Bågenholm, A., Tjuus, T., Blidner, E. (1990) 'Autism under age 3 years: a clinical study of 28 cases referred for autistic symptoms in infancy.' *Journal of Child Psychology and Psychiatry*, **31**, 921–934.

Johnson, M.H., Siddons, F., Frith, U., Morton, J. (1992) 'Can autism be predicted on the basis of infant screening tests?' *Developmental Medicine and Child Neurology*, **34**, 316–320.

Le Couteur, A., Rutter, M., Lord, C., Rios, P., Robertson, S., Holdgrafer, M., McLennan, J. (1989) 'Autism diagnostic interview: a standardized investigator-based instrument.' *Journal of Autism and Developmental Disorders*, **19**, 363–387.

Links, P.S., Stockwell, M., Abichandi, F., Simeon, J. (1980) 'Minor physical anomalies in childhood autism: Part I. Their relationship to pre- and perinatal complications.' *Journal of Autism and Developmental Disorders*, **10**, 273–285.

Lord, C., Rutter, M., Goode, S., Heemsbergen, J., Jordan, J., Mawhood, L., Schopler, E. (1989) 'Autism diagnostic observation schedule: a standardized observation of communicative and social behavior.' *Journal of Autism and Developmental Disorders*, **19**, 185–212.

Ornitz, E. (1988) 'Autism: a disorder of directed attention.' *Brain Dysfunction*, **1**, 309–322.

Ornitz, E., Gurhrie, D., Farley, A.J. (1978) 'The early symptoms of childhood autism.' *In:* Serban, G. *Cognitive Defects in the Development of Mental Illness*. New York: Brunner/Mazel.

Sauvage, D., Hameury, L., Adrien, J.L., Larmande, C., Perrot-Beaugerie, A., Barthélémy, C., Peyraud, A. (1987) 'Signes d'autisme avant deux ans. Evaluation et signification.' *Annales de Psychiatrie*, **3**, 418–424.

Schaffer, H.R., Emerson, P.E. (1964) 'The development of social attachments in infancy.' *Monographs of the Society for Research in Child Development*, **94**, 1–77.

Short, A.B., Schopler, E. (1988) 'Factors relating to age of onset in autism.' *Journal of Autism and Developmental Disorders*, **18**, 207–216.

Smith, D.E., Miller, S.D., Stewart, M., Walter, T.C., McConnel, J.V. (1988) 'Conductive hearing loss in autistic learning-disabled and normal children.' *Journal of Autism and Developmental Disoders*, **1**, 53–65.

Stone, W.L., Lee, E.B., Ashford, L., Brissie, J., Hepburn, S.L., Coonrod, E.E., Weiss, B.H. (1999a) 'Can autism be diagnosed accurately in children under 3 years?' *Journal of Child Psychology and Psychiatry*, **40(2)**, 219–226.

Stone, W.L., Ousley, O.Y., Hepburn, S.L., Hogan, K.L., Brown, C.S. (1999b) 'Patterns of adaptive behavior in very young children with autism.' *American Journal of Mental Retardation*, **104(2)**, 187–199.

Teitelbaum, P., Teitelbaum, O., Nye, J., Fryman, J., Maurer, R.G. (1998) 'Movement analysis in infancy may be useful for early diagnosis of autism.' *Proceedings of the National Academy of Science*, USA, November 10, **95(23)**, 13982–7.

Walker, H. (1976) 'The incidence of minor physical anomalies in autistic children.' *In:* Coleman, M. *The Autistic Syndromes*. Amsterdam: North-Holland, pp. 95–116.

Watkins, J.M., Asarnow, R.F., Tanguay, P.E. (1988) 'Symptom development in childhood onset schizophrenia.' *Journal of Child Psychology and Psychiatry*, **29**, 865–878.

Wing, L. (1971) 'Perceptual and language development in autistic children: a comparative study.' *In:* Rutter, M. *Infantile Autism: Concepts, Characteristics and Treatment*. London: Churchill-Livingstone, pp. 173–197.

—— (1980) *Early Childhood Autism*. Oxford: Pergamon Press.

Wolman, S.R., Campbell, M., Marchi, M.L., Deutsch, S.I., Gershon, T.M. (1990) 'Dermatoglyphic study in autistic children and controls.' *Journal of the American Academy of Child and Adolescent Psychiatry*, **29**, 878–884.

5
CLINICAL COURSE IN CHILDHOOD AND ADOLESCENCE

Autism, like other developmental disorders, shows changes with respect to prevailing symptomatology with age (Rutter 1978, Wing 1980, Ornitz 1983, Waterhouse *et al.* 1984, Frith 1989, 1991, Wing 1989, Gillberg 1990, Wing 1996, Nordin and Gillberg 1998). This needs repeated emphasis, especially since many children with autism develop in rather different directions. Children who could scarcely be distinguished behaviorally at age 18 months may, by the age of 10 years, have developed completely different personalities and symptoms. This is one of the reasons why early recognition and observation are essential for establishing a precise diagnosis. Several years later it may even be impossible to say that the child ever had autism. We have followed several children who, before 5 years of age, showed all the characteristics of Kanner autism, but who ten years later were only a little odd, had some peculiarities of spoken language, but were socializing with several age peers. By the time these children had reached the age of 7 to 10 years, most people would find it hard to believe that they had ever suffered from autism. One of the current authors has followed a boy with classic Kanner autism – who also developed uncomplicated epilepsy (controlled by carbamazepine for several years) – who, for various reasons, did not receive appropriate educational interventions, but who, nevertheless, was considered "indistinguishable from normal" by age 10 years. The same observation has been made by Gillberg *et al.* (1990) and Stone *et al.* (1999) in follow-up studies of children diagnosed as having autism at under 3 years of age, and by Chess (1977) in her follow-up of children with autism who had suffered rubella embryopathy. It is possible that it is children such as these who are reported to have been cured by various kinds of intervention.

Infancy and the first few years of life
Home videos and medical history data from parents and other caregivers suggest that non-specific symptoms such as lack of initiative, hyperactivity, sleep problems and feeding difficulties are often the first to be recognized. That such problems are frequent "first symptoms" in autism was also suggested by two systematic studies (Dahlgren and Gillberg 1989, Gillberg *et al.* 1990). These studies further indicated that certain other symptoms might possibly be more specifically associated with autism. These included abnormal responses to sensory stimulation, autistic aloneness and various abnormalities of behavior and play. These issues are discussed in more detail in Chapter 3.

Some of the DSM/ICD diagnostic characteristics for autism are difficult to apply to very young children. These include poor peer relationships, limited conversational skills and stereotyped language. It is difficult, if possible at all, to judge the quality of peer relations in children with mental ages below 24 months; and language abnormalities cannot be readily assessed in children who have not yet acquired useful spoken language (Stone *et al.* 1999).

It is not unusual for children with autism to develop several single words before the age of 2 years and then to stop using them soon after. It is as though the capacity for spoken language is there, but, because an understanding of the meaning of communication is lacking, there is no inherent "drive" for further development.

About 15 per cent of all children with autism develop seizures in the first few years of life (and another 20 per cent have seizure onset later in life, usually in adolescence). Infantile spasms may have their onset around age 5–18 months and may appear to trigger the development of autistic withdrawal. In other instances it is clear that the autistic symptoms were already present when the epilepsy appeared. Other children have other kinds of seizures, which, like infantile spasms, may or may not signal underlying medical disorders such as tuberous sclerosis or Rett syndrome.

The preschool years
From about age 2 to 6 years, the typically autistic behavior patterns are usually most clearly evident. One explanation for this is the fact that many of the children with autism described by Kanner belonged in that age group, and thus the stereotype of "Kanner syndrome" is to some extent associated with children of that age.

A diagnosis of autism can be made with a considerable degree of confidence if the child is about 30 months of age or older (Gillberg *et al.*1990, Stone *et al.*1999). In younger children the diagnosis may well be suspected, but it is often a good idea to postpone the definitive diagnostic decision – but not necessarily the medical work-up – until the child is about 30 months old and/or has a mental age of about 18 months or more.

For most families, the preschool years (and, in some cases, the adolescent years) are the hardest to cope with. The fearful temper tantrums associated with the more extreme forms of insistence on sameness are usually at a peak during this period. Also, most children with autism, after they have started walking unsupported (which they often do on time or only a few months late), become very difficult to manage in that they may be hyperactive, destructive or constantly engaging in repetitive activities, such as endlessly listening to tape recordings or occupying themselves with the tape recorder as a technical device. A particular object, such as a set of keys, fascinates some, and the child will be furious if deprived of it. Motor stereotypies are an extremely common, but not invariable, feature.

Around age 2 years, most normal children have developed some kind of communicative, spoken language, and begin to show a greater interest in other children. The child with autism usually fails to do any of these things, and so is, for the first time, recognized as definitely abnormal. Many normal children – and children with autism – experience the birth of a sibling at about this age. It has become popular to attribute the withdrawal of some children with autism to the psychological trauma supposedly connected with this birth. A careful history-taking will reveal, however, that the child has already displayed abnormal characteristics, and it is only the demands on normal development, which they cannot live up to, and the comparison with a normal sibling, which make their abnormalities so much more conspicuous.

In some cases of autism it seems that normal development precedes a period of regression to an autistic state at about the age of 18 to 30 months. It is still unclear what proportion of all autism cases they represent. Some authors would prefer to group them with the cases of childhood disintegrative disorder (Baird *et al.* 1991). Others maintain that it is possible to separate cases with late onset autism from those with disintegrative disorders (Volkmar and Cohen 1989). As has already been argued in Chapter 2, there is reason to hypothesize that at least some of these cases may be congenital in spite of the fact that obvious symptoms emerge only after a period of seemingly normal development. In other cases, however, it is clear that the autistic syndrome developed after some particular postnatal brain affliction, such as herpes encephalitis (DeLong *et al.* 1981, Gillberg 1986, I.C. Gillberg 1991) or epilepsy (Rapin 1995). Rett syndrome (in girls) and tuberous sclerosis should be particularly high on the list of possible underlying medical disorders in children who show the combination of severe autistic symptoms, developmental delay/mental retardation and early onset epilepsy.

During the later preschool years, the child with autism quite often shows active avoidance of other children. In all cases there are severe problems in interacting normally – *i.e.* in a reciprocal fashion – with other children. The child may be perceived as suffering from "extreme autistic aloneness."

Autistic "withdrawal" may not be the most striking feature in autism. Some children appear more "perplexed" and appear not to be able to make sense of the world around them. They may seem to accept proximity to other people, and quite a number actually show, in various odd ways, that they want to interact with other people: they just do not know how to. Others still are passive and friendly so long as no demands for change of routine are made. These three broad groups of children with autism (that is, the "aloof," the "active but odd" and the "passive") correspond roughly to similarly named subgroups of adults who were diagnosed in early childhood as suffering from autism (Wing 1996).

Some of the more high-functioning children with autism develop useful spoken language during the preschool years, although the majority have very little comprehensible speech before the age of 4 to 5 years. Those who do develop early language skills have a way of talking *at* rather than *with* other people. They appear not to be able to understand that they are talking "to the inside" of people and not merely repeating phrases which do not require an answer or require only one specific standard reply.

Early school years
During the early school years (about the age of 6 to 12 years) most children with autism, if in an understanding and appropriate environment, gradually become less difficult to manage. The social aloofness usually subsides to some extent, and they become more cooperative. A proportion (perhaps a third) remain quite severely withdrawn throughout childhood. Nevertheless, the vast majority no longer totally avoid other children, even though they cannot relate to them in a manner appropriate to their age.

The degree of development of spoken language at age 5 to 6 years is one of the most significant factors affecting outcome (Rutter 1983, Nordin and Gillberg 1998). Two children with autism who might appear equally behaviorally deviant at around age 3 years may be very different from each other at 7 years: one could appear almost as deviant as at age 3, and without useful language skills; while the other could appear "odd" but in possession of useful speech and much less deviant than during the preschool years.

On the whole, hyperactivity and temper tantrums are not as frequent during the school years as earlier, and therefore parents, siblings and teachers usually have a relatively calmer period. However, in our experience, this will depend to some extent on whether or not the child has been correctly diagnosed as suffering from autism at the earlier age. Fewer families now live "in the dark" for years, not knowing what is wrong with their child and constantly oscillating between fear, "perplexity" and hope. Families receiving an early diagnosis and adequate educational programs, involving the parents, report better coping strategies and fewer problems than those who are given the diagnosis later (Bågenholm and Gillberg 1991).

Sleep problems no longer tend to take on such dramatic guises, and, although children with autism sometimes still have a greatly reduced need for sleep, they may be able to occupy themselves at night and leave other family members to rest.

There are, of course, exceptions to this rule, and some children with autism, especially those with severe mental retardation (and perhaps also some of the very high-functioning cases), have major behavior problems throughout the school years.

Puberty and adolescence

Several studies have shown clearly that the adolescent period may be critical in many cases. Epilepsy, deterioration, aggravation of symptoms and additional psychiatric problems are the most common complications accompanying autism in adolescence.

IMPROVEMENT IN ADOLESCENCE

A minority of children do improve perceptibly during the teenage period (Kanner 1971). These are usually relatively high-functioning children who have also shown positive development during the early school years (Szatmari *et al.* 1989, Nordin and Gillberg 1998). Many others go through their teens with no more major behavior problems than are usually associated with puberty in normal children.

One Japanese study (Kobayashi *et al.*1992) found a relatively high proportion (43 per cent) of individuals with autism who improved in adolescence.

PHYSICAL CHANGES

Among those with mental retardation and borderline intellectual functioning, rather marked physical changes sometimes occur, so that bright-looking children with autism may come out of puberty looking more "dull." Very occasionally this can be due to an underlying medical disorder such as tuberous sclerosis or neurofibromatosis which may produce skin problems and other physically visible changes only after infancy and childhood.

EPILEPSY

Many youngsters with autism who have not been affected by seizures in childhood will develop epilepsy before adulthood. It seems that 30 to 40 per cent of all people with autism develop epilepsy before the age of 30 years (Rutter 1970, Gillberg and Steffenburg 1987, Olsson *et al.* 1988). At least half of this group have seizure onset around the time of puberty. The risk of epilepsy is higher among people with autism and mental retardation, but the rate is also high in those of normal intelligence (Gillberg *et al.* 1987, Olsson *et al.* 1988).

There has been much controversy about whether to include children with obvious brain dysfunction in the category of infantile autism. Although the view has become less common during the last decade, some would still argue for the exclusion of those with major neurological impairment. The onset of epilepsy in adolescents with autism who previously demonstrated no signs of neurological dysfunction (and even in children without previous EEG abnormalities) demonstrates the impossibility of such a position. At present, there is still no way of predicting in early childhood (the time when autism is most often diagnosed) just who will experience seizures later in life. However, girls seem to run a slightly higher risk than boys (Gillberg and Steffenburg 1987).

DETERIORATION

Brown (1969), Rutter (1970) and Gillberg and Schaumann (1981) have all described cases of autism with deterioration in adolescence. According to these studies, an estimated 10 to 30 per cent of children with autism can be expected to show cognitive and behavioral deterioration in puberty, accompanied by regression and a reappearance of many of the symptoms typical of the preschool period (Gillberg 1984b).

In the follow-up studies by Gillberg and Steffenburg (1987), 22 per cent of the whole group showed deterioration (12 per cent of the male and 50 per cent of the female group). In the series of "infantile psychosis" followed by Brown (1969), 34 per cent of those for whom adequate information was available did less well during puberty than during the early school years, and 6 per cent became so disturbed that they required admission to hospital. In the Rutter (1970) study, 12 per cent of the subjects with "childhood psychosis" deteriorated progressively during adolescence. Several of these simultaneously developed neurological signs and symptoms such as seizures and paralysis of the legs. The development of seizures was also commonly encountered in the Gillberg and Steffenburg (1987) study. However, seizures usually occurred only after a year or two of obvious behavioral deterioration. In the latter study there was also a marked tendency for periodicity in the gradual downhill development. Von Knorring and Hägglöf (1993) have also reported on deterioration in autism, as have the Japanese group who found both a high rate of improvement *and* a high rate of deterioration in adolescence (Kobayashi *et al.* 1992). The rate of adolescent deterioration was 32 per cent in the latter study.

The overall conclusion to be drawn on the basis of the various outcome studies published so far is that 12 to 32 per cent of all children with autism deteriorate in adolescence, either behaviorally or cognitively – sometimes both. In these cases there is regression and reappearance of many of the symptoms typical of the preschool period.

Unfortunately, so far, prospective neurobiological studies of deteriorating autism cases have not been reported. Gillberg and Schaumann (1981) and Gillberg and Steffenburg (1987) have suggested that high maternal age, female sex and a family history of affective disorders might increase the risk of deterioration in puberty in autism.

AGGRAVATION OF SYMPTOMS NOT FOLLOWED BY DETERIORATION

At the onset of puberty – or a year before or after – there is often a dramatic aggravation of symptoms such as self-destructiveness, aggressiveness, restlessness and hyperactivity. In the Göteborg studies, such aggravation has been observed in about half of all subjects with autism or autistic-like conditions. Between 40 and 50 per cent of those who show aggravation appear to go on to develop frank deterioration (see above), but the remainder, after a few years, begin to improve again. Again, there is a marked tendency for periodicity in some cases, with a return to "normal" for weeks or months, and then new periods of exacerbation of negative behavioral symptoms. This seems to be particularly common if there is a family history of affective disorder. There is accumulating evidence that autism may be associated with a family history of affective disorder (Tsai *et al.* 1981, Gillberg 1984b, DeLong and Dwyer 1988, Bailey *et al.* 1998), and it is possible that there is a specific subgroup with autism and bipolar disorder.

The pubertal symptom aggravation, whether accompanied by deterioration or not, very often prompts some kind of medication (usually prescribed by adult psychiatrists who may know little about autism). In one study, before puberty, less than a quarter of children with autism had been given a medication affecting the nervous system, whereas at age 16 to 23 years, three out of four were given such treatment (Gillberg and Steffenburg 1987).

While most medications prescribed in the pubertal period appear to do little to alter the negative course, our clinical impression has been that lithium can sometimes be effective in controlling pubertal behavioral/"mood" swings in autism (Gillberg 1989, see also Campbell 1989).

It is important to point out that some of the "pubertal symptom aggravation" may also be the effect of (a) the sheer physical growth and strength of the person with autism, and hence (b) the gradual realization on the part of teachers and parents that some of the behaviors and problems shown by the child will probably continue into adult life and will stand out as even more deviant by virtue of their more abnormal status in an adolescent/adult as compared with a child (*e.g.* problems associated with bladder or bowel function).

INACTIVITY

The marked overactivity seen in many young children with autism is often followed by a state of inactivity in adolescence (Wing 1996). There may sometimes be an extreme degree of psychomotor retardation and an almost total lack of initiative, yet no clear indications of an underlying depressive disorder (even though this may also sometimes occur). When growing up, individuals with autism – like other individuals – often lose their interest in playing with objects and engaging in playful motor activities. They have more problems than normal individuals in finding a new hobby or a new way of taking exercise, and therefore the risk of inactivity is substantial.

DEPRESSED MOOD AND DEPRESSION

Feelings of unhappiness and/or depression are often reported (Wing and Wing 1980, Newson *et al.* 1982, Ghaziuddin and Greden 1998) and may be particularly likely to occur in high-functioning autism or Asperger syndrome (Wing 1981, Tantam 1988). These better-functioning individuals may become painfully aware that they are different from other adolescents. A few develop a strong desire for friendship, but may be totally unable to establish social relationships because they lack the necessary skills.

In families with affective disorder, there is sometimes a typical episode of major depression associated with autism. This might represent a more primary depressive disorder.

Social skills groups, role-playing and videotape feedback followed by systematic training may sometimes be useful when trying to teach youngsters with autism the requirements of social interaction and conversation. Such measures may help to alleviate depressive feelings. Occasionally, individual supportive psychotherapy may also be indicated. Medication is rarely used, but tricyclic antidepressants can sometimes help in reducing depressive symptoms in autism.

CATATONIA

Wing (1996) has drawn attention to a group of relatively high-functioning individuals with autism (and Asperger syndrome) who develop pronounced catatonic features in late adolescence. In a follow-up study of individuals diagnosed in early childhood as suffering from autism or an autistic-like condition, at least 3 out of 46 cases showed moderate to severe catatonia at the age of 28–35 years (Gillberg 1999, unpublished data). A young German woman with classic autism and severe catatonia recently published an autobiography (Schäfer 1996).

PROBLEMS ASSOCIATED WITH SEXUAL MATURATION

For most individuals with autism, puberty is not associated with serious problems connected with sexual maturation. Many parents of girls with autism worry about what might happen in connection with the onset of menstruation. Often the child accepts these changes in a very matter of fact way (Wing 1980).

The growth of sexual drive, as a rule, is not accompanied by a corresponding growth in the field of social "know-how," and this often leads to embarrassing behavior. This appears to be particularly true of moderately and severely retarded boys with autism, who may expose themselves, masturbate in public and touch other people's genital regions (Gillberg 1984b). Such behavior can, of course, be very embarrassing to those confronted, including parents and siblings. Often, the sexual behavior is "interpreted," in more or less sophisticated terms, by "experts" of various professions. However, one of the simplest explanations is that the young boy with autism is simply doing one of the pleasurable things in life that he knows how to do. In autism the behavioral repertoire is very limited, and in some cases masturbation may be one of the few activities the person with autism knows how to perform. The social and planning deficits associated with autism preclude the spontaneous "arrangement" of such activities in ways that will be socially acceptable to other people. It is usually easy to diminish the extent to which the person with autism masturbates by introducing other interesting activities as a substitute. Nevertheless, masturbation activities may occasionally be very difficult to cope with, such as when bottles or other objects are inserted into the anus, or when the activity becomes "fixed" in relation to one particular person.

Some people with autism may be involved in unsolicited homo- or heterosexual contacts (Haracopos 1988) for the simple reason that they may be lacking in reticence and suspiciousness to such an extent that they may be taken advantage of sexually.

Problems associated with sexual maturation need to be handled with consistency, common sense and not too much emotion. Medication is usually not indicated.

Summary

The developmental changes that occur in children with autism from early childhood through adolescence are sometimes dramatic and may be either positive or negative or a mixture of both. There appear to be at least three subgroups which may present with slightly different symptoms already in the first few years of life: the aloof; the active but odd; and the passive. Unspecific symptoms are often present in the first few years, whereas the typical syndrome of autism crystallizes in the later preschool years. The early school years are often a period of amelioration. Adolescence may bring further improvement, but also, in some cases, a tragic set-back with deterioration. Epilepsy can be associated with regressive changes both in the first few years of life and in adolescence.

REFERENCES

Bågenholm, A., Gillberg, C. (1991) 'Psychosocial effects on siblings of children with autism and mental retardation: a population-based study.' *Journal of Mental Deficiency Research*, **35**, 291–307.

Bailey, A., Palferman, S., Heavey, L., Le Couteur, A. (1998) 'Autism: the phenotype in relatives.' *Journal of Autism and Developmental Disorders*, **28**, 369–392.

Baird, G., Baron-Cohen, S., Bohman, M., Coleman, M., Frith, U., Gillberg, C., Howlin, P., Mesibov, G., Peeters, T., Ritvo, E., Steffenburg, S., Taylor, D., Waterhouse, L., Wing, L., Zappella, M. (1991) 'Autism is not necessarily a pervasive developmental disorder.' (Letter) *Developmental Medicine and Child Neurology*, **33**, 363–364.

Brown, W.T. (1969) 'Adolescent development of children with infantile psychosis.' *Seminars in Psychiatry*, **1**, 79–89.

Campbell, M. (1989) 'Pharmacotherapy in autism: an overview.' *In:* Gillberg, C. (Ed.) *Diagnosis and Treatment of Autism*. New York: Plenum Press, pp. 203–218.

Chess, S. (1977) 'Follow-up report on autism in congenital rubella.' *Journal of Autism and Childhood Schizophrenia*, **7**, 68–81.

Dahlgren, S.O., Gillberg, C. (1989) 'Symptoms in the first two years of life. A preliminary population study of infantile autism.' *European Archives of Psychiatry and Neurological Sciences*, **238**, 169–174.

DeLong, G.R., Dwyer, J.T. (1988) 'Correlation of family history with specific autistic subgroups: Asperger's syndrome and bipolar affective disease.' *Journal of Autism and Developmental Disorders*, **18**, 593–600.

DeLong, G.R., Beau, S.C., Brown, F.R. (1981) 'Acquired reversible autistic syndrome in acute encephalopathic illness in children.' *Archives of Neurology*, **38**, 191–194.

Frith, U. (1989) 'Autism and "theory of mind."' *In:* Gillberg, C. (Ed.) *Diagnosis and Treatment of Autism.* New York: Plenum Press, pp. 33–52.

—— (1991) '"Autistic psychopathy" in childhood. Hans Asperger.' *In:* Frith, U. (Ed.) *'Autistic Psychopathy' in Childhood. Hans Asperger.* Translated and annotated by U. Frith. Cambridge: Cambridge University Press, pp. 37–92.

Ghaziuddin, M., Greden, J. (1998) 'Depression in children with autism/pervasive developmental disorders: a case–control family history study.' *Journal of Autism and Developmental Disorders,* **28**, 111–115.

Gillberg, C. (1984a) 'Infantile autism and other childhood psychoses in a Swedish urban region. Epidemiological aspects.' *Journal of Child Psychology and Psychiatry,* **25**, 35–43.

—— (1984b) 'Autistic children growing up: problems during puberty and adolescence.' *Developmental Medicine and Child Neurology,* **26**, 125–129.

—— (1986) 'Brief report: Onset at age 14 of a typical autistic syndrome. A case report of a girl with herpes simplex encephalitis.' *Journal of Autism and Developmental Disorders,* **16**, 369–375.

—— (1989) 'The first evaluation: treatment begins here.' *In:* Gillberg, C. (Ed.) *Diagnosis and Treatment of Autism.* New York: Plenum Press, pp. 139–150.

—— (1990) 'Autism and pervasive developmental disorders.' *Journal of Child Psychology and Psychiatry,* **31**, 99–119 (published erratum appears in *Journal of Child Psychology and Psychiatry,* **32**(1): 213).

Gillberg, C., Schaumann, H. (1981) 'Infantile autism and puberty.' *Journal of Autism and Developmental Disorders,* **11**, 365–371.

Gillberg, C., Steffenburg, S. (1987) 'Outcome and prognostic factors in infantile autism and similar conditions: a population-based study of 46 cases followed through puberty.' *Journal of Autism and Developmental Disorders,* **17**, 273–287.

Gillberg, C., Steffenburg, S., Jakobsson, G. (1987) 'Neurobiological findings in 20 relatively gifted children with Kanner-type autism or Asperger syndrome.' *Developmental Medicine and Child Neurology,* **29**, 641–649.

Gillberg, C., Ehlers, S., Schaumann, H., Jakobsson, G., Dahlgren, S.O., Lindblom, R., Bågenholm, A., Tjuus, T., Blidner, E. (1990) 'Autism under age 3 years: a clinical study of 28 cases referred for autistic symptoms in infancy.' *Journal of Child Psychology and Psychiatry,* **31**, 921–934.

Gillberg, I.C. (1991) 'Autistic syndrome with onset at age 31 years. Herpes encephalitis as one possible model for childhood autism.' *Developmental Medicine and Child Neurology,* **33**, 920–924.

Haracopos, D. (1988) *Hvad med mig?* Svendborg, Denmark: Andonia.

Kanner, L. (1971) 'Follow-up study of eleven children originally reported in 1943.' *Journal of Autism and Childhood Schizophrenia,* **1**, 119–145.

Kobayashi, R., Murata, T., Yoshinaga, K. (1992) 'A follow-up study of 201 children with autism in Kyushu and Yamaguchi areas, Japan.' *Journal of Autism and Developmental Disorders,* **22**, 395–411.

Newson, E., Dawson, M., Everard, P. (1982) *The Natural History of Able Autistic People: The Management and Functioning in a Social Context. Summary of Report to DHSS.*

Nordin, V., Gillberg, C. (1998) 'The long-term course of autistic disorders: update on follow-up studies.' *Acta Psychiatrica Scandinavica,* **97**, 99–108.

Olsson, I., Steffenburg, S., Gillberg, C. (1988) 'Epilepsy in autism and autistic-like conditions: a population-based study.' *Archives of Neurology,* **45**, 666–668.

Ornitz, E.M. (1983) 'The functional neuroanatomy of infantile autism.' *International Journal of Neuroscience,* **19**, 85–124.

Rapin, I. (1995) 'Acquired aphasia in children.' *Journal of Child Neurology,* **10**, 267–270.

Rutter, M. (1970) 'Autistic children: infancy to adulthood.' *Seminars in Psychiatry,* **2**, 435–450.

—— (1978) 'Diagnosis and definition.' *In:* Rutter, M., Schopler, E. (Eds) *Autism. A Reappraisal of Concepts and Treatment.* New York: Plenum Press, pp. 1–25.

—— (1983) 'Cognitive deficits in the pathogenesis of autism.' *Journal of Child Psychology and Psychiatry,* **24**, 513–531.

Schäfer, S. (1996) *Stjärnor, linser och äpplen. Att leva med autism.* Stockholm: Cura.

Stone, W.L., Lee, E.B., Ashford, L., Brissie, J., Hepburn, S.L., Coonrod, E.E., Weiss, B.H. (1999) 'Can autism be diagnosed accurately in children under 3 years?' *Journal of Child Psychology and Psychiatry,* **40**(2), 219–226.

Szatmari, P., Bartolucci, G., Brenner, R., Bond, S., Rich, S. (1989) 'A follow-up study of high-functioning autistic children.' *Journal of Autism and Developmental Disorders,* **19**, 213–225.

Tantam, D. (1988) 'Asperger's syndrome.' *Journal of Child Psychology and Psychiatry,* **29**, 245–255.

71

Tsai, L.Y., Stewart, M.A., August, G. (1981) 'Implication of sex differences in the familial transmission of infantile autism.' *Journal of Autism and Developmental Disorders*, **11**, 165–173.

Volkmar, F.R., Cohen, D.J. (1989) 'Disintegrative disorder or "late onset" autism?' *Journal of Child Psychology and Psychiatry*, **30**, 717–724.

von Knorring, A.-L., Hägglöf, B. (1993) 'Autism in Northern Sweden. A population based follow-up study: psychopathology.' *European Child and Adolescent Psychiatry*, **2**, 91–97.

Waterhouse, L., Fein, D., Nath, J., Snyder, D. (1984) *Pervasive Schizophrenia Occurring in Childhood: A Review of Critical Commentary*. Washington, DC: American Psychiatric Association.

Wing, J.K., Wing, L. (1980) 'Provision of services.' *In:* Wing, L. (Ed.) *Early Childhood Autism*. Oxford: Pergamon Press.

Wing, L. (1980) *Early Childhood Autism*. Oxford: Pergamon Press.

—— (1981) 'Asperger's syndrome: a clinical account.' *Psychological Medicine*, **11**, 115–129.

—— (1989) 'Autistic adults.' *In:* Gillberg, C. (Ed.) *Diagnosis and Treatment of Autism*. New York: Plenum Press, pp. 419–432.

—— (1996) *The Autism Spectrum*. London: Constable.

6
ADULTS WITH AUTISM

So far, relatively few reports on adults with autism have been published (Kanner 1973, Gillberg 1983, 1992a, Wing 1983, 1989, Gillberg and Steffenburg 1987, Rumsey and Hamburger 1988, Szatmari *et al.* 1989, Kobayashi *et al.* 1992, von Knorring and Hägglöf 1993) and there have been a few interesting congress reports that have not been formally published at the time of going to press with this edition (*e.g.* Goode *et al.* 1994). Systematic longitudinally collected data on adult individuals diagnosed in childhood as suffering from Asperger syndrome have yet to be reported. Nevertheless, there is growing concern for the continuing psychosocial and psychiatric needs of adults who were diagnosed as suffering from disorders in the autism spectrum in childhood (Schopler and Mesibov 1983, Wing 1996).

Those who do well as adults
It has long been recognized that a small proportion of persons with autism develop into normal – or sometimes highly original, though not psychiatrically ill – adults. In most follow-up studies (reviewed in Gillberg 1991 and Nordin and Gillberg 1998) they constitute no more than a few per cent of all persons with autism. They have usually shown positive development very early in childhood, but, occasionally, the amelioration may not come until the pubertal years. Individuals such as these are often regarded as related to "cures" of various kinds rather than as examples of different developmental pathways. However, even though some studies reporting on the effects of intensive behavioral therapy (*e.g.* Lovaas 1987) have claimed superior results, with almost half of all individuals being cured, there is not enough evidence to suggest that interventions in themselves can so dramatically alter the course of autism that it would be reasonable to speak of a true cure.

If one concentrates on only the high-functioning individuals with autism – and perhaps particularly on those diagnosed as suffering from Asperger syndrome – then the proportion of individuals with a very good outcome increases. Quite a number of such patients actually have a fair prognosis and may be able to hold down good jobs, live independent lives and even marry and raise children (Szatmari *et al.* 1989). Nevertheless, a number of individuals in this group have major psychiatric problems, which are briefly discussed below.

Wing's three broad groups of adults with autism
Wing (1983) outlined three major groups of adults previously diagnosed with childhood autism: the "aloof" group, the "passive" group and the "active but odd" group. Empirical support for this subgrouping has also been provided by studies in Göteborg (Gillberg and Steffenburg 1987).

The "aloof" group comprises those individuals who retain many or some of the characteristics of autistic aloneness. They will still prefer to be alone and even to withdraw actively from the nearness of other human beings. It may not be as obviously apparent in adult age, but the aloofness shows in the company of others in that individuals with autism do not readily react to other people's questions or approaches. They may quietly withdraw to the seclusion of their own room, where they may play records or just sit and rock incessantly to and fro. If disturbed, they may forcefully push the intruder out of the room, after first having appeared oblivious to the other person's presence for several minutes. Adults in this group cause problems mostly when demands are made. They may be quite easy to "handle" if they are left completely to themselves. On the other hand, leaving them alone quickly leads to the deterioration of both acquired and self-help skills.

The "passive" group may also, at a glance, appear aloof. However, approaches by both strangers and familiar people are accepted in a quite friendly manner. They may have "automatic" imitation skills which enable them to participate in some social activities without appearing extremely odd, so long as reciprocal social interaction is not demanded. As a group, the passive people with autism are those who have the most skills and are most likely to be able to lead relatively independent lives. Changes of routine, especially if introduced in abrupt ways, may be very upsetting to this group, as well as to the aloof and active groups. Because of the overall friendly attitude of the passive people with autism, disturbed behavior in connection with change may be especially alarming. Unless those living with or caring for these individuals are well informed, tragic mistakes may be made, such as expulsion from a secure group or admission for psychiatric treatment in an emergency ward.

The "active but odd" group is by far the most difficult. On the surface, adults in this group appear to be totally unlike those in the other two groups, but there is the same lack of reciprocity in all three. The active group tend to approach other people with physical touching if mute, or constant repetitive questioning if speaking. The endless monologues or questioning may seem rather harmless, but anyone who has been confronted with it for any length of time, and learned that answering leads to even further repetitions of the same questions, knows how wearing and frustrating this behavior is.

Within these three groups there is, of course, considerable variation. Some persons may show characteristics of more than one "type," and personality differences naturally play an essential role in all cases.

Periodicity in autism

There are several clinical accounts (Coleman 1976, Wing 1983, Gillberg 1984) and a few systematic studies (*e.g.* Gillberg and Steffenburg 1987) acknowledging a periodic intensification of symptoms in the autistic syndromes. This periodicity may be particularly prominent in puberty (Komoto *et al.* 1984b). However, after thorough interviewing of the parents, it is often evident that it has been present from the onset in infancy or early childhood. Several authors (see above) have suggested that affective illness might be more common in the families of children with autism than in families of normal children.

There is direct or indirect evidence that this might be the case, from several different sources (Lotter 1967, Rutter and Bartak 1971, Folstein and Rutter 1977, DeLong and Dwyer 1988, Steffenburg 1991). Early authors generally tended to attribute conditions such as recurrent depression in the parents to reactions against the situation with the affected child. Later writers have considered genetic factors instead. It is likely that a hereditary trait of periodicity exists in some cases of autism in which parents and other relatives have shown major affective disorders.

Overall outcome

There have been a small number of follow-up studies reporting on the overall outcome for children diagnosed as suffering from autism, childhood psychosis or autistic-like conditions. Studies published up to the mid-1970s were closely examined by Lotter (1978). Only a handful of these studies – from the USA (Eisenberg 1956, DeMyer *et al.* 1973), and from the UK (Creak 1963, Rutter 1970, Lotter 1974) – have presented enough detail to allow conclusions to be drawn. The studies all yielded remarkably similar results, in spite of the fact that only one (Lotter 1974) was population-based. In the 1980s, only one more population-based follow-up study was published (Gillberg and Steffenburg 1987), and this showed results that were consistent with those from the previous studies. In all of the studies published, a poor or very poor outcome with regard to social adjustment (characterized by limited independence in social relations) was seen in 61 to 73 per cent of cases followed up to pre-adolescence or early adult life. A good outcome (with near normal or normal social life and acceptable functioning at work or school, in spite of certain difficulties in social relationships and oddities in behavior) was seen in 5 to 17 per cent of cases. In the studies mentioned, 39 to 54 per cent of subjects had been placed in institutions at follow-up.

According to a recent review of the outcome literature in autism, mortality in the 2 to 30 years age group is slightly, but significantly, increased (Gillberg 1992a). Even though it is hard to compare mortality rates across Western countries, it appears that mortality in this age group might be increased from about 0.6 per cent in the general population to almost 2 per cent in autism. The higher mortality rate could be accounted for by the association of autism with certain severe medical conditions, such as tuberous sclerosis.

A few (clinic-based) studies of high-functioning people with autism (Rumsey and Hamburger 1988, Szatmari *et al.* 1989) suggest that their outcome may be considerably better, yet severely restricted as compared with people without autism.

All of the follow-up studies mentioned above, as well as another from the USA (Goldfarb 1970), agree that the absence of communicative speech at age 5 to 6 years is indicative of a worse overall long-term outcome. However, the single best predictor of outcome is IQ rating at the time of diagnosis in childhood (Rutter 1970, Gillberg and Steffenburg 1987). Educational functioning in childhood also has relatively good predictive power (DeMyer *et al.* 1973). Other prognostic variables include a lack of reaction to sound in infancy or early childhood (poor outcome), and milder forms of behavior problems, more schooling and acquisition of specific skills (better outcome).

It might appear from the foregoing discussion that making a reliable prognosis on the basis of diagnostic data obtained at about the age of 5 to 6 years would be fairly easy. However, there are several problems.

Difficulties associated with IQ testing are very common. In the preschool years it may be difficult to test a child with autism at all. Detailed knowledge of the child and special testing skills or experience with autism on the part of the psychologist reduce the problems of testing to a minimum. Freeman (1976) has argued that it is usually possible to accomplish reliable testing of a preschool child with autism. Also, DeMyer *et al.* (1973) showed that a simple index of educational attainments was a stable predictor of educational outcome. Such measures (*e.g.* the currently widely-used Psychoeducational Profile or PEP (Schopler *et al.* 1980) plus a Vineland interview (Doll 1965)) could be added to the test battery in order to strengthen the predictive validity of the IQ factor. Furthermore, it seems that IQ is predictive of overall long-term outcome only for those with ratings <50. Almost all of those who have an IQ <50 before age 5 to 6 years are likely to have a poor, or very poor, prognosis. For those with higher IQ it is much more difficult to make a reliable prediction of outcome. On the whole, though, IQ remains as stable throughout childhood for children with autism as for normal or mentally retarded children (Rutter 1983).

Speech as a prognostic indicator is useful for group effects but not always for individual children. Even in those who show no intelligible speech at 5 years (about half of the group with classical autism) there may later be major speech development and a fair overall outcome. Occasionally one comes across a child who unexpectedly starts to talk or communicate at age 10 or even later. One person with a typical history of autism, and medical record data to substantiate the diagnosis, said nothing for 27 years and then started to write long communicative sentences using a pocket-size typewriter (Sanua 1981).

A considerable minority of children who show deterioration in puberty constitute another problem. As yet we have no way of knowing in advance who they are. It is possible that high maternal age, female sex and a family history of affective disorder might all point in the direction of pubertal aggravation of symptoms and possibly deterioration, but, so far, nothing definite is known in this respect.

On the bright side is the as yet unexplained tendency for a small minority of children with autism to develop in a very promising way, with or without treatment.

Summary

For the most part, we must retain a cautious attitude when discussing outcome in autism with the parents. The majority of children with autism will show deviancies and psychiatric impairments throughout life, but others will improve enough to make it possible to lead an (almost) independent adult life. The problem with the individual child is that there is no sure way of knowing to which of these two groups he or she will later belong. In the future it will become increasingly more common to make a prognosis according to the known associated medical diagnosis. It is already clear that outcome in autism with tuberous sclerosis is different from that in autism associated with the fragile X syndrome

(Gillberg 1992b). A comprehensive state-of-the-art medical work-up will contribute to the refinement of appropriate diagnosis and prognosis in autism.

REFERENCES

Coleman, M. (1976) *The Autistic Syndromes*. Amsterdam: North-Holland.

Creak, E.M. (1963) 'Childhood psychoses: a review of 100 cases.' *British Journal of Psychiatry*, **109**, 84–89.

DeLong, G.R., Dwyer, J.T. (1988) 'Correlation of family history with specific autistic subgroups: Asperger's syndrome and bipolar affective disease.' *Journal of Autism and Developmental Disorders*, **18**, 593–600.

DeMyer, M.K., Barton, S., DeMyer, W.E., Norton, J.A., Allen, J., Steele, R. (1973) 'Prognosis in autism: a follow-up study.' *Journal of Autism and Childhood Schizophrenia*, **3**, 199–246.

Doll, E. (1965) *Vineland Social Maturity Scale (Revised)*. Circle Pines, Minnesota: American Guidance Service, Inc.

Eisenberg, L. (1956) 'The autistic child in adolescence.' *American Journal of Psychiatry*, **112**, 607–612.

Folstein, S., Rutter, M. (1977) 'Infantile autism: a genetic study of 21 twin pairs.' *Journal of Child Psychology and Psychiatry*, **18**, 297–321.

Freeman, B.J. (1976) 'Evaluating autistic children.' *Journal of Pediatric Psychology*, **1**, 18–21.

Gillberg, C. (1983) 'Psychotic behaviour in children and young adults in a mental handicap hostel.' *Acta Psychiatrica Scandinavica*, **68**, 351–358.

—— (1984) 'Autistic children growing up: problems during puberty and adolescence.' *Developmental Medicine and Child Neurology*, **26**, 125–129.

—— (1991) 'Outcome in autism and autistic-like conditions.' *Journal of the American Academy of Child and Adolescent Psychiatry*, **30**, 375–382.

—— (1992a) 'The Emanuel Miller Memorial Lecture 1991: Autism and autistic-like conditions: subclasses among disorders of empathy.' *Journal of Child Psychology and Psychiatry*, **33**, 813–842.

—— (1992b) 'Subgroups in autism: are there behavioural phenotypes typical of underlying medical conditions?' *Journal of Intellectual Disability Research*, **36**, 201–214.

Gillberg, C., Steffenburg, S. (1987) 'Outcome and prognostic factors in infantile autism and similar conditions: a population-based study of 46 cases followed through puberty.' *Journal of Autism and Developmental Disorders*, **17**, 273–287.

Goldfarb, W. (1970) 'A follow-up investigation of schizophrenic children treated in residence.' *Psychosocial Process*, **1**, 9–64.

Goode, S., Rutter, M., Howlin, P. (1994) 'A 20-year follow-up of children with autism.' Paper presented at the 13th Biennial Meeting of ISSBD, Amsterdam.

Kanner, L. (1971) 'Follow-up study of eleven children originally reported in 1943.' *Journal of Autism and Childhood Schizophrenia*, **1**, 119–145.

—— (1973) 'Historical perspective on developmental deviations.' *Journal of Autism and Childhood Schizophrenia*, **3(3)**, 187–198.

Kobayashi, R., Murata, T., Yoshinaga, K. (1992) 'A follow-up study of 201 children with autism in Kyushu and Yamaguchi areas, Japan.' *Journal of Autism and Developmental Disorders*, **22(3)**, 395–411.

Komoto, J., Usui, S., Otsuki, S., Terao, A. (1984a) 'Infantile autism and Duchenne muscular dystrophy.' *Journal of Autism and Developmental Disorders*, **14**, 191–195.

Komoto, J., Usui, S., Hirata, J. (1984b) 'Infantile autism and affective disorder.' *Journal of Autism and Developmental Disorders*, **14**, 81–84.

Lotter, V. (1967) 'Epidemiology of autistic conditions in young children. II. Some characteristics of the parents and children.' *Seminars in Psychiatry*, **1**, 163–173.

—— (1974) 'Factors related to outcome in autistic children.' *Journal of Autism and Childhood Schizophrenia*, **4**, 263–277.

—— (1978) 'Follow-up studies.' *In:* Rutter, M., Schopler, E. (Eds) *Follow-up Studies*. New York: Plenum Press, pp. 475–495.

Lovaas, O.I. (1987) 'Behavioral treatment and abnormal educational and intellectual functioning in young autistic children.' *Journal of Consulting and Clinical Psychology*, **55**, 3–9.

Nordin, V., Gillberg, C. (1998) 'The long-term course of autistic disorders: update on follow-up studies.' *Acta Psychiatrica Scandinavica*, **97**, 99–108.

77

Rumsey, J.M., Hamburger, S.D. (1988) 'Neuropsychological findings in high-functioning men with infantile autism, residual state.' *Journal of Clinical and Experimental Neuropsychology*, **10**, 201–221.

Rutter, M. (1970) 'Autistic children: infancy to adulthood.' *Seminars in Psychiatry*, **2**, 435–450.

—— (1983) 'Cognitive deficits in the pathogenesis of autism.' *Journal of Child Psychology and Psychiatry*, **24**, 513–531.

Rutter, M., Bartak, L. (1971) 'Causes of infantile autism: some considerations from recent research.'*Journal of Autism and Childhood Schizophrenia*, **1**, 20–32.

Sanua, V.D. (1981) 'Cultural changes and psychopathology in children: with special reference to infantile autism.' *Acta Paedopsychiatrica*, **47**, 133–142.

Schopler, E., Mesibov, G. (Eds) (1983) *Autism in Adolescents and Adults*. New York: Plenum Press.

—— (Eds) (1988) *Diagnosis and Assessment in Autism*. New York: Plenum Press.

Schopler, E., Reichler, R.J, Bashford, A., Lansing, M.D., Marcus, L.M. (1980) *Psychoeducational Profile – Revised (PEP-R)*. Austin, Texas: Pro-Ed.

Steffenburg, S. (1991) 'Neuropsychiatric assessment of children with autism: a population-based study.' *Developmental Medicine and Child Neurology*, **33**, 495–511.

Szatmari, P., Bartolucci, G., Brenner, R., Bond, S., Rich, S. (1989) 'A follow-up study of high-functioning autistic children.' *Journal of Autism and Developmental Disorders*, **19**, 213–225.

von Knorring, A.-L., Hägglöf, B. (1993) 'Autism in Northern Sweden. A population based follow-up study: psychopathology.' *European Child and Adolescent Psychiatry*, **2**, 91–97.

Wing, L. (1983) 'Diagnosis, clinical description and prognosis.' *In:* Wing, L. (Ed.) *Early Childhood Autism*. Oxford: Pergamon Press.

—— (1989) 'Autistic adults.' *In:* Gillberg, C. (Ed.) *Diagnosis and Treatment of Autism*. New York: Plenum Press, pp. 419–432.

—— (1996) *The Autism Spectrum*. London: Constable.

7
ADDITIONAL BEHAVIORS SEEN IN INDIVIDUALS WITH AUTISM

This chapter will deal with those behaviors seen in children with autism that are not basic behaviors which are part of the autistic syndrome, but may also be seen in other disorders as well. Although these behaviors are not core symptoms, some of them can be quite troubling in the management of the child.

Food faddism

Some children with autism eat a very restricted diet; they may insist on eating the same food every day in a repetitive fashion. Some even refuse to move beyond a particular baby food. Although the underlying reason for this feeding dysfunction is not definitely established, there are several possible explanations.

One likely explanation is the great need for sameness that is seen in so many other areas of the life of a child with autism. Children with autism may become obsessive about food. Another possible explanation is that they have some type of gastrointestinal immaturity or disorder which leads to abdominal pain with new foods (see Chapter 10). A third explanation relates to the refined sense of taste/smell in these children; they sometimes even use smell to identify a new person who walks into a room, instead of the visual/auditory methods that the rest of us use. Such children may indeed be gourmets and, as such, very selective about their food. A rather unlikely explanation highlights the link between opioid peptides and food intake (Mercer and Holder 1997), even though there is some evidence of opioid dysfunction in autism (see Chapter 13).

The consequences of food faddism can be very serious. There is a case in the literature of an 8-year-old boy who only ate French fries and water for several years. He ended up with rickets, periorbital swelling, xerophthalmia and corneal abrasions secondary to vitamin A and D deficiencies (Clark *et al.* 1993). Some of the vitamin deficiencies described in Chapter 13 may well be secondary to peculiar dietary habits in certain children.

There are programs of behavioral therapy set up to deal with this problem. Also, in any particular child, it is sometimes possible to test hypotheses regarding etiology with pharmacological therapies. There is the case of a 3-year-old boy with extreme food faddism who resisted an attempt to wean him from the bottle when he was offered a cup together with increased amounts of baby food (Schwan *et al.* 1998). The child's response was a decrease in intake, along with a refusal to eat any baby food. Then he stopped bottle-feeding altogether when one specific nipple used since birth broke, thus demonstrating an overwhelming need for sameness. The child was admitted to hospital dehydrated and anorexic; attempts at behavioral therapy were unavailing. However, two hours after his first dose of risperidone, a drug aimed at autistic behavior patterns (see Chapter 17), the child accepted baby food without resistance.

Testing another hypothesis, if there is evidence of gastrointestinal discomfort, specific drugs tied to that dysfunction (see Chapter 17) can be tried.

Self-injurious behavior (SIB)

Self-injurious behavior (SIB) is a most distressing symptom seen in some children and adults with autism. It can be mild, appearing to be an enhancement of self-stimulatory behaviors, or it can be severe, causing real harm to the self-abuser. It has been reported that SIB occurs more frequently with autism than in obsessive-compulsive disorder – based on a study of 50 adults with autism and matched obsessive-compulsive controls (McDougle *et al.* 1995). There are several ways to quantify SIB in an individual patient with autism. Examples are DSM-IV, DASH-II and the Timed Self-Injurious Behavior Scale (Brasic *et al.* 1997).

Sometimes SIB can be a clue to the underlying dysfunction of biochemistry in the patient; in other individuals, it appears non-specific. In patients with self-injurious behavior to their skin and hair (*e.g.* biting the arms or backs of hands or fingertips, pulling out the hair), abnormalities of purine metabolism have been described (Sorensen and Benke 1967, Hooft *et al.* 1968, Coleman 1974, Coleman *et al.* 1976, Jaeken and van den Berghe, 1984). The restricted purine diet (see Chapter 17) is occasionally of help in this patient group; the specific drug to tune down the purine metabolic pathways, allopurinol, is less useful. Paroxetine, a selective serotonin reuptake inhibitor (SSRI), has been reported to bring a dramatic cessation of severe self-biting of the arms in an adolescent with autism, after a long list of other drugs had failed (Snead *et al.* 1994); biochemical studies of the patient were not reported. The failed drugs in this case included another SSRI – fluoxetine – which has been reported to be useful for self-injurious behavior in young adults with mental retardation (Ricketts *et al.* 1993).

One of the most horrifying symptoms seen in disturbed individuals is ocular self-injury, ranging from poking or hitting their own eyes to actually taking a knife and carving out their own eye. When studying patients with autism who had hypocalcinuria, Coleman (1994) found that some of them also had ocular self-abuse. Questioning an autistic patient with speech who was able to explain why he was poking his eye, the child said that he had an abnormal sensation in the eye. Correction of the hypocalcinuria to the normal levels of calcium in the urine coincided in all four patients with cessation of the ocular self-mutilation. For such patients, diets of high calcium foods are usually unable to correct the hypocalcinuria. Calcium supplements at a relatively high level have to be added (Coleman 1989).

In another type of self-injury related to biochemistry, an elderly man with PKU who had never been treated for his disease was placed on the low phenylalanine diet for PKU in an attempt to stop his self-abuse (Williams 1993). Besides resulting in improved social skills and gait, the low phenylalanine diet was clinically successful in controlling the self-abuse. However his severe self-injury, associated with leg tremor and spasm, was only reversible when plasma blood phenylalanine concentrations were titrated to near normal levels and daily phenylalanine intake was strictly controlled.

Thus, targeted metabolic treatment of the underlying condition is the ideal approach to SIB. However, if that is not possible in any individual patient, many non-specific therapies are also available. Often a combination of several approaches is the most successful, such as a combination of behavior conditioning with a pharmacological agent (Holttum *et al.* 1994). There is a wide variety of possible treatments. The non-pharmacological choices range from behavior therapy to aerobic exercise (see Chapter 18). The authors of this book object to any form of adversive therapies administered to the sensitive individuals who have autism.

Regarding pharmacological tools to stop SIB, there are a number of drugs available. A major hypothesis regarding SIB is that excessive brain opioid activity might contribute to the neurochemical basis underlying self-injury. There is a question of whether levels of beta-endorphin (beta E) change within minutes after self-injurious behavior in some patients, and whether such immediate alterations would predict that individual patient's response to opiate blockers (Sandman *et al.* 1997). A number of trials of opiate antagonists have been undertaken in studies of young children with autism. The main drug used in these studies was naltrexone, a synthetic congerer of oxymorphone with no opioid agonist properties. Comparison between studies is made unusually difficult because of the importance of different dosages in determining clinical effects, as noted by Leboyer *et al.* (1992). Overall, the research studies have generally been disappointing in regard to self-injury, as well as in regard to the core symptoms of autism such as social behavior and language/communication (as summarized in Feldman *et al.* 1999). It is possible that naltrexone may be associated with modest improvements in other behaviors, such as hyperactivity and restlessness/irritability (Campbell *et al.* 1993, Willemsen-Swinkels *et al.* 1995); in fact, Campbell has written that autistic children should have a trial of naltrexone (Campbell and Harris 1996).

Other drugs that can be tried when SIB occurs in a person with autism include clomipramine (Holttum *et al.* 1994), paroxetine (Snead *et al.* 1994), risperidone (Horrigan and Barnhill 1997, Cohen *et al.* 1998), sertraline (Hellings *et al.* 1996), sulpiride (Rothenberger 1993) and trazodone (Gedye 1991). Each individual may be responsive only to one or even to none of these drugs; these drugs do not always work (Davanzo *et al.* 1998).

Savant qualities

Sometimes children with autism have what appear to be the most remarkable skills in one limited area, while they function below the normal range in other areas of competence, particularly regarding language and communication. This combination of strengths and deficits has resulted in the label "idiot savant," a totally inaccurate and offensive term. These children are not idiots and, if they recover, neither are they savants any longer. The terms "savant" or "autistic savant" are clearly better descriptions (Bujas-Petkovic 1994). It should be noted that not all children who are savants are autistic.

A number of savant qualities have been described in children with autism. These include special skills in memory, music, mathematics, calendar calculation, drawing, painting, and a form of reading called hyperlexia. Children may have detailed, specific, in-depth knowledge of one particular subject, such as train timetables. Some autistic children with hyperlexia have been noted to have more persistent echolalia (Tirosh and Canby 1993). What they all have in common, no matter what their special skill, is a pre-occupation with, and repetitive behavior in, the restricted area of their interest (O'Conner and Hermelin 1991).

One of the most amazing skills of savants is calendar calculating. Although there is no agreement on exactly how this happens, one hypothesis about how this skill is learned elucidates much about the quality of life of children with autism. These children are truly isolated, cut off by their sensory handicaps from the ideas and emotions of other people around them. Playing with other children is beyond their social competence. Also, they may not play with toys, another important developmental experience of young children; they may line the toys up in rows instead of playing with them. They may "play" by staring at a pattern on the wall. They are alone and lonely and bored. To fill their time, the child finds an area in which to focus and, once started, returns obsessively to it again and again. Many children have a calendar on their wall and their intelligent human brain notices the variations and begins to study them. Weeks shift one day for each regular year and two days for leap years; March and November always start on the same day, and so on. After many hours of obsessive interest, the child learns the rules and regularities associated with the calendar (Young and Nettelbeck 1994). Their human isolation, combined with a tendency toward obsessive behavior, locks them into a unique pattern of self-learning. A description of such a child reads "Like a Robinson Crusoe lost in an affective desert, his only companions in solitude are called Friday or January" (Debaene 1997).

To an outside observer, the results of this memory system, built up over hundreds of hours of self-study, year after year, seem truly remarkable. All kinds of theories have been evoked to explain this, including an "innate" pattern present in the brains of these children. But how could the brain be predisposed to acquire the Gregorian calendar which has existed in its present form only since AD 1582? There is a study showing that autistic savants do not differ from carefully matched controls on measures of general short- and long-term memory, but they show a clear recall superiority for the long-term retention of calendrical material; the study showed that they also remembered calculated dates better than those that were only memorized (Heavey et al. 1999). The role of practiced memory in mathematics is easily underestimated; each of us has a number memory (the year, our address, our phone number, etc.) which we take for granted. The size of this numerical memory appears to be one of a calculating prodigy's main strengths (Debaene 1997).

Establishing a spatial number map is a fundamental operation of the human brain. Psychologists have shown that 300 hours of training spread out over two or three years are adequate to create the savant skills of mathematics in regular college students. After such training, Staszewski (1988) could demonstrate that his students took only about 30 seconds to calculate 59,451 times 86. Norris (1990) has developed a neural network computer simulation of the calendar calculations. His program, after several thousand trials, can correctly respond more than 90 per cent of the time to dates to which it has not previously been programmed. Norris says that the human brain is equipped with learning algorithms far superior to those he used in his simulation.

Calculating skills are also known to be present in mathematical geniuses. It is of interest that, not infrequently, these geniuses lose part of their calculation skills as they move on to more abstract problems of the mathematical universe. This is not unlike what happens to autistic savants, who also begin to lose their calculating skills if they are fortunate enough to recover from their autistic state and begin to focus on other topics, such as human relationships.

REFERENCES

Brasic, J.R., Barnett, J.Y., Ahn, S.C., Nadrich, R.H., Will, M.V., Clair, A. (1997) 'Clinical assessment of self-injurious behavior.' *Psychological Reports*, **80**, 155–160.

Bujas-Petkovic, Z. (1994) Special talents of autistic children (autistic-savant) and their mental functions. (In Serbo-Croatian) *Lijecnicki Vjesmik*, **116**, 26–29.

Campbell, M., Harris, J.C. (1996) 'Resolved: autistic children should have a trial of naltrexone.' *Journal of the American Academy of Child and Adolescent Psychiatry*, **35**, 246–249.

Campbell, M., Anderson, L.T., Small, A.M., Adams, P., Gonzalez, N.M., Ernst, M. (1993) 'Naltrexone in autistic children: behavioral symptoms and attentional learning.' *Journal of the American Academy of Child and Adolescent Psychiatry*, **32**, 1283–1291.

Clark, J.H., Rhoden, D.K., Turner, D.S. (1993) 'Symptomatic vitamin A and D deficiencies in an eight-year-old with autism.' *JPEN Journal of Parenteral and Enteral Nutrition*, **17**, 284–286.

Cohen, S.A., Ihrig, K., Lott, R.S., Kerrick, J.M. (1998) 'Resperidone for aggression and self-injurious behavior in adults with mental retardation.' *Journal of Autism and Developmental Disorders*, **28**, 229–233.

Coleman, M. (1974) 'A crossover study of allopurinol administration to a schizophrenic child.' *Journal of Autism and Childhood Schizophrenia*, **4**, 231.

—— (1989) 'Nutritional treatments currently under investigation.' *Clinical Nutrition*, **8**, 210–212.

—— (1994) 'Clinical presentations of patients with autism and hypocalcinuria.' *Developmental Brain Dysfunction*, **7**, 104–109.

Coleman, M., Landgrebe, M.A., Landgrebe, A.R. (1976) 'Purine autism. Hyperuricosuria in autistic children: does this identify a subgroup of autism?' *In:* Coleman, M. (Ed.) *The Autistic Syndromes*. Amsterdam: North-Holland.

Davanzo, P.A., Belin, T.R., Widawski, M.H., King, B.H. (1998) 'Paroxetine treatment of aggression and self-injury in persons with mental retardation.' *American Journal of Mental Retardation*, **102**, 427–437.

Debaene, S. (1997) *The Number Sense: How the Mind Creates Mathematics*. New York: Oxford University Press.

Feldman, H.M., Kolmen, B.K., Gonzaga, A.M. (1999) 'Naltrexone and communication skills in young children with autism.' *Journal of the American Academy of Child and Adolescent Psychiatry*, **38**, 587–593.

Gedye, A. (1991) 'Trazodone reduced aggressive and self-injurious movements in a mentally handicapped male patient with autism.' *Journal of Clinical Psychopharmacology*, **11**, 275–276.

Heavey, L., Pring, L., Hermelin, B. (1999) 'A date to remember: the nature of memory in savant calendrical calculators.' *Psychological Medicine*, **29**, 145–160.

Hellings, J.A., Kelley, L.A., Gabrielli, W.F., Kilgore, E., Shah, P. (1996) 'Sertraline response in adults with mental retardation.' *Journal of Clinical Psychiatry*, **57**, 333–336.

Holttum, J.R., Lubetsky, M.J., Eastman, L.E. (1994) 'Comprehensive management of trichotillomania in a young autistic girl.' *Journal of the American Academy of Child and Adolescent Psychiatry*, **33**, 577–581.

Hooft, C., Van Nevel, C., de Schaepdryer, A.F. (1968) 'Hyperuricosuric encephalopathy with hyperuricaemia.' *Archives of Diseases in Childhood*, **43**, 734–737.

Horrigan, J.P., Barnhill, L.J. (1997) 'Risperidone and explosive aggressive autism.' *Journal of Autism and Developmental Disorders*, **27**, 313–323.

Jaeken, J., van den Berghe, G. (1984) 'An infantile autistic syndrome characterized by the presence of succinylpurines in body fluids.' *Lancet*, **2**, 1058–1061.

Leboyer, M., Bouvard, M.P., Launay, J.M., Tabuteau, F., Waller, D., Dugas, M., Kerdelhue, B., Lensing, P., Panksepp, J. (1992) 'Brief report: A double-blind study of naltrexone in infantile autism.' *Journal of Autism and Developmental Disorders*, **22**, 309–319.

McDougle, C.J., Kresch, L.E., Goodman, W.K., Naylor, S.T., Volkmar, F.R., Cohen, D.J., Price, L.H. (1995) 'A case-controlled study of repetitive thoughts and behavior in adults with autistic disorder and obsessive-compulsive disorder.' *American Journal of Psychiatry*, **152**, 772–777.

Mercer, M.E., Holder, M.D. (1997) 'Food cravings, endogenous opioid peptides and food intake: a review.' *Appetite*, **29**, 325–352.

Norris, D. (1990) 'How to build a connectionist idiot (savant).' *Cognition*, **35**, 277–291.

O'Conner, N., Hermelin, B. (1991) 'Talents and preoccupations in idiots-savants.' *Psychological Medicine*, **21**, 959–964.

Ricketts, R.W., Goza, A.B., Ellis, C.R., Singh, Y.N., Singh, N.N., Cooke, J.C. 3rd (1993) 'Fluoxetine treatment of severe self-injury in young adults with mental retardation.' *Journal of the American Academy of Child and Adolescent Psychiatry*, **32**, 865–869.

Rothenberger, A. (1993) 'Psychopharmacological treatment of self-injurious behavior in individuals with autism.' *Acta Paedopsychiatrica*, **56**, 99–104.

Sandman, C.A., Hetrick, W., Taylor, D.V., Chicz-DeMet, A. (1997) 'Dissociation of POMC peptides after self-injury predicts responses to centrally acting opiate blockers.' *American Journal of Mental Retardation*, **102**, 182–199.

Schwann, J.S., Klass, E., Alonso, C., Perry, R. (1998) 'Risperidone and refusal to eat.' (Letter) *Journal of the Academy of Child and Adolescent Psychiatry*, **37**, 572–573.

Snead, R.W., Boon, F., Presbeerg, J. (1994) 'Paroxetine for self-injurious behavior.' *Journal of the American Academy of Child and Adolescent Psychiatry*, **33**, 909–910.

Sorensen, L.B., Benke, P.J. (1967) 'Biochemical evidence for a distinct type of primary gout.' *Nature*, **213**, 1122–1123.

Staszewski, J.J. (1988) 'Skilled memory and expert mental calculation.' *In:* Chi, M., Glaser, R., Farr, M.J. (Eds) *The Nature of Expertise*. Hilldale, NJ: Erlbaum.

Tirosh, E., Canby, J. (1993) 'Autism with hyperlexia: a distinct syndrome?' *American Journal of Mental Retardation*, **98**, 84–92.

Willemsen-Swinkels, S.H., Buitelaar, J.K., Nijhof, G.J., van England, H. (1995) 'Failure of naltrexone hydrochloride to reduce self-injurious and autistic behavior in mentally retarded adults. Double-blind placebo-controlled studies.' *Archives of General Psychiatry*, **52**, 766–763.

Williams, K. (1993) 'Benefits of normalizing plasma phenylalanine: impact on behavior and health. A case report.' *Journal of Inherited Metabolic Diseases*, **21**, 785–790.

Young, R.L., Nettelbeck, T. (1994) 'The "intelligence" of calendrical calculators.' *American Journal of Mental Retardation*, **99**, 186–200.

8
THE EPIDEMIOLOGY OF AUTISM AND ITS SPECTRUM DISORDERS

The prevalence of autistic disorder

The rate of autistic disorder is often reported as being in the 2–5 in 10,000 range (Lord *et al.* 1994, Fombonne 1996), even though the actual evidence supporting this claim is weak. There is a view among many professionals in the field of developmental disorders that they are seeing increasing numbers of children with all types of autism spectrum disorders at all levels of ability (Bax 1994). It has recently been proposed (Wing 1996) that autism spectrum disorders (that is, autism and autistic-like conditions) might be as prevalent as 1 in 100 children. The possibility that there may be an increasing prevalence has relevance for provision of services, and implications for causes and for prevention and treatment of autism.

This chapter will review the evidence regarding the prevalence of autistic disorder (including narrowly delineated Kanner syndrome), Asperger syndrome, Heller syndrome (disintegrative disorder) and other autism spectrum disorders. The review covers, in detail, the years 1966 (when the first autism epidemiological study was published) through 1997. A preliminary analysis of the studies published in 1998 is also included, but separately because it is uncertain at the time of going to press with this volume whether all relevant studies from that year have yet been indexed in accessible databases. In addition, the following criteria had to be met for inclusion in the review:

1 Target population consisting of a temporally and geographically well-defined cohort.
2 Screening performed among a wide range of children and not just among those diagnosed as having an autism spectrum disorder in specialized clinic registers or parent association registers.
3 Final case identification performed after individual clinical examination of suspected cases and not just based on record (medical, psychological or educational) information.
4 Specified/accepted diagnostic criteria for autism spectrum disorders used.

Only English language papers or papers containing detailed English abstracts were included. In all studies, the number of identified individuals with autism as well as the number of individuals in the screened populations were detailed. For each subgroup of studies, all autism cases were pooled and the number was divided by the pooled number of individuals in the screened populations to provide an estimate of the *mean prevalence* and allow the calculation of exact *95 per cent confidence intervals (CI)* (Poisson distribution). This was done in order to ensure that studies using small populations would not unduly inflate prevalence estimates. In the statistical analysis, the optimal test for comparisons of Poisson distributions (Lehmann 1959) was used.

Ten epidemiological studies did not meet full inclusion criteria. They are listed in Table 8.1.

TABLE 8.1
Studies not meeting full criteria for inclusion in the review

Authors/country	Reasons for exclusion
Treffert 1970/USA	Only information from computer printouts on cases diagnosed as having childhood schizophrenia
Haga & Miyamoto 1971/Japan	Japanese with short English summary
Nakai 1971/Japan	Japanese with short English summary
Tanino 1971/Japan	Japanese with short English summary
Yamasaki et al. 1971/Japan	Japanese with short English summary
McCarthy et al. 1984/Ireland	Sample identified on the basis of asking child psychiatrists and other relevant staff the names of children who had been diagnosed as having autism
Steinhausen et al. 1986/Germany	Only university clinic for child psychiatry and centre providing program for children with autism were searched
Cialdella & Mamelle 1989/France	Final diagnosis not based on clinical examination
Aussilloux et al. 1989/France	Diagnosis based only on case notes of children known to specific services
Fombonne & du Mazaubrun 1992/France	Diagnosis based only on case notes of children known to specific services

One study, by Steffenburg and Gillberg (1986), although meeting full inclusion criteria, was omitted from further analysis because the results overlapped with those of a later study performed by the same group (Gillberg et al. 1991a), which was included in the estimates of mean prevalence (see below).

The range of reported rates in these excluded studies was 0.9 to 10.8 in 10,000 individuals.

TRENDS OVER TIME: SUBDIVISION OF DATA SET
Twenty-two studies met full criteria for inclusion in the review. Altogether, 18 of these were non-US studies published from 1966 (the year of publication of the first-ever population study of autism) through 1997. This 32-year period was subdivided into four 8-year periods covering: 1966–1973 (2 studies); 1974–1981 (1 study); 1982–1989 (7 studies); and 1990–1997 (8 studies). Two non-US studies published in 1998 were

analyzed separately (see above). Two US studies published in 1987 and 1989 were also analyzed separately, because the findings of these studies stood out as atypical.

THE FIRST NON-US STUDIES (1966–1973)

Two studies (Lotter 1966, Brask 1972) meeting criteria for inclusion in the review were performed in the period from 1966 to 1973 (see Table 8.2).

TABLE 8.2
Non-US studies published 1966–1997 divided into eight-year periods – confidence limits in brackets

Authors/country/criteria	Population rate, n/10,000		n	(M:F)	Population
Studies performed 1966–1973					
*Lotter 1966/UK/Kanner	4.5	(3.1–6.2)	35	(23:9)	78,000
*Brask 1972/Denmark/Kanner	4.3	(2.6–6.6)	20	(12:8)	46,500
All studies 1966–1973 (n = 2)	**4.4**	**(3.3–5.8)**	**55**	**(35:17)**	**124,500**
Studies performed 1974–1981					
*Wing & Gould 1979/UK/Kanner	4.9	(2.9–7.8)	17	(16:1)	34,700
All studies 1974–1981 (n = 1)	**4.9**	**(2.9–7.8)**	**17**	**(16:1)**	**34,700**
Studies performed 1982–1989					
*Hoshino et al. 1982/Japan/Kanner	5.0	(4.1–6.0)	109	(98:11)	217,600
Ishii & Takahashi 1982/Japan/ DSM-III similar	16.0	(12.1–20.8)	56	(48:8)	35,000
*Bohman et al. 1983/Sweden/Rutter	5.6	(4.0–7.7)	39	(24:15)	69,600
*Gillberg 1984/Sweden/Rutter-DSM-III	4.0	(3.0–5.2)	51	(33:18)	128,600
Bryson et al. 1988/Canada/DSM-III-R	10.1	(6.2–15.4)	21	(15:6)	20,800
Tanoue et al. 1988/Japan/DSM-III	13.8	(11.6–16.4)	132	(106:26)	95,400
Sugiyama & Abe 1989/Japan/DSM-III	13.0	(7.4–19.5)	16	(?)	12,300
All studies 1982–1989 (n = 7)	**7.7**	**(7.0–8.5)**	**424**	**(324:84)**	**579,300**
Studies performed 1990–1997					
Gillberg et al. 1991/Sweden/DSM-III-R	9.5	(7.4–11.9)	74	(55:19)	78,100
Wignyosumarto et al. 1992/Indonesia/ CARS	11.7	(4.3–25.6)	6	(4:2)	5,100
Deb & Prasad 1994/Scotland/DSM-III-R	9.0	(7.2–11.0)	91	(69:22)	101,800
Baron-Cohen et al. 1996/UK/ICD-10	6.3a		10	(?)	16,000
Nordin & Gillberg 1996/Sweden/ DSM-III-R	9.0b	(5.1–14.9)	15	(10:5)	16,600
Webb et al. 1997/UK/DSM-III-R	9.2c	(6.3–12.9)	33	(29:4)d	35,900
Honda et al. 1996/Japan/ICD-10	21.1	(12.6–33.5)	18	(13:5)	8,500
Arvidsson et al. 1997/Sweden/ICD-10	31.0	(11.6–68.4)	6	(5:1)	1,900
All studies 1990–1997 (n = 8)	**9.6**	**(8.4–10.8)**	**253**	**(185:58)**	**263,900**

* denotes study that included individuals born before 1970; all other studies included only individuals born in 1970 or later. Please note that the Lotter figures are as reported in his original paper, even though 23 + 9 does not equal 35.

a Baron-Cohen et al. study did not screen children with severe and profound mental retardation, so true total population rate likely to be considerably higher

b Nordin & Gillberg study did not screen all non-retarded children, so true total population rate possibly higher

c 5.4 per 10,000 for previous seven-year period

d estimated on basis of overall male:female ratio

Victor Lotter's classical study was a landmark in autism research and has served as a model for most of the best studies in the field (Lotter 1966). In a two-stage population study, he first screened all 8–10-year-old children attending schools in the county of Middlesex in England in the mid-1960s, and then examined personally those who raised some suspicion of being affected by autism. He found 4.5 in 10,000 children having autism, with slightly less than half of that group showing "nuclear autism" – that is, meeting the criteria for Kanner autism in very marked form.

The mean prevalence from this period was 4.4 (CI 3.3–5.8) in 10,000.

THE LATE 1970s (1974–1981)

Only one autism prevalence study meeting full inclusion criteria was published during the period from 1974 to 1981 (see Table 8.2). Wing and Gould (1979) tried to locate all individuals with social impairment in Camberwell, London. Among this broader group, using the same criteria as Lotter's study, 4.9 (CI 2.7–7.8) per 10,000 had autism, with slightly less than half of these showing "nuclear autism" (see above).

THE 1980s (1982–1989)

This period witnessed the beginning of the use of DSM-III criteria, leading on to DSM-III-R (and eventually DSM-IV and ICD-10 criteria). It also saw the start of a trend toward higher rates of autism. The mean prevalence was 7.7 (CI 7.0–8.4) per 10,000.

Three of the seven studies in this subgroup included some children who had been born before 1970, and all of these showed considerably lower rates – consistent with the studies in the two previous subgroups, which also included some children born before 1970.

THE 1990s (1990–1997)

All of the eight studies published in the 1990s showed higher autism rates than the studies in the first two subgroups. The mean prevalence for this period was 9.6 (CI 8.4–10.8) per 10,000.

For a few of these studies, important groups in the general population had been excluded from screening. The Scottish study (Deb and Prasad 1994) screened only those children and adolescents with learning disability, and reported prevalence was regarded as a minimum. Another study (Nordin and Gillberg 1996) screened for autism only in individuals with mental or physical disability – only some of whom were in the normal or low-normal range of intellectual abilities. Yet another study excluded individuals with severe and profound mental retardation from the screening procedure (Baron-Cohen *et al.* 1996). All three studies are likely to have provided underestimates of the true general population autism prevalence. Given previous estimates of 30–50 per cent of children with autism having severe or profound retardation (Lord and Rutter 1994), the true population rate of autism in the Baron-Cohen *et al.* (1996) study would have to be at least 10–12 in 10,000.

There is a trend toward higher prevalence in some of the latest studies (Webb *et al.* 1997, Kadesjö *et al.* 1999), which report rates in excess of 20 in 10,000 children.

NON-US STUDIES FROM THE LATE 1990S

Two non-US studies published in the 1990s have arrived at very different prevalence estimates for ICD-10 childhood autism. A Norwegian study found 3.8 in 10,000 3–14-year-olds in 1992 (Sponhcim and Skjeldal 1998), and a Swedish study reported 60 in 10,000 7-year-olds (also in 1992), with 24 in 10,000 fitting the full clinical picture of Kanner syndrome (Kadesjö et al. 1999). The Norwegian study included a population screening of some 65,000 children, whereas the Swedish study only screened some 800 children. The Norwegian study did not include IQ-testing; there were very few cases of high-functioning autism; and also there were unusual sex ratios in the low- and high-functioning groups. The Swedish study, although referring to a very small population, included more intensive case-finding, IQ-testing and ADI-R interviews (Lord et al. 1994).

THE TWO US STUDIES

Two major US autism prevalence studies (Burd et al. 1987, Ritvo et al. 1989), meeting criteria for inclusion in the review, have been published, both of which were performed in the 1980s (see Table 8.3).

TABLE 8.3
US studies – confidence limits in brackets

Authors/state/criteria	Rate n/10,000	n	(M:F)	Population
Burd et al. 1987/Dakota/DSM-III	3.3 (2.5–4.2)	59	(43:16)	181,000
Ritvo et al. 1989/Utah/DSM-III	3.6 (2.8–4.5)	66	(52:14)*	184,800
Both studies	**3.4 (2.9–4.1)**	**125**	**(95:30)**	**365,800**

* estimated on basis of overall male:female ratio in study

These studies were based on relatively large populations and do not suffer from the risk of chance findings. However, given the well-known difficulty of performing population studies in the US, where populations are mobile and no comprehensive community health care exists, there is a risk of false negatives. The two US studies provided similar estimates of autism prevalence. The rate of autism in these two studies is markedly different from that of the seven non-US studies performed in the same period (p<0.001). It also differs markedly from that of the most recent non-US studies (p<0.001). There is actually even a trend toward the rate being lower than in the very early non-US studies.

ANNUAL RATES OF INCREASE

There was an estimated yearly increase – highly statistically significant – of almost 4 per cent from 1966 through 1997.

MALE:FEMALE RATIOS

The male:female ratios varied from 2.1:1 to 3.9:1 (except in the Wing and Gould study (1979) and the Webb et al. study (1997), where the ratios of males:females were 16:1 and 7.3:1 respectively) with no clear cohort/calendar year trend.

Most studies of autism report a boy:girl ratio of 3:1 or 4:1 (see Rutter 1985). It appears that in cases exactly fitting Kanner's description, this ratio may be considerably higher: Wing and Gould (1979) reported a 16:1 ratio and Gillberg *et al.* (1991a) a 13:1 ratio in the groups with the most typical Kanner-type profiles. Nevertheless, the population-based studies reported lower ratios when all levels of IQ were included and nuclear and non-nuclear cases were pooled. There has been a tendency for some of the Scandinavian studies to show particularly "low" boy:girl ratios. Thus, a ratio of 1.5:1 was reported in a study of twins with autism by Steffenburg *et al.* (1989). The reasons for these discrepant sex ratios are unclear.

In Asperger syndrome, the boy:girl ratio tends to be even higher than in classical autism. However, the population-based studies do not support such a difference (see Chapter 3).

Wing (1981), and others before and after, have documented that the over-representation of boys with autism is less pronounced in the severely mentally retarded group. Thus, in her group of 74 children with the triad, the boy:girl ratios were 1.1:1, 1.3:1 and 14.2:1 in the IQ ranges of 0–19, 20–49 and >50, respectively. Similar, though less pronounced, trends have been reported by most authors in the field. These trends could suggest that, whereas boys are (genetically?) much more prone to developing autism, more severe brain damage would be required for the development of autism in girls.

YEARS OF BIRTH
The 5 studies that included some children born before 1970 yielded much lower rates than the 13 studies that included only children born in 1970 and later (see Table 8.4).

TABLE 8.4
Non-US studies comprising some individuals born before 1970 compared with those studies comprising only individuals born in 1970 and later – confidence limits in brackets

| | Studies comprising individuals born: | |
	before 1970	in 1970 and later
Number of studies	5	13
Total number of individuals with autism	271	478
Male:female ratio	206:62 = 3.3:1	354:98 = 3.6:1
Total population screened	575,000	427,400
Mean prevalence (per 10,000 population)	**4.7 (4.1–5.3)**	**11.2 (10.2–12.2)**

TRENDS WITHIN GEOGRAPHICAL AREAS
Only the Göteborg group has performed repeated population-based studies within the same geographical area. The studies in this region showed an increase in the Göteborg area from 4.0 in 10,000 in 1980 (Honda *et al.* 1996), to 7.6 in 10,000 in 1984 (Steffenburg and Gillberg 1986), and to 11.5 in 10,000 in 1988 (Gillberg *et al.* 1991a). (The figures given in the tables for the last of these studies are slightly lower; they include not only the region of Göteborg but also the adjacent county of Bohuslän.) The rate of autistic disorder in children with IQs in the 50–70 range in this region remained constant throughout the

studies (around 1.9 to 2.0 in 10,000). More children with IQs in the 20–49 range and IQs >70 were identified in the later study. These findings suggest that the children with mild mental retardation and autism were the most likely to appear very obviously autistic in the way Kanner described, and that awareness of the way autism presents in the more retarded and non-retarded individuals has increased over the eight-year period from 1980 through 1988.

In the study from 1988, there was a dramatic increase in the number of children with autism born to mothers who had migrated to Sweden from faraway regions. There was a disproportionate rate of such children in the autism group as compared with the general population.

A total of nine studies from Japan are known to the present authors. Four of these were excluded from the analyses presented here because of the language difficulty (they were published in Japanese, with only brief English summaries). However, judging from the dates of publication, they probably used criteria based on Kanner's descriptions. One of the included papers from Japan used these criteria and found a prevalence of 5.0 per 10,000. The four other Japanese papers, published between 1982 and 1996, using DSM-III or ICD-10 criteria, have all found higher rates, varying from 13.0 to 21.1 in 10,000. These studies used intensive methods of case-finding, some including examinations at different ages in child welfare clinics attended by the great majority of all families in the population.

IMPACT OF DIAGNOSTIC SYSTEM USED

The first epidemiological study was published by Lotter in 1966 and used diagnostic criteria that were intended to identify Kanner's classic variant of autism. These criteria were designed for Lotter by his Ph.D. supervisors, John Wing and Neil O'Conner. At that time, these three researchers were of the firm belief that Kanner's classic autism was a unique and separate condition and that the criteria for the study should be very narrow. No child was included unless they had the two criteria emphasized by Kanner and Eisenberg (1956), namely profound lack of affective contact, at least up to age 5 years, and elaborate repetitive routines. Lotter gradually found that the borderlines were much less clear than anticipated, and thus began the process of learning that eventually led to the formulation of the hypothesis of a spectrum of autistic disorders (Wing and Gould 1979). This brief historical account has been included here to emphasize that the rate of 4.5 per 10,000 found by Lotter was based on criteria that were markedly narrower than those subsequently adopted by the DSM or ICD systems.

Kanner's criteria, or approximations of them, were used in three more of the earliest studies (Brask 1972, Wing and Gould 1979, Hoshino et al. 1982). These all gave results ranging from 4.3 to 5.0 (see Table 8.4). Bohman et al. (1983) used Rutter criteria (1978) which were also based on Kanner's descriptions, and found a prevalence of 5.6 per 10,000.

In order to investigate the relationship between criteria based on Kanner's autism and the ICD-10 criteria for "childhood autism" and "atypical autism," the data from the Wing and Gould (1979) study were reanalyzed. The ratings on the Handicaps, Behaviour and

Skills (HBS) schedule, written reports on past and present behavior, additional information from the first follow-up (Wing 1980a), and an on-going second follow-up, were available. ICD-10 research criteria, as described in the manual (WHO 1993), were applied, using this information. Among the children who were mobile, the prevalence for childhood autism was 14.3 per 10,000. This included the 4.9 per 10,000 with Kanner syndrome. A further 8.9 per 10,000 had atypical autism. Almost all of the studies from the 1986–1995 period (including the two US studies) used DSM-III (APA 1980) or DSM-III-R (APA 1987) criteria. Most of the studies after 1996 have used ICD-10 (WHO 1993)/DSM-IV (APA 1994) or DSM-III-R criteria.

The five Swedish studies (Bohman *et al.* 1983, Gillberg 1984, Gillberg *et al.* 1991a, Nordin and Gillberg 1996, Arvidsson *et al.* 1997) provide another opportunity to look at the influence of the set of diagnostic criteria used for diagnosing autism on the actual prevalence of the disorder. All of the Swedish studies have been performed by researchers who have discussed case-identification in detail, or who have performed inter-rater reliability studies of the diagnosis of autism together. The Swedish studies have been performed in several different regions, but the organization of services and population coverage are similar throughout the country. The two studies from Göteborg (Gillberg 1984, Gillberg *et al.* 1991a) have been performed by the same small group of researchers, and all cases have been diagnosed according to all of the Rutter, DSM-III, and DSM-III-R criteria for autism. The studies by Arvidsson *et al.* (1997) and the 1999 paper by Kadesjö *et al.* (1999) applied Kanner, DSM-III-R and ICD-10/DSM-IV criteria.

In these Swedish studies, the rates were lower with Kanner criteria than if DSM-III, DSM-III-R or ICD-10 criteria were used. For instance, Kanner autism was reported in about half of the cases meeting DSM-III and DSM-III-R criteria in the 1984 and 1986 Göteborg studies, and in only 30–40 per cent of the cases meeting ICD-10 criteria in the two latest Swedish studies (Arvidsson *et al.* 1997, Kadesjö *et al.* 1999). However, there is no convincing evidence that the higher prevalence figures reported since about 1985 are associated with the use of one of the versions of DSM (III, III-R or IV) or with ICD-10 criteria, or with any other diagnostic system used.

Other disorders in the autism spectrum
The studies that have been published (Gillberg and Gillberg 1989, Ehlers and Gillberg 1993, Petrusdóttir *et al.* 1994, Kadesjö *et al.* 1999) suggest that these disorders – including Asperger syndrome – occur at a minimum rate of 26–36 in 10,000 children (plus about as many with social impairment but not meeting full criteria for Asperger syndrome). More details about Asperger syndrome can be found in Chapter 3. The reported rate of Heller syndrome (childhood disintegrative disorder) has been extremely low, with estimates of 0.05 to 0.1 in 10,000 children (Burd *et al.* 1987, Gillberg and Steffenburg 1987).

Sibling rank
There is still no clear consensus with regard to birth order of children with autism. Early studies (Despert 1951, Kanner 1954, Rimland 1964) suggested a high number of first-born children, but later reports (Lotter 1967, Wing 1980b) have yielded conflicting results. On

balance, it seems reasonable to assume that the Tsai and Stewart (1983) position of more first- and late-born (fourth or later) children in autism may turn out to be correct. Jones and Szatmari (1988) have proposed that so-called genetic stoppage might be in operation in autism. Genetic stoppage implies that, if a child with a severe disability such as autism is born into a family, it often leads to the parents deciding either to refrain from having further children, or to limit themselves to having only one more (hopefully healthy) child.

Social class

From as early as Kanner's first account of autism (1943), there has been a notion – which has sometimes taken on mythological qualities – that children with autism come from the upper social classes (see Chapter 1, p. 1). Kanner, in all probability, saw a highly selected population of children with autism. Wing (1980b), Andersson and Wadensjö (1981), Gillberg and Schaumann (1982), Bohman et al. (1983), Steffenburg and Gillberg (1986), Lögdahl (1989), Cialdella and Mamelle (1989) and Gillberg et al. (1991a), in population studies of autism, all found no indication whatsoever of a trend toward upper social class in autism. Brask (1972), on the basis of her epidemiological sample, reported no upper-social class bias. Lotter (1967) is the only student of autism epidemiology who has found a slight social-class bias. Taken together, the bulk of the evidence does not favor a high social-class bias in autism. It is hoped that the endless, often pointless, arguments about social class in autism will come to an end. There is nothing very substantial to suggest that autism has anything to do with social class. That clinic-based samples may be biased in favor of higher social class is uninformative regarding social class in autism generally. The possibility remains that, among the relatively brighter children with autism, social class might be somewhat higher. This, in turn, might mean no more than that, among the normal child population, high intelligence and high social class show some correlation.

Mental retardation

All studies to date agree that the vast majority of children with autism and autistic-like conditions are also mentally retarded (see Rutter 1983) and test reliably in the IQ range <70 (Clark and Rutter 1979, Rutter 1983). Between 70 and 90 per cent of the children included in various studies are described as clearly mentally retarded, whereas only about 10 per cent are of average (or in rare instances, above-average) intelligence.

Many Kanner autism cases, in spite of severe overall mental retardation, have an "islet" of special ability, which does not represent a signal symptom of hidden superior talents, but is rather to be taken as the only intact functioning area in an otherwise extremely deviant child (Shah and Frith 1983). Our concepts relating to the combination of autism and mental retardation may have to change considerably over the next decade if, as currently seems quite likely, the Asperger phenotype becomes "incorporated" in the inclusive category of autism. Asperger syndrome is probably substantially more common than Kanner autism, and, since mental retardation is rare in Asperger syndrome (Gillberg and Gillberg 1989), the pooled Kanner/Asperger group would no longer show mental retardation in the majority of cases, although still at an increased level compared with the general population.

Epilepsy

One-quarter to one-third of all people with autism develop seizures at some time before adulthood (see Chapter 12). Infantile spasms and complex partial seizures are possibly more frequent than in other populations.

Other disorders

There are several references in the literature (*e.g.* Keeler 1958, Fraiberg 1977, Rapin 1979, Wing 1981) to the high incidence of blindness and deafness in autism. However, there is little in the way of scientific evidence to support this view, and, although clinically credible, claims for a connection between visual/auditory deprivation and autism await definitive scientific study. A longitudinal study in the New York area by Rapin found 61 cases of autism among 1,150 hearing-impaired children (5.3 per cent), but the authors of this report (Jure *et al.* 1991) cautioned that this did not represent data on the prevalence of autism in hearing-impaired children generally, as Rapin's sample was drawn from three clinically-biased populations. According to a recent study by Steffenburg (1991), it appears that visual and hearing deficits may be very common in autism, even though blindness and deafness appear to be rare.

Dysphasia may also be common in autism, but empirical evidence is lacking so far. That there is considerable overlap between certain kinds of speech–language disorder and autism is not a matter of dispute, but it is unclear where the boundaries are (Bishop 1989). For instance, so-called semantic–pragmatic disorders often overlap with Asperger syndrome, and the majority of people with Asperger syndrome would probably be classified as suffering from a semantic–pragmatic disorder.

Epidemiological and clinical studies strongly suggest that tuberous sclerosis, neurofibromatosis, fragile X syndrome, Rett syndrome and Moebius syndrome may all be associated with autism in a 'stronger than chance' fashion. Steffenburg (1991), in a population-based study, demonstrated that more than one in four people with nuclear autism had an associated known medical syndrome, in many cases revealed only after extensive neurobiological/medical work-up. Table 8.5 lists those disorders that have been reported in various epidemiological studies as being associated with autism, thereby pointing toward a neurobiological basis for the development of autism.

Conclusions based on review of epidemiological studies

From the various strands of evidence presented in this chapter, it appears that using strict criteria based on Kanner's descriptions gives significantly lower rates of autism than if DSM or ICD criteria are applied. It is very likely that the low rates found in the earliest studies reported in the 1960s and 1970s – which gave rise to the often-quoted prevalence of 2–5 in 10,000 – are due to the use of these criteria.

On the other hand, there is no evidence suggesting reliable differences among the rates found in the studies using DSM-III, DSM-III-R, DSM-IV or ICD-10 criteria. It is therefore legitimate to pool cases diagnosed with these different systems. All of the studies included were based on clinical judgement after review of a specific set of diagnostic criteria.

TABLE 8.5
Medical disorders shown to be associated with autism in epidemiological studies

Medical condition	Reference
Cytomegalovirus infection	Stubbs 1976
Duchenne muscular dystrophy	Komoto *et al.* 1984
Encephalitis	Greenebaum and Lurie 1948
Fragile X syndrome	Hagerman 1989
Hemophilus influenzae meningitis	Ritvo *et al.* 1989
Herpes simplex encephalitis	Gillberg 1986
Hypomelanosis of Ito	Zappella 1992
Hypothyroidism	I.C. Gillberg *et al.* 1992
Lactic acidosis	Coleman and Blass 1985
Maternal rubella	Chess *et al.* 1971
MCA/MR syndromes	Steffenburg 1991
Moebius syndrome	Ornitz *et al.* 1977
Mucopolysaccharidosis	Knobloch and Pasamanick 1975
Neurofibromatosis	Gillberg and Forsell 1984
Other autosomal chromosome anomalies	Hagerman 1989
Other sex chromosome anomalies	Hagerman 1989
Partial tetrasomy 15 syndrome	Gillberg *et al.* 1991b
Phenylketonuria	Friedman 1969
Purine disorders	Coleman *et al.* 1976
Rett syndrome	Coleman *et al.* 1988
Sotos syndrome	Zappella 1990
Tuberous sclerosis	Hunt and Shepherd 1993
West syndrome	Riikonen and Amnell 1981
Williams syndrome	Reiss *et al.* 1985

Note: All the conditions included have been reported either in (a) at least one population study plus at least one clinical study, or in (b) at least three clinical studies of autism

Even omitting the studies using Kanner's criteria, a trend toward increasing numbers can be seen, apart from in the two studies carried out in the USA. Not a single one of the 11 post-1985 studies from outside the US has reported a minimum rate under 6.3 in 10,000, and 10 of the 11 have yielded minimum rates of 9 in 10,000 or more. The US studies stand out as yielding markedly atypical findings. Whether this is a function of the greater difficulty with coverage in epidemiological studies in the US, or whether it indicates real geographical differences in the prevalence of autistic disorder, cannot be settled by the present review.

One possibility is that the rise in reported rates is spurious. The studies with the highest rates – in excess of 20 in 10,000 – were performed on very small populations, and the findings, therefore, must be interpreted with particular caution. However, they were clearly among the most in-depth studies ever performed with respect to autism case-finding, partly counterbalancing the drawback of a small population. The rates of autism in the new study by Kadesjö *et al.* (1999) – also on a very small population – and in another Swedish epidemiological study (Landgren *et al.* 1996) – not specifically geared to analyzing the prevalence of autism – support the notion that the rates tend to be even higher than about 1 in 1,000. The fact that *all* of the smaller-scale studies have found high rates cannot be immediately dismissed as a likely reflection of chance findings: one would expect that, by chance, some small-scale studies would come up with low rates and others with high rates.

Another possibility to be considered is that the rise is due to greater awareness of autism, and that the prevalence has always been higher than early studies suggested. The effect of the change from Kanner's criteria to the DSM and ICD systems has already been mentioned. It is significant that applying ICD-10 criteria to the children in the Camberwell study carried out in the early 1970s (Wing and Gould 1979) gave a prevalence of 14.3 in 10,000 for childhood autism. However, more recent studies give rates even higher than this. The studies in Göteborg seem to suggest that awareness that autism exists in severely retarded and in more able autistic individuals has increased over the eight-year period from 1980 through 1988.

There may be a real increase in prevalence, at least in Europe and Japan. One reason to be considered is the effect of migration. A trend toward children of parents who have migrated over long distances having autism and mental retardation more often than other children was noted in the Göteborg studies, and has been noted by several authors including Lotter (1974), Wing (1980b), Akinsola and Fryers (1986), Tanoue *et al.* (1988) and Gillberg and Gillberg (1996). Several factors could have contributed to this high rate, including: maternal viral infections in pregnancy (because of lack of maternal immunity to culture-specific infectious agents); metabolic disorder triggered by environmental factors in the new country; indirect associations of maternal immigrant status and paternal Asperger syndrome (for instance, men with Asperger syndrome – with increased risk of fathering children with autism and with difficulty finding a native partner – might have children by women from faraway countries, who might not immediately identify the social oddities or might ascribe them to difference in culture); and factors not yet explored (Gillberg and Gillberg 1996).

Other explanations that have been suggested, with greater or lesser credibility, include pollution, multiple inoculations (including MMR/mumps, measles, rubella) (Montgomery *et al.* 1997) and increased survival of premature infants (Ek *et al.* 1998). There is, at the present time, no clear evidence for or against any of these hypotheses.

Summary
It is not possible, at the time of writing, to determine whether or not the observed increase in prevalence of autism is real or simply reflects better ascertainment. It seems clear that autism, as defined according to DSM-III-R and ICD-10 criteria, is considerably more common than 2–5 in 10,000 children, and that the most reasonable, conservative estimate is about 1 in 1,000 children. This prevalence figure was calculated, after review of the different studies included, by dividing the sum of all identified autism cases by the sum of all individuals screened. This way of estimating the prevalence is conservative in that it does not allow findings from small-scale population studies to heavily influence/inflate the rate. It is of considerable interest that the five non-US studies that included some children born before 1970 yielded a mean prevalence of 4.7 in 10,000, whereas the 13 non-US studies that included only children born 1970 or later produced a corresponding rate of 11.2 in 10,000. This finding could be taken to suggest that there has indeed been a

marked increase in the rate of autism in younger populations of children. However, such a conclusion has to be tempered by the fact that the five early studies mostly used Kanner's criteria, whereas most of the 13 later studies did not. The figure of 1 in 1,000 refers to autistic disorder/childhood autism only, and does not include autism spectrum disorders such as Asperger syndrome, disintegrative disorder or atypical autism/PDDNOS. It is clear that the numbers would be much higher were these categories to be included in autism prevalence estimates. However, so far, no really large-scale studies of prevalence in these disorders have been performed, and it is too early to ascertain how common they actually are, or whether or not prevalence rates are stable across regions. Nevertheless, the few studies that have been published all suggest prevalence figures that are much higher than those for autism, which would indicate that the prevalence of autism spectrum disorders – including childhood autism, Asperger syndrome, disintegrative disorder and atypical autism – is at least 4 to 5 in 1,000 children.

Autism should no longer be conceptualized as an extremely rare disorder. The higher prevalence rate needs to be communicated to administrators, service providers and boards of research funds, so that appropriate resources may be allocated. Quoting the old prevalence figures, when a dozen recent studies show double or triple rates, runs counter to the best interests of children, adults and families affected by autism.

REFERENCES

Akinsola, H.A., Fryers, T. (1986) 'A comparison of patterns of disability in severely mentally handicapped children of different ethnic origins.' *Psychological Medicine*, **16**, 127–133.

APA (American Psychiatric Association) (1980) *Diagnostic and Statistical Manual of Mental Disorders*. Washington, DC: APA.

—— (1987) *Diagnostic and Statistical Manual of Mental Disorders. 3rd Edn (Revised)*. Washington, DC: APA.

—— (1994) *Diagnostic and Statistical Manual of Mental Disorders (4th Edn)* Washington, DC: APA.

Andersson, L., Wadensjö, K. (1981) 'Early childhood psychoses in Malmöhus län – a descriptive study.' (In Swedish) Research report. Lund: Socialavdelningen.

Arvidsson, T., Danielsson, B., Forsberg, P., Gillberg, C., Johansson, M., Källgren, G. (1997) 'Autism in 3–6-year-old children in a suburb of Göteborg, Sweden.' *Autism*, **1**, 163–173.

Aussilloux, C., Collery, F., Roy, J. (1989) 'Epidémiologie de l'autisme infantile dans le départment de l'Herault.' *Revue Française de Psychiatrie*, **7**, 24–28.

Baron-Cohen, S., Cox, A., Baird, G., Swettenham, J., Nightingale, N., Morgan, K., Drew, A., Charman, T. (1996) 'Psychological markers in the detection of autism in infancy in a large population.' *British Journal of Psychiatry*, **168**, 158–163.

Bax, M. (1994) Editorial – Autism. *Developmental Medicine and Child Neurology*, **36**, 659–660.

Bishop, D.V.M. (1989) 'Autism, Asperger's syndrome and semantic–pragmatic disorders. Where are the boundaries?' *British Journal of Disorders of Communication*, **24**, 107–121.

Bohman, M., Bohman, I.L., Björk, P., Sjöholm, E. (1983) 'Childhood psychosis in a northern Swedish county: some preliminary findings from an epidemiological survey.' *In:* Schmidt, M.H., Remschmith, H. (Eds) *Epidemiological Approaches in Child Psychiatry*. Stuttgart: Georg Thieme, pp. 164–173.

Brask, B.H. (1972) 'A prevalence investigation of childhood psychosis.' *Barnepsykiatrisk forening: Nordic Symposium on the Comprehensive Care of the Psychotic Children*, 145–153.

Bryson, S.E., Clark, B.S., Smith, I.M. (1988) 'First report of a Canadian epidemiological study of autistic syndromes.' *Journal of Child Psychology and Psychiatry*, **29**, 433–445.

Burd, L., Fisher, W., Kerbeshian J. (1987) 'A prevalence study of pervasive developmental disorders in North Dakota.' *Journal of the American Academy of Child and Adolescent Psychiatry*, **26**, 704–710.

——— (1989) 'Pervasive disintegrative disorder: are Rett syndrome and Heller dementia infantilis subtypes?' *Developmental Medicine and Child Neurology*, **31**, 609–616.

Chess, S., Korn, S.J., Fernandez, P.B. (1971) *Psychiatric Disorders of Children with Congenital Rubella*. New York: Brunner/Mazel.

Cialdella, P., Mamelle, N. (1989) 'An epidemiological study of infantile autism in a French department (Rhone): a research note.' *Journal of Child Psychology and Psychiatry*, **30**, 165–175.

Clark, P., Rutter, M. (1979) 'Task difficulty and task performance in autistic children.' *Journal of Child Psychology and Psychiatry*, **20**, 271–285.

Coleman, M., Blass, J.P. (1985) 'Autism and lactic acidosis.' *Journal of Autism and Developmental Disorders*, **15**, 1–8.

Coleman, M., Landgrebe, M., Landgrebe, A. (1976) 'Purine autism.' *In*: Coleman, M. (Ed.) *The Autistic Syndromes*. Amsterdam: North-Holland.

Coleman, M., Brubaker, J., Hunter, K., Smith, G. (1988) 'Rett syndrome: a survey of North American patients.' *Journal of Mental Deficiency Research*, **32**, 117–124.

Deb, S., Prasad, K.B. (1994) 'The prevalence of autistic disorder among children with learning disabilities.' *British Journal of Psychiatry*, **165**, 395–399.

Despert, J.L. (1951) 'Some considerations relating to the genesis of autistic behaviour in children.' *American Journal of Orthopsychiatry*, **21**, 335–350.

Ehlers, S., Gillberg, C. (1993) 'The epidemiology of Asperger syndrome. a total population study.' *Journal of Child Psychology and Psychiatry*, **34**, 1327–1350.

Ek, U., Fernell, E., Jacobsson, L., Gillberg, C. (1998) 'Relation between blindness due to retinopathy of prematurity and autistic spectrum disorders: a population-based study.' *Developmental Medicine and Child Neurology*, **40**, 297–301.

Fombonne, E. (1996) 'Is the prevalence of autism increasing?' *Journal of Autism and Developmental Disorders*, **26**, 673–676.

Fombonne, E., du Mazaubrun, C. (1992) 'Prevalence of infantile autism in four French regions.' *Social Psychiatry and Psychiatric Epidemiology*, **27**, 203–210.

Fraiberg, S. (1977) *Insights from Behind. Comparative Studies of Blind and Sighted Infants*. New York: Basic Books.

Friedman, E. (1969) 'The autistic syndrome and phenylketonuria.' *Schizophrenia*, **1**, 249–261.

Gillberg, C. (1984) 'Infantile autism and other childhood psychoses in a Swedish urban region. Epidemiological aspects.' *Journal of Child Psychology and Psychiatry*, **25**, 35–43.

——— (1986) 'Brief report: Onset at age 14 of a typical autistic syndrome. A case report of a girl with herpes simplex encephalitis.' *Journal of Autism and Developmental Disorders*, **16**, 369–375.

Gillberg, C., Forsell, C. (1984) 'Childhood psychosis and neurofibromatosis – more than a coincidence?' *Journal of Autism and Developmental Disorders*, **14**, 1–8.

Gillberg, C., Schaumann, H. (1982) 'Social class and infantile autism.' *Journal of Autism and Developmental Disorders*, **12**, 223–228.

Gillberg, C., Steffenburg, S. (1987) 'Outcome and prognostic factors in infantile autism and similar conditions: a population-based study of 46 cases followed through puberty.' *Journal of Autism and Developmental Disorders*, **17**, 273–287.

Gillberg, C., Steffenburg, S., Schaumann, H. (1991a) 'Is autism more common now than 10 years ago?' *British Journal of Psychiatry*, **158**, 403–409.

Gillberg, C., Steffenburg, S., Wahlström, J., Gillberg, I.C., Sjöstedt, A., Martinsson, T., *et al.* (1991b) 'Autism associated with marker chromosome.' *Journal of the American Academy of Child and Adolescent Psychiatry*, **30**, 489–494.

Gillberg, I.C., Gillberg, C. (1989) 'Asperger syndrome – some epidemiological considerations: a research note.' *Journal of Child Psychology and Psychiatry*, **30**, 631–638.

——— (1996) 'Autism in immigrants. A population-based study from a Swedish rural and urban area.' *Journal of Intellectual Disability Research*, **40**, 24–31.

Gillberg, I.C., Gillberg, C., Kopp, S. (1992) 'Hypothyroidism and autism spectrum disorders.' *Journal of Child Psychology and Psychiatry*, **33**, 531–542.

Greenebaum, J.V., Lurie, L.A. (1948) 'Encephalitis as a causative factor in behavior disorder in children: analysis of 78 cases.' *Journal of the American Medical Association*, **136**, 923–930.

Haga, H., Miyamoto, Y. (1971) 'A survey on the actual state of so-called autistic children in Kyoto prefecture.' *Japanese Journal of Child Psychiatry*, **12**, 160–167.

Hagerman, R.J. (1989) 'Chromosomes, genes and autism.' *In*: Gillberg, C. (Ed.) *Diagnosis and Treatment of Autism*. New York: Plenum Press, pp. 105–132.

Honda, H., Shimizu, Y., Misumi, K., Niimi, M., Ohashi, Y. (1996) 'Cumulative incidence of childhood autism in children in Japan.' *British Journal of Psychiatry*, **169**, 228–235.

Hoshino, Y., Kumashiro, H., Yashima, Y., Tachibana, R., Watanabe, M. (1982) 'The epidemiological study of autism in Fukushima-ken.' *Folia Psychiatrica Neurologica Japonica*, **36**, 115–124.

Hunt, A., Shepherd, C. (1993) 'A prevalence study of autism in tuberous sclerosis.' *Journal of Autism and Developmental Disorders*, **23**, 323–339.

Ishii, T., Takahashi, O. (1982) 'Epidemiology of autistic children in Toyota City, Japan. Prevalence.' *World Child Psychiatry Conference*, Dublin, Ireland.

Jones, M.B., Szatmari, P. (1988) 'Stoppage rules and genetic studies of autism.' (Published erratum appears in *Journal of Autism and Developmental Disorders* (1988) **18**(3): 477.) *Journal of Autism and Developmental Disorders*, **18**, 31–40.

Jure, R., Rapin, I., Tuchman, R.F. (1991) 'Hearing-impaired autistic children.' *Developmental Medicine and Child Neurology*, **33**, 1062–1072.

Kadesjö, B., Gillberg, C., Hagberg, B. (1999) 'Brief report: Autism and Asperger syndrome in seven-year old children. A total population prevalence study.' *Journal of Autism and Developmental Disorders*. Accepted.

Kanner, L. (1943) 'Autistic disturbances of affective contact.' *Nervous Child*, **2**, 217–250.

—— (1954) 'To what extent is early childhood autism determined by constitutional inadequacies?' *Proceedings of the Association for Research in Nervous and Mental Diseases*, **33**, 378–385.

Kanner, L., Eisenberg, L. (1956) 'Early infantile autism: 1943–1955.' *American Journal of Orthopsychiatry*, **26**, 55–65.

Keeler, W.R. (1958) 'Autistic patterns and defective communication in blind children with retrolental fibroblasia.' *In:* Hoch, P.H., Zubin, J. (Eds) *Psychopathology of Communication*. New York: Grune & Stratton, pp. 64–83.

Knobloch, H., Pasamanick, B. (1975) 'Some etiologic and prognostic factors in early infantile autism and psychosis.' *Journal of Pediatrics*, **55**, 182–191.

Komoto, J., Usui, S., Otsuki, S., Terao, A. (1984) 'Infantile autism and Duchenne muscular dystrophy.' *Journal of Autism and Developmental Disorders*, **14**, 191–195.

Landgren, M., Pettersson, R., Kjellman, B., Gillberg, C. (1996) 'ADHD, DAMP and other neurodevelopmental/neuropsychiatric disorders in six-year-old children. Epidemiology and comorbidity.' *Developmental Medicine and Child Neurology*, **38**, 891–906.

Lehmann, E.L. (1959) *Testing Statistical Hypotheses*. New York: Wiley.

Lögdahl, K. (1989) 'The prevalence of autism in a Swedish county.' Eskilstuna: Report to Sörmland County Authorities.

Lord, C., Rutter, M. (1994) 'Autism and pervasive developmental disorders.' *In:* Rutter, M., Taylor, E., Hersov, L. (Eds) *Child and Adolescent Psychiatry. Modern Approaches*. Oxford: Blackwell Scientific, pp. 569–593.

Lord, C., Rutter, M., Le Couteur, A. (1994) 'Autism Diagnostic Interview – Revised: A revised version of a diagnostic interview for caregivers of individuals with possible pervasive developmental disorders.' *Journal of Autism and Developmental Disorders*, **24**, 659–685.

Lotter, V. (1966) 'Epidemiology of autistic conditions in young children.' *Social Psychiatry*, **1**, 124–137.

—— (1967) *The Prevalence of the Autistic Syndrome in Children*. London: University of London Press.

—— (1974) 'Factors related to outcome in autistic children.' *Journal of Autism and Childhood Schizophrenia*, **4**, 263–277.

McCarthy, P., Fitzgerald, M., Smith, M. (1984) 'Prevalence of childhood autism in Ireland.' *Irish Medical Journal*, **77**, 129–130.

Montgomery, S.M., Morris, D.L., Pounder, R.E., Wakefield, A.J. (1997) 'Measles vaccination and inflammatory bowel disease.' *Lancet*, **350**, 1774.

Nakai, M. (1971) 'Epidemiology of autistic children in Gifu-ken.' *Japanese Journal of Child Psychiatry*, **12**, 262–266.

Nordin, V., Gillberg, C. (1996) 'Autism spectrum disorders in children with physical or mental disability or both. Part I: Clinical and epidemiological aspects.' *Developmental Medicine and Child Neurology*, **38**, 297–313.

99

Ornitz, E.M., Guthrie, D., Farley, A.J. (1977) 'The early development of autistic children.' *Journal of Autism and Childhood Schizophrenia*, **7**, 207–229.

Petrusdóttir, G., Sigurdsson, S., Karlsson, M.M., Axelsson, J. (1994) 'The epidemiology of autism and Asperger syndrome in Iceland: a summary of a pilot study.' Proceedings of the 9th International Congress on Circumpolar Health 93, 1993, June 20–25, Reykjavik, Iceland. *Arctic Medical Research*, **53**(Suppl. 2): 464–466.

Rapin, I. (1979) 'Effect of early blindness and deafness on cognition.' *In:* Katzman, R. (Ed.) *Congenital and Acquired Cognitive Disorders*. New York: Raven, pp. 189–245.

Reiss, A.L., Feinstein, C., Rosenbaum, K.N., Borengasser-Caruso, M.A., Goldsmith, B.M. (1985) 'Autism associated with Williams syndrome.' *Journal of Paediatrics*, **106**, 247–249.

Riikonen, R., Amnell, G. (1981) 'Psychiatric disorders in children with earlier infantile spasms.' *Developmental Medicine and Child Neurology*, **23**, 747–760.

Rimland, B. (1964) *Infantile Autism*. Englewood Cliffs, NJ: Prentice-Hall.

Ritvo, E.R., Freeman, B.J., Pingree, C., Mason-Brothers, A., Jorde, L., Jenson, W.R., McMahon, W.M., Petersen, P.B., Mo, A., Ritvo, A.R. (1989) 'The UCLA–University of Utah epidemiologic survey of autism: prevalence.' *American Journal of Psychiatry*, **146**, 194–199.

Rutter, M. (1978) 'Diagnosis and definition of childhood autism.' *Journal of Autism and Childhood Schizophrenia*, **8**, 139–161.

—— (1983) 'Cognitive deficits in the pathogenesis of autism.' *Journal of Child Psychology and Psychiatry*, **24**, 513–531.

—— (1985) 'Infantile autism and other pervasive developmental disorders.' *In:* Rutter, M., Hersov, L. (Eds) *Child and Adolescent Psychiatry: Modern Approaches*. Oxford: Blackwell Scientific, pp. 545–566.

Shah, A., Frith, U. (1983) 'An islet of ability in autistic children: a research note.' *Journal of Child Psychology and Psychiatry*, **24**, 613–620.

Sponheim, E., Skjeldal, O. (1998) 'Autism and related disorders: epidemiological findings in a Norwegian study using ICD-10 diagnostic criteria.' *Journal of Autism and Developmental Disorders*, **28**, 217–227.

Steffenburg, S. (1991) 'Neuropsychiatric assessment of children with autism: a population-based study.' *Developmental Medicine and Child Neurology*, **33**, 495–511.

Steffenburg, S., Gillberg, C. (1986) 'Autism and autistic-like conditions in Swedish rural and urban areas: a population study.' *British Journal of Psychiatry*, **149**, 81–87.

Steffenburg, S., Gillberg, C., Hellgren, L., Andersson, L., Gillberg, I.C., Jakobsson, G., Bohman, M. (1989) 'A twin study of autism in Denmark, Finland, Iceland, Norway and Sweden.' *Journal of Child Psychology and Psychiatry*, **30**, 405–416.

Steinhausen, H.C., Göbel, D., Breinlinger, M., Wohlleben, B. (1986) 'A community survey of infantile autism.' *Journal of the American Academy of Child and Adolescent Psychiatry*, **25**, 186–189.

Stubbs, E.G. (1976) 'Autistic children exhibit undetectable hemagglutination-inhibition antibody titers despite previous rubella vaccination.' *Journal of Autism and Childhood Schizophrenia*, **6**, 269–274.

Sugiyama, T., Abe, T. (1989) 'The prevalence of autism in Nagoya, Japan: a total population study.' *Journal of Autism and Developmental Disorders*, **19**, 87–96.

Tanino, Y. (1971) 'An investigation into infantile autism and autistic children in Toyama prefecture.' *Japanese Journal of Child Psychiatry*, **12**, 150–159.

Tanoue, Y, Oda, S., Asano, F., Kawashima, K. (1988) 'Epidemiology of infantile autism in Southern Ibaraki, Japan: differences in prevalence rates in birth cohorts.' *Journal of Autism and Developmental Disorders*, **18**, 155–166.

Treffert, D.A. (1970) 'Epidemiology of infantile autism.' *Archives of General Psychiatry*, **22**, 431–438.

Tsai, L.Y., Stewart, M.A. (1983) 'Etiological implication of maternal age and birth order in infantile autism.' *Journal of Autism and Developmental Disorders*, **13**, 57–65.

Webb, E.V.J., Lobo, S., Hervas, A., Scourfield, J., Fraser, W.I. (1997) 'The changing prevalence of autistic disorder in a Welsh health district.' *Developmental Medicine and Child Neurology*, **39**, 150–152.

WHO (World Health Organization) (1993) *The ICD-10 Classification of Mental and Behavioural Disorders. Diagnostic Criteria for Research*. Geneva: WHO.

Wignyosumarto, S., Mukhlas, M., Shirataki, S. (1992) 'Epidemiological and clinical study of autistic children in Yogyakarta, Indonesia.' *Kobe Journal of Medical Science*, **38**, 1–19.

Wing, L. (1980a) *Handicap, Behaviour and Skills Schedule*. London: MRC Social Psychiatry Unit.

—— (1980b) 'Childhood autism and social class: a question of selection.' *British Journal of Psychiatry*, **137**, 410–417.

—— (1981) 'Sex ratios in early childhood autism and related conditions.' *Psychiatry Research*, **5**, 129–137.

—— (1996) 'Autism spectrum disorder.' (Editorial.) *British Medical Journal*, **312**, 327–328.

Wing, L., Gould, J. (1979) 'Severe impairments of social interaction and associated abnormalities in children: epidemiology and classification.' *Journal of Autism and Developmental Disorders*, **9**, 11–29.

Yamasaki, K., Yamashita, I., Suwa, N., Kuroda, T., Iwabuchi, J., Imamura, S., Miyamoto, M., Fujino, T., Ito, N., Sugaya, K. (1971) 'Survey on the morbidity rate of "autistic children" in the Hokkaido district.' *Japanese Journal of Child Psychiatry*, **12**, 141–149.

Zappella, M. (1990) 'Autistic features in children affected by cerebral gigantism.' *Brain Dysfunction*, **3**, 241–244.

—— (1992) 'Hypomelanosis of Ito is common in autistic syndromes.' *European Child and Adolescent Psychiatry*, **1**, 170–177.

9
NEUROPSYCHOLOGY IN AUTISM AND ITS SPECTRUM DISORDERS

Recent years have witnessed a veritable explosion in the fields of cognitive psychology and neuropsychology in relation to autism. Several of the most interesting developments in all autism research have emerged from neuropsychological and cognitive psychological studies of young children with autism, of adult high-functioning men with autism, and of children and adults with Asperger syndrome. Systematic studies of three concepts – mentalizing, central coherence and executive function – have changed the conceptual framework in autism research. The pioneering work of Hermelin and O'Conner (1970) is still influential and has, in fact, inspired some of the most important recent studies – for example, the Frith group study. There is now a considerable autism literature document-ing deficits in (1) mentalizing or theory of mind, (2) drive for central coherence and (3) executive functions. Autistic disorder shows a fairly characteristic pattern on neuro-psychological tests such as the Wechsler scales (Frith 1989), the Tower of Hanoi or Tower of London tests, and other assessments of so-called executive function (Ozonoff and Miller 1995). Individuals with autism often fail on specific mentalizing tests – such as the "Sally-Anne" and "Smarties" tasks (Happé 1994) – and on tasks aimed at measuring drive for central coherence – such as elaborate versions of the WISC/WAIS (Wechsler 1974, 1981) block design subtest (Happé 1996). Not all people with autism are impaired in all of these fields, but there is usually evidence of dysfunction in at least one of the areas outlined. In addition, the most severely affected group in the autism spectrum, the one diagnosed as suffering from autistic disorder, shows global cognitive deficits which range from mild to profound.

During the 1980s the new hypotheses about the basic dysfunctions in autism soon came to dominate the way clinicians and researchers conceptualized the core autistic dys-functions, and by the early 1990s it was taken almost for granted that theory of mind deficits were at the root of autism and accounted for most of the variance in clinical presentation. However, it soon became clear that theory of mind deficits are not specific to autism, nor can they explain all of the clinical and neuropsychological problems encountered even in the narrowly defined Kanner variant of the syndrome. At the turn of the millennium, it has become generally accepted that several neuropsychological mecha-nisms are impaired in autism, and that mentalizing is just one of them. Nevertheless, theory of mind *is* deficient in autism, and its relation to (and overlap with) other neuro-psychological impairments – including executive dysfunction and weak central coherence – remains to be established.

Global cognitive deficits

The early studies by Lockyer and Rutter (1970) have been rediscovered and followed-up by new work which looks at both the "cognitive level" and "cognitive profile" in autism and autistic-like conditions. In spite of assertions to the contrary, it has been documented for decades that many children with classic autism are also mentally retarded (that is, they test reliably below IQ 70 on conventional IQ tests (Clark and Rutter 1979)). How large the proportion of children with autism who also show mental retardation actually is has varied somewhat according to different studies, but most authors agree that the figure is in the range of 65 to 85 per cent (Lotter 1967, Wing and Gould 1979, Bohman *et al.* 1983, Gillberg 1984, Gillberg and Steffenburg 1987, Sponheim and Skjeldal 1998). Recent studies suggesting a much higher prevalence rate for Asperger syndrome (usually with IQ >70) – possibly equivalent with high-functioning autism – than for autism "proper" (I.C. Gillberg and Gillberg 1989, Ehlers and Gillberg 1993, Kadesjö *et al.* 1999) could imply that the rate of clear mental retardation in autism spectrum disorders (including classic autism and Asperger syndrome), although much higher than in the general population, might be in the 10–25 per cent range instead. Be that as it may, most authorities agree that, even within the range of "normal intellectual functioning," children with autism (and Asperger syndrome) all show cognitive problems.

Defining features of autism (notably social, communication and symbolic play deficits) make it clear that various cognitive functions associated with these deficits are likely to be particularly affected. The longstanding debate as to whether autism is *either* "cognitive or social" tends to miss the point. The issue is not really *whether* autism is cognitive or social but rather *how* the social and cognitive deficits can be conceptualized as emerging from one common "primary" dysfunction. However, with regard to neuropsychological views of autism, the semantic squabble over "cognitive" on the one hand and "social" on the other still has far-reaching consequences in that the former is regarded as "cortical" (new brain) and the latter as "subcortical" (old brain) dysfunction. The overall point here is that there is a danger that the way in which we use words ("cognitive," "language," and "social," for instance) might substantially influence the way in which we conceptualize autism as *primarily* one thing or the other, when in fact it may be neither. For example, much emphasis has been put on language (supposedly more "cognitive" than "social") as a "primary" deficit in autism, even though there is now good evidence that people with autism can have excellent (at least formal expressive) language skills (Wing 1981a, Gillberg *et al.* 1987, Rumsey and Hamburger 1988), and that language deficits often associated with autism (*e.g.* pronominal reversal) might be conceptualized as delay rather than deviance (Oshima-Takane and Benaroya 1989) and as "communicative" and "pragmatic" rather than "linguistic" and "semantic." This emphasis has led to expectations that neuroimaging techniques – aimed at visualizing specialized cerebral cortical areas – would be successful in disclosing the common neurobiological denominator in autism. So far such studies have, by and large, been disappointing.

Cognitive impairment is usually thought of as a global phenomenon: it is expected that all cognitive functions will be affected in a child with cognitive impairment. This is a gross oversimplification even in children who are mentally retarded but do not show autism (*e.g.* those with Down syndrome and Williams syndrome, two mental retardation syndromes with clearly different cognitive profiles). In autism it is essential that the cognitive impairment be recognized as showing in (sometimes extremely) uneven cognitive profiles (Frith 1989, Happé 1994). Verbal abilities are usually poorer than performance skills; comprehension is quite often much more impaired than word production; fine motor skills may be better than gross motor skills; and a variety of measures reflecting rote memory skills demonstrate good or even superior results while working memory may be impaired (Wing 1981a, Ohta 1987).

The typical classic autism profile on the WISC is one with relatively very good results on block design, but poor or very poor results on comprehension and picture arrangement (Lockyer and Rutter 1970, Ohta 1987, Rumsey and Hamburger 1988, Frith 1989, Siegel *et al.* 1996, Ehlers *et al.* 1997). It has been suggested (Frith 1989, Happé 1994, Nydén *et al.* 1999) that a "cognitive profile" of this kind might be diagnostic of autism or at least highly suggestive of autism.

In a number of children, adolescents and adults with autism there is, in addition, "an islet of special ability" (Shah and Frith 1983). Around 1 in 2 people with autism have an area of functioning which stands out as exceptionally good compared with other areas. In a very few cases (about 5 per cent according to O'Conner and Hermelin 1988, fewer still according to the present authors), there may exist extraordinary "savant skills" (Treffert 1989), such as shown by Raymond (Dustin Hoffman) in the Barry Levinson film *Rain Man*. Such "autistic savants" usually show extremely superior rote memory abilities, musical giftedness or mathematical skills. Similar, though not quite such striking, giftedness (not so striking because of the overall better cognitive level) is also seen in cases with autism spectrum disorders (*e.g.* Asperger syndrome (Wing 1981b)).

It appears that many children with autism rely on visuospatial rather than temporal processing (Hermelin and O'Conner 1970), and that meaningful information tends to be less often correctly identified (Aurnhammer-Frith 1969). Many children with autism show excellent skills with jigsaw puzzles but cannot even conceive of the notion of time. This is unlike normal children who tend to extract as many meaningful clues as possible in trying to solve problems. Also, whereas normal children will make use of several clues, children with autism will often depend on one single piece of information when attending to a task.

The picture is different in Asperger syndrome, where most individuals have IQs above 70 and their verbal scores often exceed those on the performance side. There are often WISC/WAIS troughs on picture arrangement (possibly as a marker of mentalizing deficits) and object assembly (a possible indication of weak central coherence), and quite commonly also in areas that are usually dysfunctional in attention disorders and "right hemisphere dysfunction" disorders (*e.g.* arithmetic, digit span and digit symbol) (Ehlers *et al.* 1997).

Specific theories relating to the proposed underlying core deficits in autism and its spectrum disorders

In the 1980s and 1990s, the focus of neuropsychological studies in autism shifted gradually from language and other conservative measures of cognition to the description and delineation of social and pragmatic deficits. Several distinct theories have emerged which have been subjected to systematic scientific study. For the sake of brevity, they will here be referred to as the "affective theory" (Hobson 1986a and 1986b), the "meta-representation theory" (Baron-Cohen 1988), the "central coherence theory" (Frith 1989, Happé 1994) and the "executive function theory" (Ozonoff and Strayer 1997). Many studies testing these hypotheses have been published in the last decade. There have also been many neuropsychological studies not clearly related to these theories, but which have nevertheless contributed to a better understanding of the basic dysfunctions involved in the development of autistic syndromes.

The Affective Theory

The affective theory goes back to Kanner's original assertion that children with autism have "inborn disturbances of *affective* contact" (our italics), and Piaget's theories. In the affective theory, autism is seen as stemming from an affective deficit which is primary and irreducible and involves a dysfunction in the ability to perceive other people's mental states as reflected in their bodily expressions. This primary affective dysfunction underlies the social and communication problems. Support for the theory has been generated by a number of interesting experiments concerned with various aspects of emotion recognition in children with autism (Hobson 1986a and 1986b, Hobson *et al.* 1988). However, the studies by Marian Sigman and her group (Sigman and Ungerer 1984, Sigman *et al.* 1986) have demonstrated convincingly that some attachment behaviors – *e.g.* eye contact and reaching after tickling – are usually preserved in autism. Such behaviors can all be seen as primarily "affective" variables. Also, most authorities agree that children with autism may have well-developed primary emotions such as anger and gladness.

The Meta-representational Theory

The meta-representational theory – which is sometimes also referred to as the "cognitive theory" (to distinguish it from the affective theory) – argues rather differently that mental states with content (such as "invisible" knowing and believing, and not "obvious" happiness and anger) are not directly observable but have to be inferred.

The ability to impute mental states with content to other people has been referred to as a "theory of mind" (Premach and Woodruff 1978). This "theory" is present in normal children from at least 4 years of age (Hogrefe *et al.* 1986), but could be in operation much earlier, perhaps even before the age of 1 year (Leslie 1987). The specific cognitive peaks and troughs encountered in autism (low scores on comprehension and picture arrangement, and high on block design on the WISC; low scores on hearing and speech and practical reasoning, and high on motor and performance on the Griffiths) could be taken to indicate the lack of a core capacity for coherence in autism. Uta Frith (1989) and her collaborators (Baron-Cohen *et al.* 1985, Baron-Cohen 1990) have proposed a theory to account for the basic psychological features of autism. They hypothesize that underlying the behavioral symptoms of autism is a central disorder of empathy, characterized by inability or decreased capacity to conceive of other people's mental states (such as knowing and believing). If a deficit of this kind exists, then it could explain the lack of coherence and need for coherence in autism. If you do not understand that behind people's actions are thought-out purposes and wilful planning, then much of what people do will stand out as incomprehensible. What they say will be even more "uncommunicative" – if you do not understand that spoken words are a "message from the mind," then spoken language may be something you learn to imitate but not a tool for communication.

Not having a well-developed theory of mind will lead to extreme deficits in reciprocal social interaction, in communication and in "creative" imagination. However, not having a theory of mind does not necessarily affect memory skills or visuospatial skills, areas in which many people with autism excel. Feats of rote memory and skill in doing jigsaw puzzles are fairly common in autism. These are skills that are not dependent on having a theory of mind. Such skills are reflected in high scores on block design and performance. The meta-representational theory predicts that only specific social capacities will be constantly restricted in autism (that is, those that require a concept of other people's wishes, beliefs and thoughts, *e.g.* reciprocal social interactions or "emphatic" relation-ships), whereas other social capacities may be spared (for instance, those that only require perception of the observable world, *e.g.* face recognition). The theory further predicts that the pragmatics of existing language skills in a child with autism will be specifically impaired. A number of simple, yet thought-provoking, experiments have been performed to test this theory (see Baron-Cohen 1989a for a review). In one of these experiments, two dolls, Sally and Anne, were presented to normal children, children with Down syndrome and children with autism. In Sally's basket there was a marble, but in Anne's box there was nothing. Sally then "left the room," which meant that she could no longer see what was going on. In the meantime, Anne moved the marble to her box. When Sally "came back," the children participating in the study were asked: "Where will Sally look for the marble?" Children with Down syndrome and normal children said she would look where it was when she left the room (a false but reasonable belief), whereas most of the children with autism said she would look in the box, where it actually was (a true but unreasonable belief). Children with autism under the age of 11 years and with a mental age under 6 years constantly fail this task according to Baron-Cohen (1990). One way to account for this finding – and similar findings from other experiments – would be the lack of a theory of mind – if the child cannot understand that Sally has a mind (a belief/thought about the marble being where it once was), the child will believe only what he or she sees or hears.

There is now general agreement that young children with autism – across the board of intellectual functioning and severity – have severe problems in the area of mentalizing or "theory of mind" (Frith 1989, Baron-Cohen 1995). They have severe problems taking another person's social point of view, and, at least when young or of low mental age, in understanding that other people have thoughts and beliefs and other mental states that do not necessarily show on the outside in mimicry or gesture. There has been some doubt as to whether the mentalizing deficits are linked to autism or mental retardation or low language competence (Prior *et al.* 1990), since a number of individuals with autism pass theory-of-mind tests. It now appears that older, mildly retarded or normally intelligent individuals with autism pass such tests in a majority of all cases, and that those diagnosed as having Asperger syndrome do so even from around early school age. It appears that the emergence of mentalizing skills may be greatly delayed in autism, and that in the most severely handicapped group, with severe and profound levels of mental retardation, such skills may never develop at all (Baron-Cohen 1995). Reaction times to so-called false-belief tasks tend to be delayed in autism even in those individuals who actually formally pass the tasks *per se* (Bowler 1997). Young children can be trained successfully in theory-of-mind skills (Howlin *et al.* 1998), but such training does not appear to affect their everyday social behavior. Unfortunately, there is good correspondence between poor theory-of-mind skills and impairments in everyday social behavior (Hughes *et al.* 1997).

There is now also a growing literature showing that difficulties in understanding mental states are not specific to autism but also occur in other conditions, such as schizophrenia (Frith and Corcoran 1996) and "social immaturity" (Muris *et al.* 1998). These findings do not contradict the broader concept of autism, but are compatible with findings that schizophrenia may be anteceded by autistic-type problems (Asarnow *et al.* 1988), and that the broader phenotype of autism may well include variants reflecting mainly as social immaturity (Le Couteur *et al.* 1996). These findings also fit in well with the theory that genes and environmental hazards, acting in concert, only rarely produce the (arbitrarily defined) "syndrome" of autism, but more often cause "spectrum" problems and "similar" problems/disorders, depending on which genes/hazards and neuropsychological functions are most severely affected.

Originally conceptualized as an all-or-nothing phenomenon (Baron-Cohen *et al.* 1985), theory-of-mind skills are now regarded as the result of gradual emergence and moulding of developmentally more primitive skills such as "eye-direction detection" (Baron-Cohen 1995) and joint attention (Sigman *et al.* 1983). Both of these functions appear to be impaired very early in the lives of children with autism (Baron-Cohen 1995, Mundy and Crowson 1997).

The meta-representational theory provides a plausible account for the developmental changes in the clinical picture of autism across time and IQ levels. Impairments in "first order belief attribution" (*e.g.* "I think he thinks") may be typical of the most severely disabled people with autism, whereas impairments of "second order belief attribution" (*e.g.* "I think he thinks she thinks") may typify high-level cases of those currently referred to as Asperger syndrome (see also Baron-Cohen 1989b). A proposed deficient theory of mind in autism has the merit of making comprehensible to parents and professionals alike some of the mystifying features of autism. A theory of this kind has the great merit of being testable at several levels and also of providing a clinically relevant model for the development of autism.

Gillberg (1992) has suggested that poorly developed theory-of-mind skills might be equivalent to having poor empathy (although not necessarily to having poor sympathy), and has launched the concept of "disorders of empathy" for the broader group of individuals who have mentalizing deficits. He has argued that in an older person who had such problems as a child there may be an inability to react quickly enough to social stimuli and, hence, the striking quality of lack of intuition and common sense. His model also suggests that the ability to mentalize may be normally distributed in the general population, and that individuals diagnosed as having an autism spectrum disorder may either represent cases on the lowermost tail of the normal distribution curve, or have severely deficient empathy skills because of an acquired brain lesion hitting neural circuitries that subserve empathy.

THE CENTRAL COHERENCE THEORY

The notion of weak central coherence in autism can be distilled from the very first studies by Beate Hermelin and Neil O'Conner. There is mounting support for the notion that individuals with autism are characterized by their "weak drive for central coherence" (Happé 1994). Such a deficit biases them toward processing information at an analytic rather than global level, and they have difficulty in switching from details to concepts of whole gestalts or vice versa. Both children and adults with autism and Asperger syndrome perform better on the so-called "Embedded Figures Test" than do normal controls (Jolliffe and Baron-Cohen 1997), but they do not differ significantly from each other. Counting abilities differentiate children with autism from those with moderate learning difficulties and from normally developing children (Jarrold and Russell 1997). These findings, along with the well-known tendency for individuals with autism to score relatively high or very high on the block design subtest of the WISC or WAIS (Frith 1989) – and the suggestion that those with Asperger syndrome score low on the object assembly subtest (Ehlers *et al.* 1997) – have been taken as evidence of "lack of a drive for" or "weak" central coherence in autism and autistic-like conditions.

THE EXECUTIVE FUNCTION THEORY

Executive function is a collective term for all those faculties that are needed for the individual to work in a motivated fashion toward a goal that may not be reached instantly. Good executive functions require good focusing skills, time concepts, sequential thinking, and motivation. Clinical experience has long suggested that such qualities are often poorly developed in autism. There is widespread acceptance that executive functions – usually believed to reflect prefrontal brain activity – are dysfunctional in autism and its spectrum disorders, most notably Asperger syndrome (Ozonoff and Strayer 1997). However, the issue of whether or not there are *specific* executive function deficits in autism, has yet to be resolved. One study, comparing school-age children with a variety of neuropsychiatric disorders to normal children, found that high-functioning autism, ADHD and dyslexia were all markedly different from normality, but not significantly different from each other in terms of executive functions (Nydén *et al.* 1999). Children – and adults – with autism show impairments in respect of working memory, ability to inhibit, plan, organize, and shift flexibly from one cognitive set to another (Dawson 1996). Attentional abilities – accepted by some researchers as markers of executive function, but considered by others to be a different set of neuropsychological/cognitive functions – are impaired with regard to orienting, disengaging and selection, but the "sustained attention" category is usually spared.

Other neuropsychological characteristics of autism

Several other neuropsychological domains have been studied in the pathogenesis of autism. Some of these may be seen to represent functions overlapping or even synonymous with those referred to in the previous three sections. Deficits in social perception, in symbolic play and in memory are examples of such domains. Other functions that have been suggested as being impaired in autism comprise motor performance, some visually related abilities (in spite of the fact that other aspects of visuospatial functions appear to be spared or even hyperfunctioning in many cases of autism), facial recognition and interhemispheric transfer. These areas appear to be slightly more clearly separated from executive functions, mentalizing and drive for central coherence. Language is a tricky area in autism research, given that communication deficits (verbal and non-verbal) are a defining feature of the syndrome. Nevertheless, there is evidence that the non-verbal communication deficit resulting from impairment in mentalizing ability might be of greater importance than specific language dysfunction in autism, meaning that the language deficits observed in the syndrome may also best be interpreted in the light of knowledge that has accumulated on the basis of research into theory of mind.

SOCIAL PERCEPTION, SYMBOLIC PLAY AND ATTENTIONAL DEFICITS

In a well-controlled study, children with autism were unimpaired on social perception tasks that involved only one cue (Pierce *et al.* 1997), but failed when more cues were involved. The findings were interpreted as possibly reflecting attentional rather than primarily social deficits. Symbolic play and memory were delayed rather than deviant in an experimental setting in which children with autism and children matched for receptive language and others matched for non-verbal IQ were compared to each other (McDonough *et al.* 1997). These findings – sharply contrasting with the impairments in these areas found when children with autism are observed in naturalistic settings – again were taken to suggest attentional deficits in autism: distractions typically occur in naturalistic settings but experimental settings tend to minimize disruptions of this kind. However, even in highly structured settings with a familiar partner at home, attentional deficits and low affective responsiveness tend to persist, albeit at a less striking level than in unstructured situations (Joseph and Tager-Flusberg 1997).

Adults with autism were much delayed compared with normal controls in orienting their attention on a traditional spacial cueing task. This sluggishness of shifting attention between and within modalities was interpreted as a sign of cerebellar dysfunction (Townsend *et al.* 1996).

MOTOR DEFICITS

There is a small literature on motor problems in autism and autistic-like conditions, including Asperger syndrome (*e.g.* DeMyer 1975, Gillberg 1989, Ghaziuddin *et al.* 1992). It now seems clear that such disorders are associated with minor–moderate motor problems. It is unclear whether there is anything in the motor domain that might separate Asperger syndrome from high-functioning autism (Gillberg 1998). Motor imitation is impaired in autism (Heimann *et al*. 1995, Stone *et al*. 1997a), but whether or not this deficiency is responsible for the clumsy and ill-coordinated movements is not known. Coordination problems are often most evident in the high-functioning individuals with autism/Asperger syndrome, but this might be because the most high-functioning people have a greater repertoire of activities and, hence, get to show their awkward and clumsy motor skills much more often and in many more settings than those who are lower functioning (who are usually not *perceived* as motor clumsy, even though, on formal testing, they may well be) (Miyahara *et al*. 1997).

VISUOSPATIAL PROBLEMS AND STRENGTHS
It has been known for more than half a century that children with autism have some relatively superior visuospatial skills (Kanner 1943). Whether this should be seen as merely reflecting an area of intact functioning – and hence an impression that such skills are "superior" to other impaired functions – or as an association with a more fundamental characteristic of the core impairment in autism, is debatable. The lack of, or delayed, development of an eye-direction detector (see above) could be taken as a symptom of impaired visuospatial functioning, but is probably best understood in the context of a joint attention–theory of mind framework. It is quite possible that individuals with autism have similar attention deficits in the auditory domain.

Specific localizing neuropsychological dysfunctions in autism
MEDIAL TEMPORAL LOBE AND DORSOLATERAL FRONTAL LOBE DYSFUNCTION
Dawson and coworkers compared young children with autism with developmentally matched groups of children with Down syndrome and with typical development on neuropsychological tests purportedly tapping specific medial temporal lobe functions and dorsolateral frontal lobe functions. Children with autism scored persistently worse than the other two groups, and severity of autistic symptoms was strongly correlated with poor performance on the medial temporal lobe task (Dawson *et al*. 1998).

INTERHEMISPHERIC TRANSFER DYSFUNCTION
The prevalence of non-right-handedness is increased in autism (Gillberg 1983). A SPECT study revealed autism to be associated with low regional cerebral blood flow in the left hemisphere, particularly in sensorimotor and language areas (Chiron *et al*. 1995). This was regardless of handedness, which was often "non-right" in autism. The results support anomalous hemispheric specialization or interhemispheric transfer dysfunction in autism.

One study examined the potential contribution of right hemisphere dysfunction to the communicative impairments of autism (Ozonoff and Miller 1996). Pragmatic language measures, sensitive to right hemisphere damage, were administered to non-retarded adults with autism and to controls matched on age and intellectual ability. Individuals with autism performed significantly less well than controls on all measures, replicating results of an earlier investigation by Rumsey and Hanahan (1990).

110

About half of all children with classic autism are functionally mute (Wing 1996). The other half have delayed and deviant language, hallmarked by reversal of pronouns, immediate and delayed echolalia, and repetitive questioning with insistence on standard answers (Rapin and Dunn 1997). There are major receptive language problems even though concrete words like nouns and verbs are usually well understood. Phonology, syntax, morphology and semantics may be impaired, but not specifically so (Tager-Flusberg 1996). Pragmatics, on the other hand, is one area of language that is always seriously impaired in autism – and in autistic-like conditions, including Asperger syndrome. Problems in non-verbal communication (pointing, showing objects, eye-gaze to regulate contact) are present from very early on in the lives of individuals with autism (Stone *et al.* 1997b). Such problems are to be expected if mentalizing deficits are at the core of the autistic syndrome. At the non-verbal level, the monotonic prosody and paucity of gesture are characteristic features that suggest right hemisphere dysfunction. At the verbal level, problems with narrative discourse (including impoverished stories), difficulties in understanding and using abstract language, and providing the appropriate level of relevant information, are striking (Loveland and Tunali 1991). The use of social conventional language, such as greetings and polite forms, is also limited (Ramberg *et al.* 1996).

The question arises as to whether people with autism also have "dysphasia" (Rapin and Dunn 1997), which would suggest left temporofrontal dysfunction. It is clear that a proportion of all individuals diagnosed as having a disorder in the "autism spectrum" do have expressive language problems that merit the diagnosis of dysphasia. However, it is equally clear that many of those with high-functioning autism and Asperger syndrome have excellent expressive language skills, and that if autism is conceptualized as a spectrum disorder, then dysphasia cannot be an inclusion criterion, but should be coded separately under developmental language disorder (Tanguay *et al.* 1998). Nevertheless, it is interesting to speculate about the links of language disorders to autism, particularly given the recent finding of genes on chromosome 7q being abnormal both in autism and severe expressive language disorders.

Preliminary conclusions

The neuropsychological profile in autism is not consistent with that seen in mental retardation or in any other general deficit syndrome. Rather it appears to involve a selective impairment in complex information processing which does not usually affect visuospatial processing. The profile is not consistent with a single primary deficit, but with a multiple primary deficit model (Minshew *et al.* 1997). Several theories have been proposed that might "explain" how the multiple primary deficits combine to produce the syndrome of autism. Among the more interesting of these is the neural circuit/neural network theory (Cohen 1994, Gustafsson 1997), which proposes that there may be inadequate cortical feature maps in autism, making it difficult for affected individuals to use previous sensory impressions when processing current information.

Is psychological testing in children and adults suffering from autism spectrum disorders useful?

It is often – though by no means always – problematic to test a young autistic child using conventional IQ tests. Problems are most likely to occur, of course, if the tester is not very well acquainted with the underlying deficits and clinical manifestations of autism. In order for it to be worthwhile testing a child with autism, testing and results on tests must have some meaning. So what are IQ tests and other tests in autism good for?

IQ tests in childhood (at normal age 5 years, for instance) have been shown to be the best available single instrument for roughly predicting outcome in autism (Rutter 1983). A very low IQ (<50) in childhood usually predicts a similar IQ and relatively poor social outcome in adult age. As has already been pointed out above, some of the IQ tests yield a typical "profile" in autism. On the WISC (for school-age children), peaks in block design (and picture assembly) and troughs in word comprehension and picture arrangement are typical. On the Griffiths developmental scale (Griffiths 1970), children with autism peak in motor and daily life activities but score very poorly on the hearing/language scales (Dahlgren-Sandberg *et al.* 1993). For these – and other – reasons, it is clear that IQ testing is essential in the work-up on any child *per se*, and for predicting outcome in a reasonably reliable way.

Results on specific tests of language performed in childhood can also help establish a fairly accurate prognosis. Useful speech at age 5 years is one of the best predictors of outcome (Gillberg 1991). In particular, it is helpful to try to pinpoint the receptive deficits (which, contrary to earlier assertions, are often even more pronounced than the expressive skill deficits), and to find out to what extent there might be added problems of "pure" dysphasia over and above any language-communicative deficits that could be accounted for by autism alone.

Finally, psychometric assessment is required because children with autism are unique individuals who do share some core deficits but who – apart from the commonalties – are quite different from each other. A detailed test of various functional capacities will help to provide a fuller picture of assets and deficits, such that a better understanding of what will be the most useful coping strategies can be achieved.

The psychometric work-up in autism and its spectrum disorders: some suggestions

Any child who is being examined for the first time under the suspicion that he or she might be suffering from autism must have a proper psychometric assessment, or, if examined in the first three years of life, must be scheduled for such assessment some years later.

Exactly which test to choose depends on a number of variables, such as age, overall and verbal development of child, tests available, the psychologist's familiarity with certain tests, etc. Also, some tests are more appropriate when evaluating autism because they have been used extensively in the scientific study of autism.

In the very young child (<5 years) with autism, the assessment by an experienced clinician often yields as much information about the child's developmental level as any developmental test. In Sweden, the Griffiths developmental scales are often used in the assessment of young autistic children. However, this test – like most other tests used with this age group – yields little detail and has very low discriminative capacity in the groups with mild, low-normal, normal, and high intelligence. Nevertheless, it can be a valuable aid in the evaluation of the severely disabled group (Dahlgren-Sandberg *et al.* 1993). Another test that may be useful with this age group is the Raven. The Leiter (Shah and Holmes 1985) is sometimes a very good instrument for evaluating non-verbal IQ in preschool children with autism. One must keep in mind the typical peaks in visual performance skills shown by children with autism, which means that superior results on the Leiter need not necessarily be a reflection of overall superior IQ.

The Vineland Social Maturity Scale can also be helpful, particularly when evaluating overall/adaptive skills. The Vineland social quotient has been shown to correlate fairly strongly with measures of IQ (Freeman *et al.* 1999).

In the school-age period, the WISC is definitely the best-documented of all tests currently available for the evaluation of cognition in autism. Every child with autism or an autistic-like condition who does not have severe or profound mental retardation (IQ >35) should, in our opinion, be given the WISC at some point after they reach school age. In countries where the Wechsler Preschool and Wechsler Adult Intelligence Scales have been standardized, they too can be used in the psychometric work-up of autism outside of the school-age period. The typical WISC profile seen in autism (and often in high-functioning or Asperger-type cases also) has been described in detail in the above section (see p. 111).

Specific language tests tend to vary from one country to another. The best approach is to have a close collaboration with a speech pathology therapist, who will be able to accumulate experience in the field of speech–language evaluation in autism. The Peabody Test may be quite useful. The current author's experience with the ITPA (Illinois Test of Psycholinguistic Abilities), on the other hand, has been that it yields relatively little information about specific communicative-language problems. In this connection it may be prudent to caution against the notion of autism as a speech–language disorder (or the idea that it is in some basic sense clearly associated with language disorders). Current concepts in autism stress the overall communicative deficits rather than specific language problems. Semantic–pragmatic problems and non-verbal communication deficits seem to be more typical of autism and autistic-like conditions than such "autism-specific language peculiarities" as echolalia and pronoun reversal. We are much in need of a good battery for testing communicative skills in the field of speech and language and – in particular – in areas such as pragmatics, semantics, mime and gesture.

For those particularly interested in detailed analyses of autism spectrum problems, all sorts of other tests may be used. The Matching Familiar Figures Test, Tower of Hanoi, Embedded Figures Test, and various tests of mentalizing abilities and social under-standing, are examples of tests which have been scientifically validated in autism.

Summary
Recent developments in autism have seen a formidable step forward for neuropsychology/cognitive psychology. Testable hypotheses suggesting that children with autism lack

a "theory of mind" and the strive for "central coherence" have been put forward and successfully put to the test. "Old truths," such as IQ being the single best predictor of outcome, have again been highlighted. Autism is no longer conceptualized as a form of psychosis but as a developmental disorder. All of these trends have led to general consensus that all children with autism and autistic-like conditions need a proper psychometric evaluation. The WISC is clearly still the best-documented psychometric instrument in the field. The next few years will tell whether autism neuropsychology will become a firm branch of autism research or not. It seems clear already at this stage that some of the most interesting constructs in the whole field of autism have been generated by cognitive psychologists.

REFERENCES

Asarnow, J.R., Ben-Meir, S. (1988) 'Children with schizophrenia spectrum and depressive disorders: a comparative study of premorbid adjustment, onset pattern and severity of impairment.' *Journal of Child Psychology and Psychiatry*, **29**, 477–488.

Aurnhammer-Frith, U. (1969) 'Emphasis and meaning in recall in normal and autistic children.' *Language and Speech*, **12**, 29–38.

Baron-Cohen, S. (1988) 'Without a theory of mind one cannot participate in a conversation.' *Cognition*, **29**, 83–84.

—— (1989a) 'The autistic child's theory of mind: a case of specific developmental delay.' *Journal of Child Psychology and Psychiatry*, **30**, 285–297.

—— (1989b) 'Do autistic children have obsessions and compulsions?' *British Journal of Clinical Psychology*, **28**, 193–200.

—— (1990) 'Autism: a specific cognitive disorder of "mind-blindness."' *International Review of Psychiatry*, **2**, 81–90.

—— (1995) *Mind Blindness. An Essay on Autism and Theory of Mind*. Cambridge, Mass.: MIT Press.

Baron-Cohen, S., Leslie, A.M., Frith, U. (1985) 'Does the autistic child have a theory of mind?' *Cognition*, **21**, 37–46.

Bohman, M., Bohman, I.L., Björk, P., Sjöholm, E. (1983) 'Childhood psychosis in a northern Swedish county: some preliminary findings from an epidemiological survey.' *In:* Schmidt, M.H., Remschmith, H. (Eds) *Epidemiological Approaches in Child Psychiatry*. Stuttgart: Georg Thieme, pp. 164–173.

Bowler, D.M. (1997) 'Reaction time to mental state and non-mental state questions and false belief tasks by high-functioning individuals with autism.' *European Child and Adolescent Psychiatry*, **6**, 160–165.

Chiron, C., Leboyer, M., Leon, F., Jambaqué, I., Nuttin, C., Syrota, A. (1995) 'SPECT of the brain in childhood autism: evidence for a lack of normal hemispheric asymmetry.' *Developmental Medicine and Child Neurology*, **37**, 849–860.

Clark, P., Rutter, M. (1979) 'Task difficulty and task performance in autistic children.' *Journal of Child Psychology and Psychiatry*, **20**, 271–285.

Cohen, I.L. (1994) 'An artificial neural analogue of learning in autism.' *Biological Psychiatry*, **36**, 5–20.

Dahlgren-Sandberg, A., Nydén, A., Gillberg, C., Hjelmquist, E. (1993) 'The cognitive profile in infantile autism – a study of 70 children and adolescents using the Griffiths Mental Development Scale.' *British Journal of Psychology*, **84**, 365–373.

Dawson, G. (1996) 'Brief report: Neuropsychology of autism: a report on the state of the science.' *Journal of Autism and Developmental Disorders*, **26**, 179–184.

Dawson, G., Meltzoff, A.N., Osterling, J., Rinaldi, J. (1998) 'Neuropsychological correlates of early symptoms of autism.' *Child Development*, **69**, 1276–1285.

DeMyer, M.K. (1975) 'The nature of the neuropsychological disability in autistic children.' *Journal of Autism and Childhood Schizophrenia*, **5**, 109–128.

Ehlers, S., Gillberg, C. (1993) 'The epidemiology of Asperger syndrome. A total population study.' *Journal of Child Psychology and Psychiatry*, **34**, 1327–1350.

Ehlers, S., Nydén, A., Gillberg, C., Dahlgren-Sandberg, A., Dahlgren, S.-O., Hjelmquist, E., Odén, A. (1997) 'Asperger syndrome, autism and attention disorders: a comparative study of the cognitive profile of 120 children.' *Journal of Child Psychology and Psychiatry*, **38**, 207–217.

Freeman, B.J., Ritvo, E.R., Yokota, A., Childs, J., Pollard, J. (1988) 'WISC-R and Vineland Adaptive Behaviour Scale scores in autistic children.' *Journal of the American Academy of Child and Adolescent Psychiatry*, **27**, 428–429.

Freeman, B.J., Del'Homme, M., Guthrie, D., Zhang, F. (1999) 'Vineland Adaptive Behavior Scale scores as a function of age and initial IQ in 210 autistic children.' *Journal of Autism and Developmental Disorders*, **29**, 379–384.

Frith, U. (1989) 'Autism and "theory of mind."' *In:* Gillberg, C. (Ed.) *Diagnosis and Treatment of Autism.* New York: Plenum Press, pp. 33–52.

Frith, U., Corcoran, R. (1996) 'Exploring "theory of mind" in people with schizophrenia.' *Psychological Medicine*, **26**, 521–530.

Ghaziuddin, M., Tsai, L.Y., Ghaziuddin, N. (1992) 'Brief report: A reappraisal of clumsiness as a diagnostic feature of Asperger syndrome.' *Journal of Autism and Developmental Disorders*, **22**, 651–656.

Gillberg, C. (1983) 'Autistic children's hand preferences: results from an epidemiological study of infantile autism.' *Psychiatry Research*, **10**, 21–30.

—— (1984) 'Infantile autism and other childhood psychoses in a Swedish urban region. Epidemiological aspects.' *Journal of Child Psychology and Psychiatry*, **25**, 35–43.

—— (1989) 'Asperger syndrome in 23 Swedish children.' *Developmental Medicine and Child Neurology*, **31**, 520–531.

—— (1991) 'Outcome in autism and autistic-like conditions.' *Journal of the American Academy of Child and Adolescent Psychiatry*, **30**, 375–382.

—— (1992) 'The Emanuel Miller Memorial Lecture 1991: Autism and autistic-like conditions: subclasses among disorders of empathy.' *Journal of Child Psychology and Psychiatry*, **33**, 813–842.

—— (1998) 'Asperger syndrome and high-functioning autism.' *British Journal of Psychiatry*, **172**, 200–209.

Gillberg, C., Steffenburg, S. (1987) 'Outcome and prognostic factors in infantile autism and similar conditions: a population-based study of 46 cases followed through puberty.' *Journal of Autism and Developmental Disorders*, **17**, 273–287.

Gillberg, C., Steffenburg, S., Jakobsson, G. (1987) 'Neurobiological findings in 20 relatively gifted children with Kanner-type autism or Asperger syndrome.' *Developmental Medicine and Child Neurology*, **29**, 641–649.

Gillberg, I.C., Gillberg, C. (1989) 'Asperger syndrome – some epidemiological considerations: a research note.' *Journal of Child Psychology and Psychiatry*, **30**, 631–638.

Griffiths, R. (1970) *The Abilities of Young Children. A Study in Mental Measurement.* London: University of London Press.

Gustafsson, L. (1997) 'Inadequate cortical feature maps: a neural circuit theory of autism.' *Biological Psychiatry*, **42**, 1138–1147.

Happé, F. (1994) 'Wechsler IQ profile and theory of mind in autism: a research note.' *Journal of Child Psychology and Psychiatry*, **35**, 1461–1471.

—— (1996) 'The neuropsychology of autism.' *Brain*, **119**, 1377–1400.

Heimann, M., Nelson, K.E., Tjus, T., Gillberg, C. (1995) 'Increasing reading and communication skills in children with autism through an interactive multimedia computer program.' *Journal of Autism and Developmental Disorders*, **25**, 459–480.

Hermelin, B., O'Conner, N. (1970) *Psychological Experiments with Autistic Children.* Oxford: Pergamon Press.

Hobson, R.P. (1986a) 'The autistic child's appraisal of expressions of emotions.' *Journal of Child Psychology and Psychiatry*, **27**, 321–342.

—— (1986b) 'The autistic child's appraisal of expressions of emotions: a further study.' *Journal of Child Psychology and Psychiatry*, **27**, 671–680.

Hobson, R.P., Ouston, J., Lee, A. (1988) 'Emotion recognition in autism: coordinating faces and voices.' *Psychological Medicine*, **18**, 911–923.

Hogrefe, G.J., Wimmer, H., Perner, J. (1986) 'Ignorance versus false belief: a developmental lag in attribution of epistemic states.' *Child Development*, **57**, 567–582.

Howlin, P., Davies, M., Udwin, O. (1998) 'Cognitive functioning in adults with Williams syndrome.' *Journal of Child Psychology and Psychiatry*, **39**, 183–189.

115

Hughes, C., Soares-Boucaud, I., Hochmann, J., Frith, U. (1997) 'Social behaviour in pervasive developmental disorders: effects of informant, group and "theory-of-mind."' *European Child and Adolescent Psychiatry*, **6**, 191–198.

Jarrold, C., Russell, J. (1997) 'Counting abilities in autism: possible implications for central coherence theory.' *Journal of Autism and Developmental Disorders*, **27**, 25–37.

Jolliffe, T., Baron-Cohen, S. (1997) 'Are people with autism and Asperger syndrome faster than normal on the Embedded Figures Test?' *Journal of Child Psychology and Psychiatry*, **38**, 527–534.

Joseph, R.M., Tager-Flusberg, H. (1997) 'An investigation of attention and affect in children with autism and Down syndrome.' *Journal of Autism and Developmental Disorders*, **27**, 385–396.

Kadesjö, B., Gillberg, C., Hagberg, B. (1999) 'Brief report: Autism and Asperger syndrome in seven-year old children. A total population prevalence study.' *Journal of Autism and Developmental Disorders*. Accepted.

Kanner, L. (1943) 'Autistic disturbances of affective contact.' *Nervous Child*, **2**, 217–250.

Le Couteur, A., Bailey, A., Goode, S., Pickles, A., Robertson, S., Gottesman, I., Rutter, M. (1996) 'A broader phenotype of autism: the clinical spectrum in twins.' *Journal of Child Psychology and Psychiatry*, **37**, 785–801.

Leslie, A.M. (1987) 'Pretence and representation: the origins of a "theory of mind."' *Psychological Review*, **94**, 412–426.

Lockyer, L., Rutter, M. (1970) 'A five to fifteen year follow-up study of infantile psychosis. IV: Patterns of cognitive ability.' *British Journal of Social and Cognitive Ability*, **9**, 152–163.

Lotter, V. (1967) *The Prevalence of the Autistic Syndrome in Children*. London: University of London Press.

Loveland, K.A., Tunali, B. (1991) 'Social scripts for conversational interactions in autism and Down syndrome.' *Journal of Autism and Developmental Disorders*, **21**, 177–186.

McDonough, L., Stahmer, A., Schreibman, L., Thompson, S.J. (1997) 'Deficits, delays, and distractions: an evaluation of symbolic play and memory in children with autism.' *Developmental Psychopathology*, **9**, 17–41.

Minshew, N.J., Goldstein, G., Siegel, D.J. (1997) 'Neuropsychological functioning in autism: profile of a complex information processing disorder.' *Journal of the International Neuropsychological Society*, **3**, 303–316.

Miyahara, M., Tsujii, M., Hori, M., Nakanishi, K., Kageyama, H., Sugiyama, T. (1997) 'Brief report: Motor incoordination in children with Asperger syndrome and learning disabilities.' *Journal of Autism and Developmental Disorders*, **27**, 595–603.

Mundy, P., Crowson, M. (1997) 'Joint attention and early social communication: implications for research on intervention with autism.' *Journal of Autism and Developmental Disorders*, **27**, 653–676.

Muris, P., Steerneman, P., Merchelbach, H. (1998) 'Difficulties in the understanding of false belief: specific to autism and other pervasive developmental disorders?' *Psychological Report*, **82**, 51–57.

Nydén, A., Gillberg, C., Hjelmquist, E., Heimann, M. (1999) 'Executive function/attention in boys with Asperger syndrome, attention disorders and reading/writing disorder.' *Autism*. In press.

O'Conner, N., Hermelin, B. (1988) 'Low intelligence and special abilities.' *Journal of Child Psychology and Psychiatry*, **29**, 391–396.

Ohta, M. (1987) 'Cognitive disorders of infantile autism: a study employing the WISC, spatial relationship conceptualization, and gesture imitation.' *Journal of Autism and Developmental Disorders*, **17**, 45–62.

Oshima-Takane, Y., Benaroya, S. (1989) 'An alternative view of pronominal errors in autistic children.' *Journal of Autism and Developmental Disorders*, **19**, 73–85.

Ozonoff, S., Miller, J.N. (1995) 'Teaching theory of mind: a new approach to social skills training for individuals with autism.' *Journal of Autism and Developmental Disorders*, **25**, 415–433.

—— (1996) 'An exploration of right-hemisphere contribution to the pragmatic impairments of autism.' *Brain and Language*, **52**, 411–434.

Ozonoff, S., Strayer, D.L. (1997) 'Inhibitory function in nonretarded children with autism.' *Journal of Autism and Developmental Disorders*, **27**, 59–77.

Pierce, K., Glad, K.S., Schreibman, L. (1997) 'Social perception in children with autism: an attentional deficit?' *Journal of Autism and Developmental Disorders*, **27**, 265–282.

Premach, D., Woodruff, G. (1978) 'Does the chimpanzee have a "theory of mind?"' *Behavioural and Brain Sciences*, **4**, 515–526.

Prior, M., Dahlstrom, B., Squires, T.-L. (1990) 'Autistic children's knowledge of thinking and feeling states in other people.' *Journal of Child Psychology and Psychiatry*, **31**, 587–601.

Ramberg, C., Ehlers, S., Nydén, A., Johansson, M., Gillberg, C. (1996) 'Language and pragmatic functions in school-age children on the autism spectrum.' *European Journal of Disorders of Communication*, **31**, 387–414.

Rapin, I., Dunn, M. (1997) 'Language disorders in children with autism.' *Seminars in Pediatric Neurology*, **4**, 86–92.

Rumsey, J.M., Hamburger, S.D. (1988) 'Neuropsychological findings in high-functioning men with infantile autism, residual state.' *Journal of Clinical and Experimental Neuropsychology*, **10**, 201–221.

Rumsey, J.M., Hanahan, A.P. (1990) *In:* Proceedings of the eighteenth annual International Neuro-psychological Society meeting, February 14–17, 1990, Kissimmee, Florida. *Journal of Clinical and Experimental Neuropsychology*, **12**, 1–109, p. 81.

Rutter, M. (1983) 'Cognitive deficits in the pathogenesis of autism.' *Journal of Child Psychology and Psychiatry*, **24**, 513–531.

Shah, A., Frith, U. (1983) 'An islet of ability in autistic children: a research note.' *Journal of Child Psychology and Psychiatry*, **24**, 613–620.

Shah, A., Holmes, N. (1985) 'The use of the Leiter International Performance Scale with autistic children.' *Journal of Autism and Developmental Disorders*, **15**, 195–203.

Siegel, D.J., Minshew, N.J., Goldstein, G. (1996) 'Wechsler IQ profiles in diagnosis of high-functioning autism.' *Journal of Autism and Developmental Disorders*, **26**, 389–406.

Sigman, M., Ungerer, J.A. (1984) 'Cognitive and language skills in autistic, mentally retarded, and normal children.' *Developmental Psychology*, **20**, 293–302.

Sigman, M., Ungerer, J.A., Russell, A. (1983) 'Moral judgment in relation to behavioral and cognitive disorders in adolescents.' *Journal of Abnormal Child Psychology*, **11**, 503–511.

Sigman, M., Mundy, P., Sherman, T., Ungerer, J. (1986) 'Social interactions of autistic, mentally retarded and normal children and their caregivers.' *Journal of Child Psychology and Psychiatry*, **27**, 647–656.

Sponheim, E., Skjeldal, O. (1998) 'Autism and related disorders: epidemiological findings in a Norwegian study using ICD-10 diagnostic criteria.' *Journal of Autism and Developmental Disorders*, **28**, 217–227.

Stone, W.L., Ousley, O.Y., Littleford, C.D. (1997a) 'Motor imitation in young children with autism: what's the object?' *Journal of Abnormal Child Psychology*, **25**, 475–485.

Stone, W.L., Ousley, O.Y., Yoder, P.J., Hogan, K.L., Hepburn, S.L. (1997b) 'Nonverbal communication in two- and three year old children with autism.' *Journal of Autism and Developmental Disorders*, **27**, 677–696.

Tager-Flusberg, H. (1996) 'Brief report: Current theory and research on language and communication in autism.' *Journal of Autism and Developmental Disorders*, **26**, 169–172.

Tanguay, P.E., Robertson, J., Derrick, A. (1998) 'A dimensional classification of autism spectrum disorder by social communication domains.' *Journal of the American Academy of Child and Adolescent Psychiatry*, **37**, 271–277.

Townsend, J., Harris, N.S., Courchesne, E. (1996) 'Visual attention abnormalities in autism: delayed orienting to location.' *Journal of the International Neuropsychological Society*, **2**, 541–550.

Treffert, D.A. (1989) *Extraordinary People.* New York: Harper & Row.

Wechsler, D. (1974) *Manual of the Wechsler Intelligence Scale for Children – Revised.* New York: The Psychological Corporation.

—— (1981) *WAIS-R Manual. Wechsler Adult Intelligence Scale – Revised.* San Antonio, Texas: The Psychological Corporation.

Wing, L. (1981a) 'Language, social and cognitive impairments in autism and severe mental retardation.' *Journal of Autism and Developmental Disorders*, **11**, 31–44.

Wing, L. (1981b) 'Asperger's syndrome: a clinical account.' *Psychological Medicine*, **11**, 115–129.

—— (1996) *The Autism Spectrum.* London: Constable.

Wing, L., Gould, J. (1979) 'Severe impairments of social interaction and associated abnormalities in children: epidemiology and classification.' *Journal of Autism and Developmental Disorders*, **9**, 11–29.

10
THE DISEASE ENTITIES OF AUTISM

In the first generation after autism was described, it was thought to be a *single disease* albeit with a rather wide spectrum of presentations. Now, at the beginning of the twenty-first century, some clinicians have moved to the other extreme, believing autism to be unique to each child as "a combination of predisposing influences and expressions of symptoms as *variable and individual as the children themselves*." In fact, the evidence now favors a concept somewhere between these two extremes.

Autism appears to be a syndrome. It is a syndrome of different and separate diseases which have a behavior pattern in common and thus must share a disability in a final common pathway of the brain which affects such behaviors. Research has begun to discover some of the underlying medical diseases that present with this distinctive pattern of behavior in young children, although there is still a long way to go.

This chapter will describe what has been uncovered to date during a search for new medical diseases presenting in children with autism. Hence these diseases are called "the disease entities of autism." In the next chapter, those children with two syndromes – an autistic syndrome and a second syndrome previously described and already well established in the medical literature – will be discussed (see Chapter 11). They are called associated medical disorders or "the double syndromes." In most of these double syndromes, the majority of the patients with the second syndrome do not meet the criteria of autism.

In some disease entities, the distinction between diseases discovered in patients with autism (this chapter) and the double syndromes of previously discovered diseases (Chapter 11) may turn out to be an artificial one. For example, among the patients with an inborn error of adenylsuccinate lyase discussed in this chapter, some meet autistic criteria and some do not. So even in disease entities initially identified in patients with autism, there is phenotypic variation reaching out beyond the autistic syndrome.

Theoretically, for a disease to be designated as a disease entity of autism, the following criteria should apply: (1) the disease should have originally been identified in patients with autism, and (2) there should be autistic symptoms in most, or at least a majority of, patients with the disease. In the future these criteria will be applied with more precision than is possible today.

There are a number of subgroups identified among patients with autism that were under consideration for inclusion in this chapter but which are not in fact listed. In some cases, they are discussed in other chapters – one example is the maternally derived aberrations of chromosome 15q (see Chapter 15). In all not included, the diagnostic criteria have yet to be clearly defined. Of the disease entities selected for this chapter, two (infantile autistic bipolar disorder and the Zappella dysmaturational subgroup with familial complex tics) appear to be related to other well-known disease entities – bipolar affective disorder and Tourette syndrome.

Infantile autistic bipolar disorder (IABD)

CRITERIA FOR DIAGNOSIS

1 Regression after initial normal development.
2 The child meets classical criteria for autism.
3 As the core autistic symptoms in the young child unfold, it becomes evident that they have a clear-cut cyclical pattern.
4 There is a positive family history of a bipolar disorder (or major depression) in first- or second-degree relatives.
5 There is an absence of dysmorphic features; there are no seizures or neurological dysfunction.

If the core autistic symptoms of a child are clearly cyclical and there is a family history of bipolar affective disorder (or major depression), the child may have infantile autistic bipolar disorder (IABD) (DeLong 1994, DeLong and Nothria 1994). It could be said that these patients have both autism and a bipolar disorder, but *they are one disease –* they are not separable. The cyclicity occurs in the autistic symptoms themselves. The characteristics of IABD include the cyclicity (the waxing and waning of the core autistic symptoms), the regression after initial normal development, affective extremes, obsessive traits and special abilities. The neurological examination of these patients shows no seizure disorder nor any identified neurological disorder (DeLong 1994). In this disease entity, there is good evidence to suggest an infantile onset of a bipolar disorder (Zappella 1996). This patient group is not common but many large clinics specializing in autism have seen a handful of IABD children.

As early as 1964, Rimland reported that children with autism were more likely to have a family history of manic-depressive disease than of schizophrenia. In 1976, Herzberg found four families with schizophrenia and two with manic-depressive psychosis in a study of 78 children with autism; however the same proportions, in relation to history of mental illness, occurred in the control group of that study. More recent family-history studies have suggested that parents of children with autism may be at increased risk for psychiatric disorders (Piven *et al.* 1991).

Beyond the narrowly defined IABD, with its clear-cut pattern of cycling of core autistic symptoms, the question exists whether there is a much more common and broader group of children with a more general affective infantile autism. Several studies have found that a major depressive disorder is more common in families of children with autism than in families of non-autistic controls. In the Smalley *et al.* (1995) study, there was a significantly higher rate of depression among first-degree relatives of children with autism, compared with the relatives of children with tuberous sclerosis complex or non-autistic seizure disorder. Also, 64 per cent of parents affected with a major depression had the onset of the first depressive episode *prior* to the birth of the autistic child. The Bolton *et al.* (1998) study of relatives of 99 autistic individuals also found that the increased risk

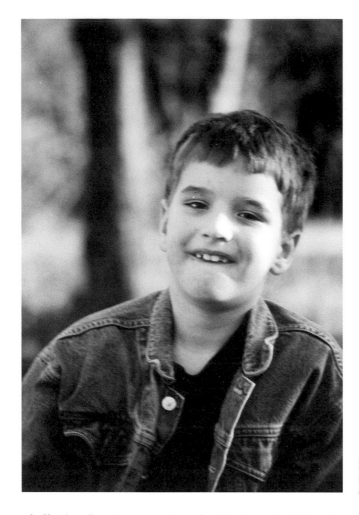

Fig. 10.1 Boy with infantile autistic bipolar disorder (IABD).

of affective disorders was not confined to the period following the birth of the child with autism. This study used direct interview data to confirm an increased rate of affective disorders (especially major depressive disorder) in first-degree relatives, although the authors indicated that they did not believe that affective disorders indicate an underlying liability to autism. Piven and Palmer (1999) also found a significantly higher rate of major depressive disorder in parents of autistic probands; however, they reported that the parents did not have the broad autism phenotype, even though they did have social phobia. In a study of siblings of boys with autism, the siblings were shown to have significantly higher scores regarding depression but not on problems of social adjustment (Gold 1993).

Also, children already suffering from autism may develop depressive symptoms later in childhood or in adult life (Clarke *et al.* 1989, Ghaziuddin *et al.* 1992, Ghaziuddin *et al.* 1995). Sometimes the depression appears to be brought about by specific unhappy life events, according to Ghaziuddin *et al.* (1995); others interpret the apparent depressive behaviors as "unblocking of autistic withdrawal" (Scifo *et al.* 1996). In their review of 17 published cases, Lainhart and Folstein (1994) have delineated the many difficulties of decoding superimposed affective disorders in individuals with autism. Bieberich and Morgan (1998) compared depression, as measured by the MN-PARS, in children with autism and Down syndrome; they found the self-regulation component more affected in children with autism. They interpreted their results as suggesting that the social cognition deficits in autism entail attentional and organizational components.

In 1998, Ghaziuddin and Greden did a case-controlled study comparing family histories of two sets of autism/PPD children: those with (13 children) and those without (10 children) clinical evidence of depression. They reported that, as in a normal population, autistic children who suffer from depression are more likely to have a family history of depression – 10 out of 13 children (77 per cent) – than autistic children without a history of current or previous depression – 3 out of 10 (30 per cent).

There is an interesting report in the literature, coming out of a population-based study, which describes comorbidity of Tourette syndrome with what the authors identify as two separate syndromes – autistic disorder and bipolar disorder (Kerbeshian and Burd 1996). They report that the developmental sequence of the syndromes in four patients was: autistic disorder, followed by Tourette syndrome, followed by bipolar disorder. Gillberg (1985) and DeLong and Dwyer (1988) have identified a family history of bipolar affective disorder in some patients with Asperger syndrome. There is also a report of a case of Asperger syndrome that presented with mania (Atlas and Gerbino-Rosen 1995).

The children with IABD appear to have a distinct clinical entity that presents within the first 30 months of life. *They should not be confused with other groups of autistic children who during childhood have a clinical course which includes depressive episodes and, sometimes, manic episodes.* These other groups of children may also have a familial load for bipolar or major depressive disorders, but it presents at a later age resulting in two separate comorbid diseases – autism and later-onset bipolar or depressive disease.

There is no biological marker as yet for IABD. Bipolar affective disorder itself affects 1–2 per cent of the population and appears to have a complex genetic nature, age-specific penetrance and variable age of onset; no biological markers or predisposing genes have been definitely identified. Whether IABD fits into the pattern as a representative of an early-age-of-onset bipolar affective disorder will only be clarified when a biological marker or genetic abnormality is located. Ross *et al.* (1993) have raised the possibility of a trinucleotide repeat disorder for some cases of bipolar affective disorder, since there is evidence for both earlier age of onset and more severe illness in the second generation of a subset of unilineal pedigrees. Trinucleotide repeat disorders have the phenomenon of "anticipation" – diseases presenting earlier and earlier in families until they present in the infantile period (at the time of presentation of IABD).

There has been one case of autism and bipolar disease (with response to lithium) who had a chromosomal deletion at chromosome 15q12 (Kerbeshian *et al.* 1990). There is preliminary evidence of maternal transmission in some patients with autism who have abnormalities of this chromosome 15q11–13 region (see Chapter 15). Recent research has also suggested an excess of maternal transmission of bipolar affective disorder in a subset of families with a high loading for that disease (McMahon *et al.* 1995, Gershon *et al.* 1996); the Gershon *et al.* study extended to several families with recurrent unipolar depression. However there are now a large number of patients with autism who have abnormalities of the chromosome 15q11-13 region (see Chapter 15) who do not have bi-polar disease. The interpretation of the single case of autism/bipolar disease by Kerbeshian *et al.* (1990) is thus far from clear; it could be a late-onset case, and whether maternal transmission will be correct or even relevant in these disease entities is unknown.

In an innovative study of parents of children with autism, Cook *et al.* (1994) found that parents who had elevated blood serotonin levels themselves had significantly higher depression scores (CES-D Scale) than parents with normal serotonin levels. However, abnormalities of serotonin, thought to be relevant to depression, are found in many, many diseases and cannot be considered as a specific biological marker (see Chapter 13).

Individuals with mania/bipolar disorder have a winter–spring excess of births (Torrey *et al.* 1997), and those with seasonal affective disorder show a peak of births in May (Castrogiovanni *et al.* 1998). This raises the question of whether there might be a second, biological environmental factor, such as a viral pandemic, in addition to any putative genetic factors, found in these complex disease entities.

Therapies currently under investigation for IABD include anti-depressants, primarily of the serotonin reuptake inhibitor class, and lithium (see Chapter 17). These patients may also respond to standard medical therapies in autism, such as valproate, carbamazepine, risperidone or buspirone. For some of these children, the prognosis for major improve-ment is favorable if early medical and educational interventions are employed.

The Zappella dysmaturational subgroup with familial complex tics
CRITERIA FOR DIAGNOSIS

1 Regression with loss of language at about 18 months after an initial normal development.
2 Classic criteria for autism when first diagnosed; hypersensitivity to auditory and tactile stimuli is marked.
3 Absence of dysmorphic facial features, normal physically, normal cranial circumference.
4 Complex tics present in patient and, usually, first-degree relatives; this feature, however, is not exclusive to this subgroup and can be observed in other children with a different course (where the autism remains stable in subsequent years).
5 Normal neurological examination, but praxic oral and manual abilities may be developmentally delayed.
6 Normal common laboratory examinations (karyotype, metabolic studies, sleep EEG).
7 Rapid improvement following motor activation, reciprocal body interaction and some physical guidance of new abilities – at times even during the first examination.
8 Rapid increase in the boy's abilities, and decrease in autistic behavior items, in the following months, reaching normal or quasi-normal abilities by 5–6 years of age.

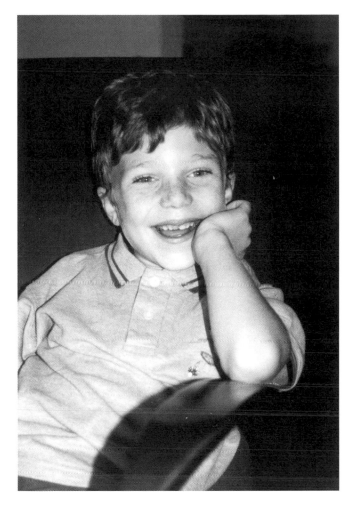

Fig. 10.2 Boy with Zappella dysmaturational syndrome.

9   This disorder can be suspected in young boys only, 2 to 4 years of age. It becomes more probable with rapid improvement obtained during treatment, but the proof of diagnosis comes with the final result.

This group of boys was identified by Michele Zappella (1994, 1996); a girl with the syndrome has yet to be identified. They are distinctive compared to other children with autism in that, if appropriately treated, they in time lose their autistic features. They resume normal or quasi-normal abilities, but after 6 years of age frequently fall into another psychopathological category, usually as ADHD; other later diagnoses such as OCD, social phobia or mood disorders are seen less frequently. They appear to have a dysmaturational disorder.

These patients may differ from Tourette/autism patients in that their early development is quite normal before the regression, there is no evidence of dysmorphism and they

123

usually have a normal outcome by age 5 to 6 years. Their complex tics include complex motor tics and vocal tics; in some patients both types are present, in others only complex motor tics. If tics are still present at the time of recovery from autistic symptoms, they usually then persist.

In an unselected study of 175 children with autism below 5 years of age attending an outpatient clinic, 10 (5.7%) of all children (and 6.7% of boys) were diagnosed with this dysmaturational syndrome (Zappella 1999).

Research into this group of patients is now underway. As one example, the percentage of D8/17 positive cells (see Chapter 13) might help to establish whether this patient group has any relationship to PANDAS (pediatric autoimmune neuropsychiatric disorders associated with streptococcal infections). Other possibilities involve DNA studies targeted to this group of boys.

These patients are quite responsive to therapy (see Chapter 17).

Purine autism
CRITERIA FOR DIAGNOSIS

1   Classical symptoms of autism.
2   Abnormal levels of uric acid (too high/too low) in urine.
3   Constipation, megalostools.
4   Gout in family members.
5   Seizures in a majority of patients.
6   Self-injury in a majority of patients.
7   Psychomotor delay in a majority of patients.

The term "purine autism" is used to describe patients with the autistic syndrome who have been found to have abnormal levels of the final end-product of all the purine pathways, uric acid, in their blood or urine. Sometimes pink or orange crystals are seen in the urine. Purine nucleotides are synthesized and degraded through a regulated series of reactions which end in the formation of uric acid (see Fig. 10.4). In the majority of patients described in the literature, the abnormal level of uric acid was only found in the urine, rarely in the blood. Thus the most accurate method of determining a uric acid abnormality involves the collection of a complete 24-hour urine in a child with autism, one of the world's most challenging tasks. Another problem is that the purine abnormality can be detected easily only during childhood; the hyperuricosuria (too much uric acid in the urine) or hypouricosuria (too little uric acid in the urine) may be modified or eliminated around the time of puberty in some patients. However, at least in the case of some patients with hyperuricosuria, studies of their fibroblasts (skin cells) showed that the rate-limiting step of purine metabolism, PRPP synthetase enzyme 1, remained abnormal after puberty (Page and Coleman 1998). There is evidence of a defect in purine nucleotide interconversion (Page and Coleman 2000).

Although it should be looked for in children with autism who have constipation combined with seizures or self-mutilation, purine autism is primarily a laboratory diagnosis. It has a long history. The first published account occurred in Japan in 1974 (Kaihara 1974).

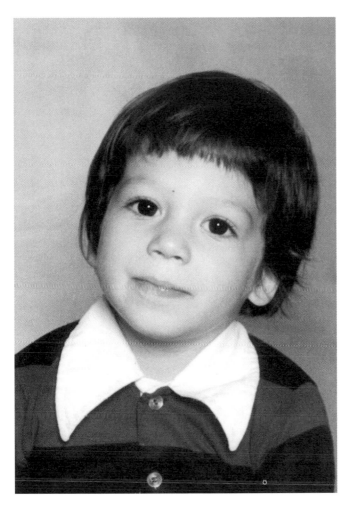

Fig. 10.3 Boy with purine autism.

The boy was an irritable baby who resisted any change in routine and never looked at people around him. By 2 years of age, the few words he had were rapidly disappearing. He lined up his toys in long straight lines instead of playing with them. He developed pica, teeth-grinding, compulsive biting of his mother's hair, and biting the tops of his fingers to the point of bleeding. He focused on tiny lines while flapping his hands. At 3 years of age, he was found to have hyperuricosuria (26 mg/kg/24 hours); the HGPRTase enzyme was normal. Many of his most disturbing habits were shown to be ameliorated by crossover studies of allopurinol, a drug that affects the purine pathway by inhibiting xanthine oxidase (see enzyme 27 in Fig. 10.4). The author found two other children with autism and hyperuricosuria in a series of 14 retarded children.

In 1976, a study of 69 children in the USA with autism, and their age- and sex-matched controls, demonstrated that 15 out of the 69 (22 per cent) children with autism and two of the control children had levels of uric acid in their urine above two standard

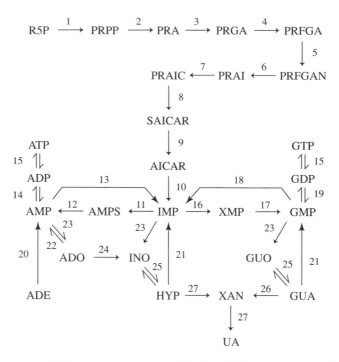

Fig. 10.4 The purine metabolic pathway. Enzymes 1, 9, 12, 23 and 24 have been reported in abnormal levels in young children with autism and/or very poor social behavior.

deviations (14 mg/kg/24 hours) (Coleman *et al.* 1976b). The mean value of 20 mg/kg/24 hours in children 3 to 12 years of age dropped to 17 mg/kg/24 hours after 13 years of age. The children were not randomly selected – the study was based on self-referral by their parents, who chose to participate in this research study. In 1982, Stubbs *et al.* looked for unusual levels of purine enzymes in 18 unselected subjects with autism; they were not tested beforehand for uric acid levels. Decreased levels of purine enzyme 24, adenosine deaminase (AD), were found at a level of significance of $p < 0.02$.

In 1984, Jeaken and van den Berghe found that three children with autism and hyperuricosuria had a deficient purine nucleotide biosynthetic enzyme 9 and 12, adenylosuccinase (also called adenylsuccinate lyase (ASL)). The children had severe psychomotor retardation in addition to their autism. In 1985, Gruber *et al.* identified decreased activity of another purine enzyme, inosinate dehydrogenase (ID), in two other patients with hyperuricosuria. In 1986, a survey of 24-hour urines in 21 children in France found 6 with hyperuricosuria, including 2 with hyperuricemia (Rosenberger-Debiesse and Coleman 1986). In 1990, a survey of 53 unselected children with autism from a private clinic found 6 (11 per cent) with hyperuricosuria; none had hyperuricemia (Nowell *et al.* 1990). Further testing of children with autism and hyperuricosuria selected from the patient group identified in the Nowell study has disclosed that the elevated excretion of uric acid in their urines was reflected in the acceleration of the rate-limiting enzyme 1 of the purine pathway, phosphoribosyl pyrophophate (PRPP) synthetase, as tested in their fibroblasts, although the underlying enzyme defect which caused this accelerated turnover has not yet been characterized (Page and Coleman 1998).

The purine nucleotide biosynthetic enzyme, adenylosuccinate lyase (ASL), has been found at deficient levels in children with autism (Jaeken and van den Berghe 1984, Stone et al. 1992). ASL catalyzes two different reactions leading to the formation of AMP and IMP; both steps involve the beta-elimination of fumarate (see Fig. 10.4). In the paper by Jaeken and van den Berghe (1984), three children with autism were described. Two were siblings whose grandparents were first cousins. Other patients have since been described (Jaeken et al. 1988), including a child who presented with epilepsy in early infancy (Maaswinkel-Mooij et al. 1997). Most cases so far have been diagnosed in Belgium and the Netherlands; the first case in the USA presented with hypotonia and had no symptoms of autism at the time of the report, when she was 15 months of age (Valik et al. 1997). In the reported families, not all members with ASL deficiency developed autistic symptoms; there is a spectrum of disease including psychomotor retardation, muscular wasting, seizures, hypotonia and/or motor delay (van den Berghe et al. 1997).

Laboratory studies have been performed on patients with ASL deficiency. PET studies in the brain of a patient have demonstrated limited glucose uptake, suggesting that the metabolic flux through the glycolytic pathway was reduced (De Volder et al. 1988). 31P-nuclear magnetic resonance spectra of a patient's muscle showed a reduction of energy reserves (Salerno and Crifò 1995). Detailed metabolic studies of cultured lymphoblasts from two of the original children reported with ASL deficiency suggested that a structurally mutated enzyme was present (Barshop et al. 1989). A single-point mutation (a Ser413Pro substitution) in the human ASL gene was then linked to mental retardation with autistic features in three affected siblings (Stone et al. 1992). However, studies of the prevalence of the mutation, as well as the experience of a number of medical practices specializing in autism, find the mutations on the ASL gene to be rare in populations of autistic children (Fon et al. 1995). A screening method for ASL deficiency has been developed using capillary electrophoresis (Gross et al. 1995). See Chapter 17 for discussion of attempts at therapy for patients with ASL deficiency.

Abnormal levels of inosinate dehydrogenase have been reported in two patients with infantile autism who had hyperuricosuria and no hyperuricemia (Gruber et al. 1985). These patients had classical symptoms of autism, constipation, psychomotor retardation and seizures. It was not clear if the abnormal enzyme levels reflected a primary enzyme defect or a secondary effect from elsewhere in the purine pathway.

As mentioned above, there is a report in the medical literature that adenosine deaminase (AD) activity is decreased in some patients with autism (Stubbs et al. 1982). An allele of AD which confers lower enzymatic activity has been found in a study of 70 patients with autism compared to 82 unrelated normal controls (De Luca *et al.* 1999). These findings possibly might be relevant regarding immunological problems in autism (see Chapter 13).

Phosphoribosylpyrophosphate (PRPP) synthetase is the rate-limiting step of purine metabolism (see Fig. 10.4). The PRPP synthetase studies in cultured fibroblasts of seven children with purine autism showed a *de novo* rate of purine synthesis elevated three- to fourfold; the underlying enzyme defect has not yet been characterized in this patient group (Page and Coleman 1998). The activity of PRPP synthetase has been determined in human erythrocytes by a method using reverse-phase high-performance liquid chromatography (Micheli *et al.* 1994). These authors tested normal adults, normal children, mentally retarded patients, autistic children and children with Rett syndrome. The enzyme activity was significantly lower in the Rett syndrome group – a double syndrome where the girls go through a temporary autistic phase. In Rett syndrome, many metabolic changes have been reported (see Chapter 11). Among these changes is a report by Rocchigiani *et al.* (1995) that enzymes of the purine pathways – PRPP synthetase, adenine phosphoribosyl transferase and hypoxanthine phosphoribosyl transferase – are at low levels in erythrocytes.

Occasionally, individual patients with autism who have other laboratory findings have been reported to have purine abnormalities. Four patients who had the classical symptoms of autism were found to have lactic acidosis and one of them also had increased levels of uric acid in the blood (hyperuricemia) and urine (hyperuricosuria) (Coleman and Blass 1985). A patient who met DSM-III criteria for autism, and had the chromosome aberration of 18q-deletion, was reported to have hyperuricemia (László *et al.* 1994). Four patients with an error in an enzyme that affects both purine and pyrimidine metabolism, elevated 5′-nucleotidase activity, were found to have decreased *de novo* synthesis of purines (Page *et al.* 1997). A girl with an error in pyrimidine metabolism, dihydropyrimidine dehydrogenase deficiency, and "solitary behavior" has been found to have hyperuricemia (Berger *et al.* 1984). (See below for a discussion of pyrimidine metabolism.)

The patients with purine autism are identified by their abnormal level of uric acid, the end-product of purine metabolism. Abnormal levels of function of several enzymes of the purine pathway have been found in this patient group, as described above. However, even with abnormal purine enzyme levels, this does not absolutely prove that the primary error in every patient lies in the purine pathway. Purines are so essential for cell function that many disease entities have abnormalities of purines as a secondary phenomenon. There are other disease entities – even the presence of a debilitating illness – that can cause increases in the purine metabolic pathway. A few of the diseases associated with purine irregularities are sickle cell disease, diseases affecting both the thyroid and parathyroid, psoriasis, sarcoidosis, pernicious anemia, lymphomas and leukemias, primary and secondary polycythemia, and non-tropical sprue.

The sister pathway of the purines, the pyrimidine pathway, often works in concert with purine metabolism; there are many examples of interconnections between purine and pyrimidine metabolic pathways (Scriver *et al.* 1995). In 1997, Page *et al.* identified four patients who had elevated levels of an enzyme, cytosolic 5'-nucleotidase, which cleaves purine and pyrimidine metabolism equally well. Their uric acids levels in the urine were low. The onset of the disease process was in infancy and all patients had language delay. The behavioral difficulties in all of the children were described as poor social ability, perseveration, severe hyperactivity and distractibility. Two of the patients were described as occasionally aggressive. One of the patients had toe-walking. Three out of the four children had skin lesions on face and trunk. They also all had seizures and paroxsysmal EEGs requiring anticonvulsant therapy. The children participated in a double-blind crossover study of uridine therapy with definite improvement in speech, behavior, frequency of infections and amount of seizure activity.

Regarding pyrimidine metabolism, a study by Minshew *et al.* (1993) using *in vivo* 31P magnetic resonance spectroscopy found a decreased level of esterified ends that include uridine diphosphosugars, a pyrimidine compound, in the dorsal prefrontal cortex of 11 high-functioning autistic patients when compared to matched normal controls. Berger *et al.* (1984) described three patients with dehydropyrimidine dehydrogenase deficiency – one had autistic features and *petit mal* seizures, another had solitary behavior and absence seizures.

It should be noted that 3 per cent of normal control children also have hyperuricosuria (Coleman *et al.* 1976b). Thus, further testing is needed before assuming that hyperurico-suria in any particular child is directly related to that child's symptoms.

Autism/steatorrhea syndrome
CRITERIA FOR DIAGNOSIS

1   Classical symptoms of autism.
2   Abdominal pain – often the child with autism is not able to adequately explain this symptom.
3   Chronic diarrhea and steatorrhea.

These children have a disease entity that causes both brain and gastrointestinal dys-function. It can be apparent from the beginning; compared to matched controls, they are more likely to have colic as well as diarrhea in the newborn period (Wiedel and Coleman 1976). Many children with autism have problems with their gastrointestinal tract; in the case of the children with the autism/steatorrhea syndrome, they have a lifelong chronic diarrhea associated with steatorrhea (increased fat in the stools). These children have stools that sometimes are a peculiar yellow color and foul-smelling. They appear to have a chronic gastrointestinal abnormality combined with their neuropsychiatric symptoms (Horvath *et al.* 1999).

Studies of this autism/steatorrhea subgroup in the past have tried to identify the cause of the abnormal bowel function in these children. Studies first focused on the possibility of celiac disease (Coleman *et al.* 1976a). In Chapter 17, the medical literature on celiac disease is reviewed with the present conclusion that, if celiac disease is found in a child with autism, it is unlikely to be related to the symptoms of autism.

Later, this subgroup was labeled as a more general "severe diarrhoea/food sensitivity" group (Coleman 1989), but this has not stood the test of time. Postulated food-related causes of autism are reviewed in Chapter 17; the case for dairy products could be construed to be somewhat stronger than the one for wheat products, but neither is well-delineated or established. Another question that was raised was regarding poor absorption of nutrients. Lis *et al.* (1976) studied a urine chromatographic sample obtained from a woman with a jejuno-ileal bypass and compared it to the urine of 19 children with autism; they report that the patient with the bypass had urine patterns very similar to those of autistic children.

In 1998, Wakefield *et al.* described intestinal abnormalities in 12 children with autism detected by endoscopy. They ranged from lymphoid nodular hyperplasia to aphthoid ulceration. Histology showed patchy chronic inflammation of the colon in 11 children, and reactive ileal lymphoid hyperplasia in 7 children. No granulomas were seen. It is interesting that ileal-lymphoid nodular hyperplasia findings similar to those in the study by Wakefield *et al.* have now been demonstrated in two children with attention deficit disorder who were allergic to various foods (Sabra *et al.* 1998); thus the nodular hyperplasia does not appear to be a specific finding limited to children with autism.

The study by Wakefield *et al.* noted that the onset of symptoms occurred after MMR (measles–mumps–rubella) immunization in most cases, although they were careful to state that they had not proved the association. Nevertheless, the report of an inflammatory bowel disease in autistic children that was possibly due to MMR vaccine stimulated a great deal of interest and was picked up by the alternative medicine movements in Britain and the United States. Of special concern was any possible effect of administrating the immunization of these particular viruses simultaneously. However, MMR vaccine (Peltola *et al.* 1998, Roberts 1998, Bower 1999, DeStefano and Chen 2000, Taylor *et al.* 1999) has not been shown to cause inflammatory bowel disease or autism. An unfortunate development is that the Wakefield report is being used to justify omitting vaccinations in many children (*BMJ* 1998), putting such children at risk for the complications of these viral diseases. In the case of rubella, that risk includes an autistic syndrome in the next generation (see Chapter 11).

That the children with autism who suffer from steatorrhea exist in a subgroup of the autistic syndrome appears highly likely; specialists in autism have noted children with steatorrhea and autism in their clinics for years. The *Journal of Pediatric Gastro-enterology and Nutrition* says "a possible association between autism and some gastrointestinal abnormalites should be given careful consideration" (Akobeng and Thomas 1999). A recent study of such children found unrecognized gastrointestinal disorders, especially reflux esophagitis and disaccharide malsabsorption (Horvath *et al.* 1999). But the specific etiological factors involved in this patient group have yet to characterized. One study has been performed of cholecystokinin 8 levels in the peripheral blood mononuclear cells of 12 children with autism and 10 with PPD; the study found normal levels compared to 11 healthy controls (Brambilla *et al.* 1997). However, in this study, there is no indication that these patients were selected because of clinical criteria such as steatorrhea; on the contrary, they were part of a larger study of autistic patients in general being studied for beta-endorphin levels. Of theoretical interest is the fact that patients with the combination of other psychiatric diseases combined with bowel disease have been shown to have cytochrome c oxidase deficiency – the MELAS syndrome with schizophrenia (Prayson and Wang 1998) and the MNGIE (mitochondrial neurogastrointestinal encephalopathy) syndrome (Hamano *et al.* 1997). To date, a patient with autism and cytochrome c oxidase deficiency has been reported (see Chapter 15).

Genetic studies on another patient with autism showed the inactivation of the gastrin-releasing peptide receptor (GRPR) gene (Ishikawa-Brush *et al.* 1997). GRPR has a wide range of activities; these include both regulation of gastrointestinal hormone release and modulation of neural activity. This gene is known to be expressed in the limbic system. GRPR is discussed further in Chapter 15. Although it has been identified as a candidate gene for autism in a patient with a translocation, as far as we know, this gene has never been studied in a child with the autism/steatorrhea syndrome.

Several research therapies have been proposed for children with autism/steatorrhea; besides food elimination diets, these include famotidine (Linday 1997) and secretin (Horvath *et al.* 1998) (see Chapter 17). Antimicrobials effective against intestinal clostridia have also been proposed in an innovative medical hypothesis (Bolte 1998).

Almost Autism: childhood disintegrative disorder/disintegrative psychosis/ Heller dementia

Sometimes, after language has developed in a completely normal child, this child may have an unexplained massive regression in language, sociability, play and apparently cognition, which has been described as late autistic regression. However, the decline begins somewhat later than in classical autism. The age of onset is between 2 and 10 years. Studies by Volkmar and Rutter (1995), Mouridsen *et al.* (1998) and Mouridsen *et al.* (1999) provide support for maintaining a diagnostic category distinct from infantile autism. Childhood disintegrative disorder has an estimated prevalence of 0.11 in 10,000. Mothers are often 30 years of age or older at time of delivery.

There is a high incidence of epilepsy in childhood disintegrative disorder. In one recent study, 77 per cent of the patients were found to have a seizure disorder (Mouridsen *et al.* 1999). The psychomotor variant accounted for 50 per cent. EEG abnormalities are significantly more common in this patient group than in infantile autism (Kurita *et al.* 1992). However, in most cases a seizure disorder does not explain the abrupt and overwhelming nature of these regressions. Trifiletti and Packard (1998) have described a set of monozygotic twins who had virtually identical clinical regressions. The twins were attending preschool, could speak in sentences and could write the entire alphabet. Then, at 3½ years of age, within the course of two weeks and without an apparent trigger, they lost all language and their social skills evaporated. Now 11 years of age, they have periodic hand-shaking and hyperventilation and no differential interest in family members, strangers or inanimate objects.

Such a group of patients cries out for sophisticated contemporary medical research to identify the underlying cause or causes of their disorder. A suggested neurological work-up for such children is provided in Russo *et al.* (1996). By definition, known degenerative disease or childhood schizophrenia rule out this diagnosis.

Conclusion

This description of the set of diseases that underlie autism or autistic-like conditions is just a beginning. These subgroups are newly defined and may well be further refined. It is likely that in the future more disease entities will be identified inside the syndrome of autism.

REFERENCES

Akobeng, A.K., Thomas, A.G. (1999) 'Inflammatory bowel disease, autism and the measles, mumps and rubella vaccine.' *Journal of Pediatric Gastroenterology and Nutrition*, **28**, 351–352.
Atlas, J.A., Gerbino-Rosen, G. (1995) 'Differential diagnosis and treatment of an inpatient adolescent showing pervasive developmental disorder and mania.' *Psychological Reports*, **77**, 207–210.
Barshop, B.A., Alberts, A.S., Gruber, H.E. (1989) 'Kinetic studies of mutant human adenylosuccinase.' *Biochimica et Biophysica Acta*, **999**, 19–23.
Berger, R., Stoker-de Vries, S.A., Wadman, S.K., Duran, M., Beemer, F.A., de Bree, P.K., Weits-Binnerts, J.J., Penders, T.J., van der Woude, J.K. (1984) 'Dihydropyrimidine dehydrogenase deficiency leading to thymine-uraciluria. An inborn error of pyrimidine metabolism.' *Clinica Chimica Acta*, **141**, 227–234.
Bieberich, A.A., Morgan, S.B. (1998) 'Brief report: Affective expression in children with autism or Down syndrome.' *Journal of Autism and Developmental Disorders*, **28**, 333–338.
Bolte, E.R. (1998) 'Autism and clostridium tetani.' *Medical Hypothesis*, **51**, 133–144.
Bolton, P.F., Pickles, A, Murphy, M., Rutter, M. (1998) 'Autism, affective and other psychiatric disorders: patterns of familial aggregation.' *Psychological Medicine*, **28**, 385–395.
Bower, H. (1999) 'New research demolishes link between MMR vaccine and autism.' *British Medical Journal*, **318**, 1643A.
Brambilla, F., Guareschi-Cazzullo, A., Tacchini, C., Musetti, C., Panerai, A.E., Sacerdote, P. (1997) 'Beta-endorphin and cholecystokinin 8 concentrations in peripheral blood mononuclear cells of autistic children.' *Neuropsychobiology*, **35**, 1–4.
(BMJ) British Medical Journal (1998) **316**, 561 (Editorial).
Castrogiovanni, P., Iapichino, S., Pacchierotti, C., Pieraccini, F. (1998) 'Season of birth in psychiatry. A review.' *Neuropsychobiology*, **37**, 175–181.
Clarke, D.J., Littlejohns, C.S., Corbett, J.A., Joseph, S. (1989) 'Pervasive developmental disorders and psychoses in adult life.' *British Journal of Psychiatry*, **155**, 692–699.
Coleman, M. (1989) 'Autism: non-drug biological treatments.' *In:* Gillberg, C. (Ed.) *Diagnosis and Treatment of Autism.* New York: Plenum Press.
Coleman, M., Blass, J.P. (1985) 'Autism and lactic acidosis.' *Journal of Autism and Developmental Disorders*, **15**, 1–8.
Coleman, M., Landgrebe, M.A., Landgrebe, A.R. (1976a) 'Celiac autism. Calcium studies and their relationship to celiac disease in autistic patients.' *In:* Coleman, M. (Ed.) *The Autistic Syndromes.* New York: Elsevier, pp. 197–208.
—— (1976b) 'Purine autism. Hyperuricosuria in autistic children: does this identify a subgroup of autism?' *In:* Coleman, M. (Ed.) *The Autistic Syndromes.* Amsterdam: North-Holland, pp. 183–195.
Cook, E.H., Jr., Charack, D.A., Arida, J., Spohn, J.A., Roizen, N.J., Leventhal, B.L. (1994) 'Depressive and obsessive-compulsive symptoms in hyperserotonemic parents of children with autistic disorder.' *Psychiatry Research*, **52**, 25–33.
DeLong G.R. (1994) 'Children with autistic spectrum disorder and a family history of affective disorder.' *Developmental Medicine and Child Neurology*, **36**, 674–678.
DeLong, G.R., Dwyer, J.T. (1988) 'Correlation of family history with specific autistic subgroups: Asperger's syndrome and bipolar affective disease.' *Journal of Autism and Developmental Disorders*, **18**, 593–600.
DeLong, G.R., Nothria, C. (1994) 'Psychiatric family history and neurologic disease in autism spectrum disorder.' *Developmental Medicine and Child Neurology*, **36**, 441–448.
De Luca, D., Bottini, N., Porfirio, C., Palminiello, S., Luccarelli, P., Curatolo, P. (1999) 'Adenosine deaminase polymorphism in autistic children.' (Abstract) *Annals of Neurology*, **46**, 529.
DeStefano, F., Chen, R.T. (2000) 'Autism and measles, mumps and rubella vaccine: no epidemiological evidence for a causal association.' *Journal of Pediatrics*, **136**, 125–126.

De Volder, A.G., Jaeken, J., van den Berghe, G., Bol, A., Michel, C., Cogneau, M., Goffinet, A.M. (1988) 'Regional brain glucose utilization in adenylosuccinase-deficient patients measured by positron emission tomography.' *Pediatric Research*, **24**, 238–242.

Fölling, A. (1934) 'Uber Ausscheidung von Phenylbenztraubensaure in den Haarn als Stoffwechselanomalie in Verbindung mit Imbessillität.' *Hoppe Seylers Z. Physiol. Chem.*, **227**, 169.

Fon, E.A., Sarrazin, J., Meunier, C., Alarcia, J., Shevell, M.I., Philippe, A., Leboyer, M., Rouleau, G.A. (1995) 'Adenylosuccinate lyase (ADSL) and infantile autism: absence of previously reported point mutation.' *American Journal of Medical Genetics*, **660**, 554–557.

Gershon, E.S., Badner, J.A., Detera-Wadleigh, S.D., Ferraro, T.N., Berrettini, W.H. (1996) 'Maternal inheritance and chromosome 18 allele sharing in unilineal bipolar illness pedigrees.' *American Journal of Medical Genetics (Neuropsychiatric Genetics)*, **67**, 202–207.

Ghaziuddin, M., Greden, J. (1998) 'Depression in children with autism/pervasive developmental disorders: a case–control family history study.' *Journal of Autism and Developmental Disorders*, **28**, 111–115.

Ghaziuddin, M., Tsai, L. (1991) 'Depression in autistic disorder.' *British Journal of Psychiatry*, **159**, 721–723.

Ghaziuddin, M., Tsai, L., Ghaziuddin, N. (1992) 'Comorbidity of autistic disorder in children and adolescents.' *European Journal of Child and Adolescent Psychiatry*, **1**, 209–213.

Ghaziuddin, M., Alessi, N., Greden, J. (1995) 'Life events and depression in children with pervasive developmental disorder.' *Journal of Autism and Developmental Disorders*, **25**, 495–502.

Gillberg, C. (1985) 'Asperger's syndrome and recurrent psychosis – a case study.' *Journal of Autism and Developmental Disorders*, **15**, 389–397.

Gold, N. (1993) 'Depression and social adjustment in siblings of boys with autism.' *Journal of Autism and Developmental Disorders*, **23**, 147–163.

Gross, M., Gathof, B.S., Kolle, P., Gresser, U. (1995) 'Capillary electrophoresis for screening of adenylosuccinate lyase deficiency.' *Electrophoresis*, **16**, 1927–1929.

Gruber, H.E., Jansen, I., Willis, R.C., Seegmiller, J.E. (1985) 'Alteration of the inosinate branchpoint enzymes in cultured human lymphoblasts.' *Biochemica et Biophysica Acta*, **846**, 135–144.

Hamano, H., Ohta, T., Takekawa, Y., Kouda, K., Shinohara, Y. (1997) 'Mitochondrial neurogastrointestinal encephalopathy presenting with protein-losing enteropathy and serum copper deficiency: a case report.' (In Japanese) *Rinsho Shinkeigaku*, **37**, 917–922.

Herzberg, B. (1978) 'The families of autistic children.' *In:* Coleman, M. (Ed.) *The Autistic Syndromes.* Amsterdam: North-Holland, pp. 151–172.

Horvath, K., Stefanatos, G., Sokolski, K.N., Wachtel, R., Nabors, L., Tildon, J.T. (1998) 'Improved social and language skills after secretin administration in patients with autistic spectrum disorders.' *Journal of the Association for Academic Minority Physicians*, **9**, 9–15.

Horvath, K., Papadimitriou, J.C., Rabsztyn, A., Drachenberg, C., Tildon, J.T. (1999) 'Gastrointestinal abnormalities in children with autistic disorder.' *Journal of Pediatrics*, **135**, 559–563.

Ishikawa-Brush, Y., Powell, J.F., Bolton, P., Miller, A.P., Francis, F., Willard, H.F., Lehrach, H., Monaco, A.P. (1997) 'Autism and multiple exostoses associated with an X;8 translocation occurring within the GRPR gene and 3' to the SDC2 gene.' *Human Molecular Genetics*, **6**, 1241–1250.

Jaeken, J., van den Berghe, G. (1984) 'An infantile autistic syndrome characterized by the presence of succinylpurines in body fluids.' *Lancet*, **2**, 1058–1061.

Jacken, J., Wadman, S.K., Duran, M., van Sprang, F.J., Beemer, F.A., Holl, R.A., Theunissen, P.M., de Cock, P., van den Berghe, G., Vincent, M.F. *et al.* (1988) 'Adenylosuccinase deficiency: an inborn error of purine nucleotide synthesis.' *European Journal of Pediatrics*, **148**, 126–131.

Kaihara, H. (1974) 'Two autistic retarded children with different inborn errors of metabolism.' *Bulletin of the Tokyo Metropolitan Rehabilitation Center for the Physically and Mentally Handicapped*, pp. 1–17.

Kerbeshian, J., Burd, L. (1996) 'Case study: comorbidity among Tourette's syndrome, autistic disorder, and bipolar disorder.' *Journal of the American Academy of Child and Adolescent Psychiatry*, **35**, 681–685.

Kerbeshian, J., Burd, L., Randal, T., Martsolf, J., Jalal, S. (1990) 'Autism, profound mental retardation and atypical bipolar disorder in a 33–year-old female with a deletion of 15q12.' *Journal of Mental Deficiency Research*, **34**, 205–210.

Kurita, H., Kita, M., Miyake, Y. (1992) 'A comparative study of development and symptoms among disintegrative psychosis and infantile autism with and without speech loss.' *Journal of Autism and Developmental Disorder*, **22**, 175–188.

133

Lainhart, J.E., Folstein, S.E. (1994) 'Affective disorders in people with autism: a review of published cases.' *Journal of Autism and Developmental Disorders*, **24**, 587–601.

László , A., Horváth, E., Eck, E., Fekete, M. (1994) 'Serum serotonin, lactate and pyruvate levels in infantile autistic children.' (Letter) *Clinica Chimica Acta*, **229**, 205–207.

Linday, L.A. (1997) 'Oral famotidine: a potential treatment for children with autism.' *Medical Hypothesis*, **48**, 381–386.

Lis, A.W., McLaughlin, D.I., McLaughlin, R.K., Lis, E.W., Stubbs, E.G. (1976) 'Profiles of ultraviolet-absorbing components of urine from autistic children.' *Clinical Chemistry*, **22**, 1528–1532.

Maaswinkel-Mooij, P.D., Laan, L.A., Onkenhout, W., Brouwer, O.F., Jaeken, J., Poorthuis, B.J. (1997) 'Adenylosuccinase deficiency presenting with epilepsy in early infancy.' *Journal of Inherited Metabolic Disease*, **20**, 606–607.

McMahon, F.J., Stine, O.C., Meyers, D.A., Simpson, S.G., DePaulo, J.R. (1995) 'Patterns of maternal transmission in bipolar affective disorder.' *American Journal of Human Genetics*, **56**, 1277–1286.

Micheli, V., Rocchigiani, M., Pompucci, G. (1994) 'An HPCL-linked assay of phosphoribosylpyrophosphate synthetase activity in the erythrocytes of adults and children with neurological disorders.' *Clinica Chimica Acta*, **227**, 78–86.

Minshew, N.J., Goldstein, G., Dombrowski, S.M., Panchalingam, K., Pettegrew, J.W. (1993) 'A preliminary 31P MRS study of autism: evidence for undersynthesis and increased degradation of brain membranes.' *Biological Psychiatry*, **33**, 762–773.

Mouridsen, S.E., Rich, B., Isager, T. (1998) 'Validity of childhood disintegrative psychosis. General findings of a long-term follow-up study.' *British Journal of Psychiatry*, **172**, 263–267.

—— (1999) 'Epilepsy in disintegrative disorder and infantile autism: a long-term validation study.' *Developmental Medicine and Child Neurology*, **41**, 110–114.

Nowell, M.A., Hackney, D.B., Muraki, A.S., Coleman, M. (1990) 'Varied MR appearance of autism: fifty-three pediatric patients having the full autistic syndrome.' *Magnetic Resonance Imaging*, **8**, 811–816.

Page, T., Coleman, M. (1998) 'De novo purine synthesis is increased in the fibroblasts of purine autism patients.' *In:* Griesmacher, A. *et al.* (Eds) *Purine and Pyrimidine Metabolism in Man IX.*, New York: Plenum Press, pp. 793–796. *Also in: Advances in Experimental Medicine and Biology*, **431**, 793–796.

—— (2000) 'Purine metabolism abnormalities in a hyperuricosuric subclass of autism.' *Biochimica et Biophysica*, **1500**, 291–296.

Page, T., Yu, A., Fontane, J., Nyhan, W.L. (1997) 'Developmental disorder associated with increased cellular nucleotidase activity.' *Proceedings of the National Academy of Sciences*, **94**, 11601–11606.

Pavone, L., Fiumara, A., Bottaro, G., Mazzone, D., Coleman, M. (1997) 'Autism and celiac disease: failure to validate the hypothesis that a link might exist.' *Biological Psychiatry*, **42**, 72–75.

Peltola, H., Patja, A., Leinikki, P., Valle, M., Davidkin, I., Paunio, M. (1998) 'No evidence for measles, mumps, and rubella vaccine-associated inflammatory bowel disease or autism in a 14-year prospective study.' (Letter) *Lancet*, **351**, 1327–1328.

Piven, J., Palmer, P. (1999) 'Psychiatric disorder and the broad autism phenotype: evidence from a family study of multiple-incidence families.' *American Journal of Psychiatry*, **156**, 557–563.

Piven, J., Chase, G.A., Landa, R., Wzorek, M., Gayle, J., Cloud, D., Folstein, S. (1991) 'Psychiatric disorders in the parents of autistic individuals.' *Journal of the American Academy of Child and Adolescent Psychiatry*, **30**, 471–478.

Prayson, R.A., Wang, N. (1998) 'Mitochondrial myopathy, encephalopathy, lactic acidosis and stroke-like episodes (MELAS) syndrome: an autopsy report.' *Archives of Pathology and Laboratory Medicine*, **122**, 978–981.

Rapin, I. (1995) 'Autistic regression and disintegrative disorder: how important is the role of epilepsy?' *Seminars in Pediatric Neurology*, **2**, 278–285.

Realmuto, G.M., August, G.J. (1991) 'Catatonia in autistic disorder: a sign of comorbidity or variable expression.' *Journal of Autism and Developmental Disorders*, **21**, 517–528.

Rimland, B. (1964) *Infantile Autism: The Syndrome and its Implications for a Neural Theory of Behavior.* Englewood Cliffs, NJ: Prentice-Hall.

—— (1998) 'Editor's Notebook: The autism-secretin connection.' *Autism Research Review International*, **12**, 3.

Roberts, R. (1998) 'MMR vaccination and autism 1998. There is no causal link between MMR vaccine and autism.' (Letter) *British Medical Journal*, **316**, 1824.

Rocchigiani, M., Sestini, S., Micheli, V., Pescoglini, M., Lacomelli, G., Hayek, G., Pompucci, G. (1995) 'Purine and pyrimidine nucleotide metabolism in the erythrocytes of patients with Rett syndrome.' *Neuropediatrics*, **26**, 288–292.

Rosenberger-Debiesse, J., Coleman, M. (1986) 'Brief report: Preliminary evidence for multiple etiologies for autism.' *Journal of Autism and Developmental Disorders*, **16**, 385–392.

Ross, C.A., McInnis, M.G., Margolis, R.L., Li, S.H. (1993) 'Genes with triplet repeats: candidate mediators of neuropsychiatric disorders.' *Trends in Neuroscience*, **16**, 254–260.

Russo, M., Perry, R., Kolodny, E., Gillberg, C. (1996) 'Heller syndrome in a pre-school boy. Proposed medial evaluation and hypothesized pathogenesis.' *European Child and Adolescent Psychiatry*, **5**, 172–177.

Sabra, A., Bellanti, J.A., Colon, A.R. (1998) 'Ileal-lymphoid-nodular hyperplasia, non-specific colitis and pervasive developmental disorder in children.' *Lancet*, **352**, 234–235.

Salerno, C., Crifò, C. (1995) 'Microassay of adenylosuccinase by capillary electrophoresis.' *Analytical Biochemistry*, **226**, 377–379.

Scifo, R., Calandra, C., Parrinello, M.A., Marchetti, B. (1996) 'Prognostic significance of depression occurrence in infantile autism.' *Minerva Pediatrica*, **48**, 495–498.

Scriver, C.R., Beaudet, A.L., Sly, E.S., and Valle, D. (Eds) (1995) *The Metabolic and Molecular Bases of Inherited Disease. 7th Edn. Vol. 2.* New York: McGraw-Hill, pp. 1655–1837.

Smalley, S.L., McCracken, J., Tanguay, P. (1995) 'Autism, affective disorders, and social phobia.' *American Journal of Medical Genetics*, **60**, 19–26.

Stone, R.L., Aimi, J., Barshop, B.A., Jaeken, J., van den Berghe, G., Zalkin, H., Dixon, J.E. (1992) 'A mutation in adenylosuccinate lyase associated with mental retardation and autistic features.' *Nature Genetics*, **1**, 59–63.

Stubbs, E.G., Litt, M., Lis, F., Jackson, R., Voth, W., Lindberg, A., Litt, R. (1982) 'Adenosine deaminase activity decreased in autism.' *Journal of the American Academy of Child Psychiatry*, **21**, 71–74.

Taylor, B., Miller, E., Farrington, C.P., Petropoulos, M.C., Favot-Mayaud, I., Li, J., Waight, P.A. (1999) 'Autism and measles, mumps, and rubella vaccine: no epidemiological evidence for a causal association.' *Lancet*, **353**, 2026–2029.

Torrey, E.F., Miller, J., Rawlings, R., Yolken, R.H. (1997) 'Seasonality of births in schizophrenia and bipolar disorder: a review of the literature.' *Schizophrenia Research*, **28**, 1–38.

Trifiletti, R.R., Packard, A.M. (1998) 'Monozygotic twins with childhood disintegrative disorder: evidence for a genetic basis.' (Abstract) *Annals of Neurology*, **44**, 574.

Valik, D., Miner, P.T., Jones, J.D. (1997) 'First U.S. case of adenylosuccinate lyase deficiency with severe hypotonia.' *Pediatric Neurology*, **16**, 252–255.

van den Berghe, G., Vincent, M.F., Jaeken, J. (1997) 'Inborn errors of the purine nucleotide cycle: adenylosuccinase deficiency.' *Journal of Inherited Metabolic Disease*, **20**, 193–202.

Volkmar, F.R, Rutter, M. (1995) 'Childhood disintegrative disorder; results of the DSM-IV autism field trial.' *Journal of the American Academy of Child and Adolescent Psychiatry*, **34**, 1092–1095.

Wakefield, A.J., Murch, S.H., Anthony, A., Linnell, J., Casson, D.M., Malik, M., Berelowitz, M., Dhillon, A.P., Thomson, M.A., Harvey, P., Valentine, A., Davies, S.E., Walker-Smith, J.A. (1998) 'Ileal-lymphoid-nodular hyperplasia, non-specific colitis and pervasive-developmental disorder in children.' *Lancet*, **351**, 637–641.

Wiedel, L., Coleman, M. (1976) 'The autistic and control population of this study.' *In:* Coleman, M. (Ed.) *The Autistic Syndromes.* Amsterdam: North-Holland.

Zappella, M. (1994) 'Bambini autistici che guariscono: l'esempio dei tic complessi familiari.' *Terapia Familiare*, **46**, 51–61.

—— (1996) 'Autismo con tic complessi familiari a evoluzione favorevole.' *Autismo infantile. Studi sull'affettività e le emozioni.* Roma: La Nuova Italia Scientifica.

—— (1999) 'Familial complex tics and autistic behavior with favorable outcome in young children.' *Infanto*, **7**, 61–66.

135

11
DOUBLE SYNDROMES

The term "double syndromes" is used to describe those patients with a dual diagnosis of a known medical syndrome plus an autistic syndrome. Double syndromes are sometimes called the associated medical conditions of autism. The comorbidity of the autistic syndrome and a second syndrome makes the diagnoses of each individual patient much more complicated. Patients with autism are said to have a double syndrome if (1) their second syndrome was a disease originally described in non-autistic patients, and if (2) the majority of individuals with the second syndrome do not have autism. The question of whether the absolute majority of patients must be non-autistic for a disease entity to be classified as a double syndrome will be clarified with time. In a very few of the diseases described in this chapter, it is possible that it may be determined in time that the majority of patients do, in fact, have autistic behavior.

A concurrence of two different syndromes in the same individual could occur by chance *or* the two syndromes could have a relationship – in any particular patient, it is hard to be sure. When there are only a handful of patients with a double syndrome described in the medical literature, the concurrence could always be a coincidence. However, population-based prevalence studies have indicated that a co-occurrence of an autistic syndrome with some of the more prevalent medical syndromes is at greater than chance expectation. Only for the purpose of looking over the medical literature on this topic, in this chapter we have included a disease entity under the double syndromes if two or more cases have been described in that literature.

What percentage of children who present with autism or autistic symptoms have a double syndrome is not known. A major epidemiological study (Gillberg and Coleman 1996) has suggested that about one in four cases is a double syndrome. It probably depends upon a number of factors, especially the issue of definition of when a person, particularly a severely retarded one, is called autistic. Another factor is the mix of disease entities within any given population, which is known to vary from country to country, as determined by infant-screening studies. The interest of physicians in a country in detecting rare diseases is also relevant, since many of the double syndromes are autism plus a rare disease. Many clinical studies or referred samples may be biased because medical conditions have been previously diagnosed and these patients were not referred to an autism center. Various percentage figures for associated medical conditions have been suggested in the larger studies – from 7 per cent to as high as 37 per cent (Ritvo *et al.* 1990, Rutter *et al.* 1994, Gillberg and Coleman 1996, Fombonne *et al.* 1997, Barton and Volkmar 1998, Fattal-Valevski *et al.* 1999). These are still quite rough estimates. For example, there is the Belgian study of adolescents and adults who had been placed in residential homes because of the diagnosis of either autism or PPDNOS. In these people, who had intelligences ranging from normal to severe mental retardation, it was found that 13 out of the 21 individuals (62 per cent) had previously undiagnosed medical diseases (Swillen *et al.* 1996).

At this early stage of understanding the double syndromes, while so much remains unknown and undoubtedly will change over time, the whole debate about the percentage of children with autism who suffer from double syndromes could be viewed as a misfocus on percentages. Instead, spending comparable professional time on accurately learning how to diagnose and treat these struggling families and their children is the priority.

In addition to the double syndromes, occasionally there are reports of triple syndromes. To further complicate the picture for a patient, comorbidity of the autistic disorder with *two* other medical conditions in the same person has now been reported, making a total of three diagnoses for those unlucky individuals. Ghaziuddin and Tsai (1991) have described a 17-year-old patient with Down syndrome, the autistic syndrome and depression. Kerbeshian and Burd (1996) have described four patients, all of whom had the autistic syndrome, the Tourette syndrome and a bipolar disorder.

One of the most difficult questions in relation to double syndromes is how to handle the cases of children with autism who later develop an adult psychiatric disease. In rare instances, autistic children when they are older develop schizophrenia, one of the bipolar disorders or a major depressive psychosis. The literature on late-onset bipolar disorders and depression is discussed under the topic of infantile autistic bipolar disorder (IABD), a disease presenting at a very early age as autism, albeit with a cyclical pattern (see Chapter 10). Besides the children with early-onset IABD, there are the patients with a comorbidity of an autistic syndrome combined at a later age with bipolar or depressive symptoms. The relevance of later-developing schizophrenia in a child with an autistic syndrome, or of schizophrenia and autism in the same family, has been a topic of interest to a number of investigators (Herzberg 1976, Asarnow and Ben-Meir 1988, Frith and Frith 1991, Gillberg 1991, Wolff 1992). It is known that these are rare occurrences.

Determining why some patients do and other patients do not have autistic symptoms inside each of the other syndromes has turned out to be of great interest to understanding the autistic syndrome in general. There is no one single mechanism that causes autism in all of these double syndromes; mechanisms that may be responsible for autistic features in patients differ from one disease entity to another. The double syndromes can help circumscribe gestational windows of time when autism might arise. They also help locate particular parts of the central nervous system where injury can cause autistic symptoms. The double syndromes also have the potential to help identify specific neuropathological factors in the developing brain which underlie the behavioral patterns of autism.

Some of the double syndromes fit together into groups. An excellent example is the phakomatoses (the neuroepidermal/neurocutaneous diseases). These are disease entities where both the brain and the skin are involved. The three most common neuroepidermal syndromes – Hypomelanosis of Ito, neurofibromatosis and tuberous sclerosis – all include a number of patients with a second autistic syndrome. There are single case reports of three rarer neuroepidermal diseases (basal cell nevus syndrome, trichothiodystrophy, xeroderma pigmentosum) in patients who also have autism. There is also a report of a child with autism and oculocutaneous albinism. A number of the second syndromes in which autism occurs are those in the group of rare disease entities classified as multiple congenital anomaly/mental retardation (MCA/MR) syndromes.

Genetic syndromes

The syndromes listed here as genetic syndromes all have strong evidence of familial factors playing a major role in their etiology. However, the fact that they are listed under the heading of "genetic" does not mean that a second factor (second somatic mutation or environmental biological factor) may not be necessary for full expression of the clinical syndrome. Today, scientists think of genetic disease expression as often a combination of several factors, including the modifying effect of other genes in any individual's genome on their primary gene mutation, as well as the effect of additional infectious, toxic and other environmental agents.

Here are the double syndromes; they may or may not have occurred by chance.

ANGELMAN SYNDROME

The Angelman syndrome is characterized by severe mental retardation with absence of speech, gait ataxia and tremulousness, microbrachycephaly, midface hypoplasia, wide-spaced mouth and teeth with protruding tongue and drooling, and a happy disposition with inappropriate laughter. Seizures begin some time between 1 and 3 years of age in many children. These patients have overwhelming hyperactivity with an attention deficit so great that in severe cases it appears to prevent facial and social clues. There is speculation that the Angelman syndrome arises during embryogenesis from a failure of an aspect of neural development in the limbic structures and the cerebellum.

Regarding the frequency of the syndrome, an American study of 285 adults with moderate to profound mental retardation found that 1.4 per cent of this cohort had the Angelman syndrome (Jacobsen *et al.* 1998). A population-based study in Sweden of almost 49,000 prepubertal school-aged children found a prevalence of 1:12,000 with Angelman syndrome; this same study found the full criteria for autistic disorder/ childhood autism in the four children identified as having Angelman syndrome (Steffenburg *et al.* 1996). This study raises the question of what percentage of patients with Angelman syndrome meet criteria for autism; such a study needs to be done.

The Angelman syndrome is thought to be due to the silencing of a maternal gene located in a segment of the long arm of the 15th chromosome (15q11–13). The syndrome is associated with the gene UBE3A. According to molecular or cytogenetic status, there are four classes of patients: maternal microdeletion of 15q11–q13; uniparental disomy (UPD); defects in a putative imprinting centre (CIM); and biparental inheritance with mutations of UBE3A (Moncla *et al.* 1999). This gene is mutated in many but not all patients with Angelman syndrome. The 6ABRB3 gene is deleted in most patients (Lalande *et al.* 1999). A small study of ten subjects with autism found no evidence so far of a functional mutation in the gene (Veenstra-VanderWeele *et al.* 1999). See chromosome 15 in Chapter 15 (pp. 240–242) for a discussion of some of the clinical effects of silencing the gene. Also, it is interesting that in the medical literature there are at least 15 cases of children and adults (summarized in Gillberg 1998) who meet strict criteria for autism and also have partial tri- or tetrasomy of the same portion of chromosome 15 (15q11–13) that functions abnormally in patients with the Angelman syndrome.

ANOREXIA NERVOSA

A small subgroup of patients with anorexia nervosa have been reported to have autistic features (Gillberg *et al.* 1996, Nilsson *et al.* 1999). This subgroup tended toward test profiles similar to those observed in autism and Asperger syndrome. Anorexia nervosa has been reported in a high-functioning, early-adolescent female with autism (Fisman *et al.* 1996) and other females (Wentz-Nilsson *et al.* 1999). A prospective ten-year outcome study of 51 cases found that 18 per cent had autism spectrum disorders (Wentz 2000). These cases raise the issue of the co-occurrence of childhood-onset disorders sharing the phenomena of obsessions and compulsions.

CHARGE ASSOCIATION

Three children with CHARGE association (coloboma, heart defect, atresia of the choanae, retarded growth and development, genital hypoplasia, ear anomalies and hearing defects) have been reported to have a concomitant autistic disorder (Fernell *et al.* 1999). Two out of three of the children were mentally retarded. The authors note that since children with the CHARGE association have many medical problems, their autistic behavior can easily be overlooked. The neural crest may be involved in the etiology of this syndrome.

COHEN SYNDROME

The Cohen syndrome is a multiple anomaly syndrome which is reported to be difficult to diagnose at a very young age (Fryns *et al.* 1996). It is phenotypically somewhat hetero- geneous. In the first year of life, hypotonia and evidence of progressive microcephaly are common. Neutropenia is present from the beginning, remains unchanged over the years and is not associated with higher susceptibility to infections. Psychomotor development appears quite slow until correction of myopia (associated with ocular anomalies such as retinal degeneration) results in some catch-up. After the age of 6 years the facial stigmata (antimongoloid slant of the eyes, prominent nasal bridge, short philtrum, prominent upper-central incisors) become more evident. The tendency to truncal obesity begins after 5 or 6 years of age. The stature is short and there are long, narrow hands and feet with elongated, tapered fingers.

Four girls with the Cohen syndrome were reported to have autistic behavior when young (Fryns *et al.* 1996). Regarding reports of older patients, a study of adolescents and adults who had been placed in residential homes because of their label of an autism spectrum disease included one case of Cohen syndrome (Swillen *et al.* 1996).

DE LANGE SYNDROME

The de Lange syndrome, also known as the Brachmann–de Lange syndrome, is a rare multiple congenital anomaly/mental retardation (MCA/MR) syndrome with characteristic facies, growth retardation and structural abnormalities of the limbs. As early as 1975,

Knobloch and Pasamanick reported that a child with the de Lange syndrome met the criteria for autism. Since then, one of the behavior phenotypes of the syndrome has been described as autistic by additional authors (Johnson *et al.* 1976, Bay *et al.* 1993, Jones 1997). A child described by Bay *et al.* (1993) met DSM-III-R criteria for autism. One of the present authors (CG) has a child with both autism and the de Lange syndrome in his practice.

DOWN SYNDROME

Down syndrome, a trisomy syndrome of the 21st chromosome, is usually not associated with autism and, indeed, is often thought of as an autism "contrast syndrome" for purposes of scientific study. A study of 371 adults with Down syndrome had a rate of autism that was no different from that of matched controls with mental retardation due to other pathologies (Collacott *et al.* 1992). Another author reported that, compared to many other syndromes associated with mental retardation, the rate of autistic behavior in Down syndrome is low (Nordin 1997).

However, the medical literature has quite a number of reports of individuals with Down syndrome who meet the criteria for autism (Knobloch and Pasamanick 1975, Campbell *et al.* 1978, Wakabayashi 1979, Wing and Gould 1979, Gillberg and Wahlström 1985, Coleman 1986, Gath and Gumley 1986, Bregman and Volkmar 1988, Lund 1988, Elia *et al.* 1990, Ritvo *et al.* 1990, Collacott *et al.* 1992, Ghaziuddin *et al.* 1992b, Li *et al.* 1993, Howlin *et al.*, 1995, Fombonne *et al.* 1997, Ghaziuddin 1997, Barton and Volkmar 1998, Kent and Hayward 1998, Capone and Lee 1999). One extremely unlucky 17-year-old has been reported to have Down syndrome, the autistic syndrome and depression (Ghaziuddin and Tsai 1991). In the cases reported in the literature, there is a predominance of males similar to the pattern seen in autism in general.

Diagnosing autistic features in a child who also has Down syndrome is not always easy. Auditory and language problems, possibly due to the recurrent otitis media that plagues Down syndrome, may be misunderstood. A child with Down syndrome who is withdrawn and irritable with poor eye contact may be developing a hidden infection, such as a bladder infection. Thus the diagnosis of the double syndrome needs to be based on a consistent pattern over a period of time and only after other etiologies of the symptoms have been ruled out. It is important to get it right, not just diagnostically, but also in planning the child's education, because a child with the double syndrome is likely to do much better in an educational program designed for autistic children than in one established for Down syndrome children. The presence of autistic features in a child with Down syndrome means that the child needs special educational and vocational programs of the type designed for children with autism. Left in a class with other children with Down syndrome, the child is unlikely to reach his or her educational potential.

There are a number of ways in which children with the double syndrome differ from children with Down syndrome alone. Many, but not all, are completely non-verbal – a rare phenomenon in Down syndrome alone. Besides the better-known symptoms of autism, such as a history of developmental regression, they are also more likely to have associated behaviors of autism such as self-injurious behavior, food faddism and sleep problems. A

140

recent study comparing 20 non-autistic with 20 autistic individuals with Down syndrome found that those with autistic features were more likely to have a lower IQ score, a greater frequency of abnormalities on neurological examination, and were more likely to have cortical hypoplasia, thinner corpus collosa and increased ventricle size compared to case controls (Capone and Lee 1999).

What causes autism in Down syndrome? Both syndromes are relatively common: the prevalence of autism is approaching 1 in less than 1000; Down syndrome has a rate of about 1 in 800. Thus, because of the relatively common frequency of the two syndromes, a double syndrome could be coincidence in any one child. Such children need two evaluations – one for Down syndrome (Rogers and Coleman 1992) and one for autism (see Chapter 16). One etiology that may cause autism in such a Down syndrome child appears to be familial factors specific to autism. Ghaziuddin (1997) studied the parents of three cases of the double syndrome and obtained a history of the broader autism phenotype of the type found in families of autistic children (see Chapter 15).

Is there any evidence that, in some patients, factors related to Down syndrome itself might predispose to autism? Infants with Down syndrome are somewhat more prone to develop infantile spasms. A report of 14 such cases found two infants with Down syndrome who had developed persistent autistic features (Silva *et al*. 1996). (Infantile spasms leading to autism are discussed in Chapter 12.) Children with Down syndrome are also more likely to develop thyroid problems (Coleman and Abassi 1984); hypothyroidism is one of the double syndromes (see later in this chapter). However, hypothyroidism is only occasionally associated with autism in an individual with Down syndrome, just as it is only occasionally associated with autism in non-Down's individuals. There is no evidence that hypothyroidism by itself is the cause of autism in a patient with Down syndrome. Lactic acidosis, a non-specific finding in some patients with autism (see Chapter 13), has been identified in a patient with autism and Down syndrome (Coleman 1986).

It should be noted that individuals with Down syndrome have many laboratory abnormalities because of the effect of a whole extra chromosome. Certain laboratory abnormalities which are compensatory should be left alone; others, such as the one indicating thyroid dysfunction, need correction. A preventive medical checklist of clinical and laboratory evaluations exists which has selected out the testing that needs to be administered in a child with Down syndrome. (Updates of the preventive medical checklist are available on a regular basis from the Down Syndrome Medical Interest Group (DSMIG) published by *Down Syndrome Quarterly*.) When administered annually throughout life, this checklist prevents possible complications of Down syndrome from developing and overtaking the cognitive and health gains achieved by individuals with Down syndrome. When abnormal laboratory tests are detected by the checklist, there should be prompt correction. In a child with both Down syndrome and autism, regular annual examinations to prevent further complications are even more important.

In summary, it seems likely that many cases of the double syndrome consisting of the autistic syndrome and Down syndrome occur by unlucky coincidence. However, the tendency toward developmental anomalies of the brain that underlies the increased incidence of infantile spasms in Down syndrome may also contribute to the development of autistic symptoms in some patients. If a child has both Down syndrome and autism, that child should be evaluated and treated medically for both syndromes. Regarding educational programming, the child should be in an autistic class.

EHLERS–DANLOS SYNDROME

The relationship of autism to Ehlers–Danlos syndrome was first discussed by Sieg (1992). Fehlow *et al.* (1993) described a fatal case of Ehlers–Danlos syndrome who had early infantile autism as well as mental retardation. The patient died at age 19 years from excessive aerophagy resulting in ectasia of the stomach, which then caused megacolon followed by a fatal ileus. Investigation of the cerebellum revealed a significant rarefication and diminuation of the Purkinje cells as well as the cells of the stratum granulare in lobules VI and VII.

FRAGILE X SYNDROME

The fragile X syndrome was first described in 1943 as a sex-linked condition with the broad physical and behavioral features of the syndrome. In 1969, Lubs described a cytogenetic abnormality in the form of a constriction close to the distal end of the long arm of the X chromosome in males afflicted with the condition and in obligate female carriers. It was noted that certain behaviors of the newly described patients resembled certain features of autism, and this led to a controversy regarding the relationship between autism and the fragile X syndrome (Cohen *et al.* 1991). Many studies later, it can now be seen that the fragile X syndrome is not a common cause of classical autism, but the number of individuals with fragile X who meet the diagnostic criteria for autism is higher than can be accounted for by chance (Feinstein and Reiss 1998).

The behavioral phenotype for the fragile X syndrome includes pronounced gaze aversion, language delay and echolalia, perseveration, hypersensitivity to sensory stimuli, tactile defensiveness, stereotypies, self-injurious behavior, preoccupations with constricted interests, need for sameness, and social anxiety, especially with peers or unfamiliar adults. However, for the majority of the patients, relationships with parents and familiar adults are characterized by strong attachments, emotional relatedness and concern for others, so, in spite of their problems in group settings, they do not appear to have a core symptom of autism. Yet a small but significant number do have autism; the actual prevalence of fragile X syndrome in individuals with autism is higher than that found in the general population (Dykens and Volkmar 1997).

The fragile X syndrome is one of the most common genetic causes of developmental disabilities, affecting approximately 1 in 2,500 to 1 in 4,000 individuals (Hagerman and Cronister (Eds) 1991). Facial features include a long, narrow face, strabismus, prominent, long ears, a thick nasal bridge, prominent jaw, and dental malocclusion. Macroorchidism after puberty is a prominent feature of this syndrome. The patients may also have excessive joint laxity, pectus excavatum, kyphoscoliosis, a single palmar crease and pes planus.

Cognitively, almost all the males and half the females with the full mutation have some degree of mental retardation. Although fragile X is unusual as an etiology in girls with autism (Meyer *et al.* 1998), a study of girls with fragile X found that they had significantly more autistic behaviors than controls (Mazzocco *et al.* 1997). One set of monozygotic female twins, with similar-sized CGG triplet repeat expansions, consisted of one girl who suffered from autism while her twin sister had mild mental retardation and marked social anxiety (Gurling *et al.* 1997). An interesting study of females with autism who were not retarded revealed deficits in executive function, measures of attention and visual–spatial defects (Mazzocco *et al.* 1993).

The mutated gene (FMR1) responsible for the fragile X karyotype produces a protein product referred to as FMRP. Based on postmortem findings, FMRP is located primarily, although not exclusively, in neuronal cells. There is evidence that FMRP is important in normal fetal brain development; there is expression of the mutated gene in proliferating and migrating cells (Abitbol *et al.* 1993); and a fetal brain examined at 23 weeks gestation was noted to already have dendritic spine abnormalities (Jenkins *et al.* 1984). Adult postmortem studies show that the hippocampus and the cerebellum appear to have particularly high expression of FMR1 (Hinds *et al.* 1993).

Males and females with the full mutation have hypoplasia of the posterior cerebellar vermis, particularly vermal lobules VI and VII. They also have enlargement of the fourth ventricle and lateral ventricles as well as abnormalities of hippocampal (Reiss *et al.* 1994) and subcortical gray (particularly the caudate nucleus) when compared to matched controls. The differences in the superior temporal gyrus and the hippocampus appear to be age-related (Feinstein and Reiss 1998).

There is perhaps no other developmental disorder where the pathogenesis from gene to the behavioral manifestations of the disease is as well described (see Chapter 15). Even so, a great more needs to be learned; in addition to the well-defined genetic abnormality, there appear to be other biological factors. Some individuals with the fragile X syndrome do not express the genetic defect in all of their cells. These cases have an active fragile X gene in some of their blood cells while other blood cells do not have the gene; they are mosaic for the mutation. In one study of affected males, Cohen *et al.* (1996) found that 41 per cent of their patient group were mosaic. The rate of adaptive skills development was 2–4 times as great in mosaic cases as in full mutation cases. Most relevantly, they noted that there was a trend for cases with autism to be more prevalent in the full mutation group.

GOLDENHAR SYNDROME (OCULO-AURICULOVERTEBRAL DYSPLASIA SPECTRUM DISORDERS)

The Goldenhar syndrome consists of an association of symptoms consisting mainly of epibulbar dermoids, preauricular appendages, microtia or other ear anomalies, and vertebral anomalies. There is a great deal of phenotypical variability. Goldenhar syndrome was categorized during the 1960s as a variant of hemifacial microsomia and is now understood as the basis of oculo-auriculovertebral dysplasia spectrum disorders. The frequency of such defects has been estimated to range from 1/3,500 to 1/26,550 live births. Chromosomal anomalies (del 5q and trisomy 18) are associated with the Goldenhar syndrome (Cohen *et al.* 1989) but the etiology in most cases is not yet established.

Landgren *et al.* (1992) have described in detail two patients with Goldenhar syndrome and moderate degrees of autistic behavior; both met current criteria for autistic disorder (American Psychiatric Association 1987). One girl presented at 7 years of age for evaluation of autistic symptoms and was then diagnosed as having Goldenhar syndrome; the other girl in the 1992 paper had a neonatal diagnosis of Goldenhar syndrome followed by a diagnosis of autistic disorder at 5 years of age. These authors reported that they have seen at least three further cases (two boys and one girl). More recently, Barton and Volkmar (1998) reported a patient with Goldenhar syndrome who met strict criteria for autism.

HYPOMELANOSIS OF ITO (INCONTINENTIA PIGMENTI ACHROMIANS)
The Hypomelanosis of Ito is the third most frequent neurocutaneous disorder. It can be defined as a syndrome providing a cutaneous epiphenomenon with a peculiar pattern of distribution, usually associated with disorders of the nervous system, skeleton and eyes. Hypopigmented areas of the skin (irregular borders, streaks, whorls, patches) are usually distributed on the trunk or limbs. In one study of young children based on 76 cases, more than half (57 per cent) were found to be mentally retarded and almost half (49 per cent) had a seizure disorder (Pascual-Castroviejo *et al.* 1998). Twelve of the 76 cases had macrocephaly while six had micocephaly; three cases of cerebellar hypoplasia were noted.

Because the Hypomelanosis of Ito is a syndrome rather than a single disease entity, there is active discussion about its present clinical delineation (Failla *et al.* 1997, Van Steensel and Steijlen 1998). For example, there have been more than ten different chromosomal aberrations found in this patient group. Regarding the central nervous system, quite a variety of brain abnormalities are described (Steiner *et al.* 1996) including neuronal migration disorders (Okuno *et al.*1997). The Hypomelanosis of Ito is classified in the Malformations of Cortical Development scheme as malformations due to abnormal neuronal and glial proliferation 1.B.3.iii.b.ii (see Chapter 14).

In 1991, two girls and a boy showing autistic behavior, and fulfilling the criteria for autistic disorder, Asperger syndrome and atypical autism, were diagnosed as having Hypomelanosis of Ito by Åkefeldt and Gillberg. Other cases have been described by Griebel *et al.* (1989), Zappella (1992a), Hermida *et al.* (1997), von Aster *et al.* (1997) and Pavone *et al.* (1997). Two pairs of twins (one monozygotic and one dizygotic) have been reported by Zappella (1993). In one series of 76 young children with Hypomelanosis of Ito, eight (10 per cent) showed autistic features (Pascual-Castroviejo *et al.* 1998).

JOUBERT SYNDROME
Joubert syndrome (JS) is a rare autosomal recessive disorder characterized by hypotonia, early hyperpnea and apnea, developmental delay, abnormal eye movements, tongue protrusion and truncal ataxia. The patients have a striking dysplasia of the superior cerebellar peduncles and vermis, as well as the isthmic segment of the brainstem. The MRI pattern resulting from these dysplasias has been called the "molar tooth" sign, which is seen in over 80 per cent of this patient group (Maria *et al.* 1997).

Two siblings with Joubert syndrome have been described with autistic features; one met DSM-III-R diagnostic criteria (Holroyd *et al.* 1991). When the authors were challenged that the behavior disorder might just be secondary to the handicaps of the syndrome, they replied that "the autistic behaviors occurring in these two children with Joubert syndrome clearly exceeded the level of dysfunction attributable to associated handicaps alone" (Holroyd and Reiss 1993). Three additional patients with DSM-IV and one with PDDNOS also have been reported (Ozonoff *et al.* 1999). Because of the marked cerebellar findings in this syndrome, it has been of interest to students of autism.

KLEINE–LEVIN SYNDROME

There is a report that two individuals with Asperger syndrome developed the Kleine–Levin syndrome (periodic hypersomnia, excessive eating, hypersexuality, irritability and apathy) during adolescence (Berthier *et al.* 1992).

LUJAN–FRYNS SYNDROME (X-LINKED MENTAL RETARDATION WITH MARFANOID HABITUS)

A type of X-linked mental retardation has been described by Lujan *et al.* (1984) and Fryns and Buttiens (1987) in males with a marfanoid habitus, craniofacial changes, hypernasal voice and hyperactive behavior. In a Belgian study of 21 adolescents and adults with autism living in residential homes, the investigators were surprised to find that as many as four of these individuals were found to have the diagnosis of X-linked mental retardation with marfanoid habitus (Swillen *et al.* 1996). Two other males with this diagnosis had previously been identified as autistic (Guerrieri and Neri 1991).

MOEBIUS SYNDROME

Congenital non-progressive bilateral facial diplegia, especially of cranial nerves VI and VII, combined with external ophthalmoplegia is a rare neurological syndrome described by Moebius as early as 1888. In addition to the cranial nerve abnormalities, limbs, chest wall, spine and soft tissues may be involved.

The Moebius syndrome is truly a syndrome with many different infectious, genetic, toxic and unknown etiologies. One etiology may be uterine contractions during the sixth and seventh week of pregnancy, including those brought on by abortifacient drugs such as egotamine and misoprostol (Pastuszak *et al.* 1998). In a postmortem examination of the brain of an infant with Moebius syndrome, mineralized foci were concentrated in paramedian wedge-shaped areas of the pontine and medullary tegmentum (Leong and Ashwell 1997). This suggested ischaemia in that zone during fetal brain development; the brainstem midline normally remains avascular for protracted periods during fetal life making it especially vulnerable to factors contributing to ischaemia.

Moebius syndrome is of particular interest to students of autism because such a high percentage of individuals with the syndrome have all or many of the symptoms typical of autism; Gillberg and Steffenburg (1987) found these symptoms present in 7 out of 17 patients. In spite of the rarity of the syndrome, a number of patients have now been recorded with the double syndrome of Moebius syndrome/autistic syndrome (Ornitz *et al.*

1977, Gillberg and Winnergard 1984, Miller *et al.* 1998). Both the present authors have such patients in their practice.

MUCOPOLYSACCHARIDOSIS

Sanfilippo's syndrome, type A (mucopolysaccharidosis III), has been reported in two siblings, one male and one female, with autism (Ritvo *et al.* 1990). Sanfilippo syndrome involves a mucopolysaccharidosis frequently associated with brain pathology, often a severe seizure disorder. Two patients with another form of mucopolysaccharidosis (Hurler's disease) have also been mentioned in the literature (Knoblock and Pasamanick 1975, Coleman (Ed.) 1976).

NEUROFIBROMATOSIS 1 (NF1)

Another of the neuroepidermal syndromes is neurofibromatosis 1. NF1 is one of the most common single-gene disorders to affect the human nervous system. Besides the nervous system, it is also associated with a wide variety of complications affecting almost every system in the body, including the eyes, endocrine system, skeleton and circulation. The major disease manifestations in the skin are:

- Café au lait spots (six or more macular spots, darker in sun-exposed areas, becoming obvious during the first two years of life; 0.5 cm or larger in prepubertal individuals, 1.5 cm or larger in postpubertal individuals).
- Skinfold freckling (axillary, inguinal, trunk, neck freckling appearing during the first five years of life).
- Cutaneous neurofibromas (usually do not develop until pre-adolescence).
- Lisch nodules (dome-shaped elevations on the iris seen with a slit lamp, which are pathognomic but may not be present until after 20 years of age (North 1998).

Because neurofibromatosis 1 is a relatively common disorder, with an estimated incidence of between 1 in 2,500 and 1 in 3,000, it is hard to be sure whether the double syndrome patients described in the literature with neurofibromatosis and autism occurred by chance or not. Supporting a chance occurrence is the observation that the peripheral, rather than the central, nervous system is the target of most neurofibromas in NF1. On the other hand, there is evidence of central nervous system involvement because epilepsy, infantile spasms (Millichap 1997), cognitive defects, intracranial tumors and hydrocephalus are known complications. One evaluation of this question addressed a study of 341 children with infantile autism and other types of childhood psychosis, seen as in-patients at two university clinics of child psychiatry during a 25-year period, and found only one case of neurofibromatosis (Mouridsen *et al.* 1992).

In 1984, Gillberg and Forsell published case reports of three children with neuro-fibromatosis and autism or autistic-like conditions. It is relevant to note that none of these children were diagnosed as having neurofibromatosis in infancy; the psychiatric symptoms had been present for many years before the underlying diagnosis of neuro-fibromatosis was made. Since then, Gaffney *et al.* (1988) have described two patients with autism. Steffenburg (1991) has described a girl with neurofibromatosis/ autism and a first-degree relative with neurofibromatosis. Pavone *et al.* (1997) have listed a 4-year-old child with neurofibromatosis/autism; Fombonne *et al.* (1997) have also identified one such patient (Williams and Hersh 1998). Since neurofibromatosis is such a relatively common condition, yet the diagnosis is often missed in the early years, the status of the double syndrome of neurofibromatosis/autism remains to be firmly established.

Neurofibromatosis 1 is inherited in an autosomal dominant pattern with 50 per cent risk of transmission to offspring. Approximately 50 per cent of cases are sporadic due to new mutations; germline mosaicism occurring in a clinically unaffected parent is likely to occur in less than 1 per cent of cases. The gene responsible for NF1 encodes a protein, neurofibromin; it shares a high-sequence homology with GAP proteins which have an important role in cell growth and differentiation. The NF1 gene, which is found on the long arm of chromosome 17 (17q11.2), is classified as a tumor suppressor gene (see Chapter 15). More than 90 mutations in the NF1 gene have been identified and no one mutation has been found to be common among affected individuals (Blaser *et al.* 1996).

Neurofibromatosis 1 is classified in the Malformations of Cortical Development scheme as malformations due to abnormal neuronal and glial proliferation 1.B.3.a.iii.b.iii (see Chapter 14).

NOONAN SYNDROME

Noonan syndrome, a rare syndrome, appears phenotypically to resemble the Turner syndrome, but the children, both boys and girls, have normal karyotypes. The most common abnormalities are short stature, characteristic facies, webbing of the neck, pectus excavatum and congenital cardiac disease. Mental retardation is more common than in the Turner syndrome.

A male with Noonan syndrome and autistic behavior has been reported (Paul *et al.* 1983). There is a paper by Ghaziuddin *et al.* (1994) describing the concordance of Noonan syndrome and autism in another case. Another patient with the double syndrome was described by Swillen *et al.* (1996). One of the authors of this book (MC) is also aware of two patients with Noonan syndrome and autism.

PEROXISOMAL DISORDERS: ZELLWEGER SYNDROME/NEONATAL ADRENOLEUKODYSTROPHY/INFANTILE REFSUM DISEASE (ZS/NALD/IRD)

The peroxisome is the most recently identified subcellular organelle. Its relationship to human disease was first discovered in 1973 by the observation of Goldfischer and colleagues that patients with the Zellweger cerebrohepatorenal syndrome (ZS) lack demonstrable peroxisomes. Since then, the amount of information about the peroxisomal disorders has increased so rapidly that the nomenclature of these disorders is still in flux. Because of the present overlap between clinical and biochemical phenotypes, the early-infantile categories of clinical symptoms are classified as a continuum – Zellweger syndrome/neonatal adrenoleukodystrophy/infantile Refsum disease (ZS/NALD/IRD) – with ZS being the most severe and IRD the least severe. Clinical symptoms vary with age and can include: 1–6 months – failure to thrive, hepatomegaly, jaundice, retinopathy, cataract; 6 months to 4 years – neurological presentation, including autistic behavior, retardation, visual and hearing impairment, osteoporosis.

In 1998, Baumgartner and colleagues described eight patients with a clinical phenotype closest to infantile Refsum disease (IRD) as follows:

> First symptoms developed between 1 and 6 months of age and were nonspecific digestive problems, osteoporosis, hepatomegaly and hypocholesterolemia. Only minor facial dysplasia was noted. Subsequently regressive changes were noted, that is, chorioretinopathy, sensorineuronal hearing loss and a kink in development followed by complete arrest and *autistic behavior* [our italics]. However, all but one were able to walk independently before the age of 3 years and explored objects bimanually; all [these] other patients are still alive, although severely handicapped (the oldest being 25 years old).

The molecular defect causing this disease entity in patients is not yet fully known. What is known is that there are elevated levels of very long chain fatty acids (VLCFA), bile acids and pipecolic acids, as well as decreased levels of docosahexaenoic acid and plasmalogens. Probably a defect in peroxismal beta oxidation causes the accumulation of VLCFAs. Liver peroxisomes on microscopy are absent or express mosaicism (Baumgartner *et al.* 1998). The prototype initial test for this syndrome is the presence of abnormally high levels of VLCFAs in plasma; cultured skin fibroblasts are the most helpful additional laboratory test. It has already been noted that the ZS-NALD-IRD continuum can be associated with at least ten distinct genes, and many families have private, individualized mutations (Moser *et al.* 1999).

When should one test for peroxisomal disorders? These peroxisomal disorders are quite rare in general and even rarer presenting as an autistic syndrome. However they should be considered in the differential diagnosis of a hypotonic infant who has a marked regression in development accompanied by the onset of autistic behavior. Major clinical criteria, defined as being present in more than 75 per cent of the children, include low/broad nasal ridge, hypotonia, impaired hearing, abnormal electroretinogram, and enlarged liver present during the first year of life. Moser and Raymond (1998) point out that therapy exists or is emerging for classic Refsum disease and possibly for some of the more mildly involved patients with infantile Refsum disease.

The peroxisomal disorders are classified in the Malformations of Cortical Development scheme as malformations due to abnormal neuronal migrations II.B.3.c.ii (see Chapter 14).

PHENYLKETONURIA (PKU)
In 1960, Dr C.E. Benda decided to try to convince child psychiatrists that a child with a known metabolic disease could appear as a psychiatric case. He took a group of psychiatrists to a ward to see several children with PKU and let them examine the children. Only after they made the diagnosis of some form of childhood psychiatric disease did he

tell them that the children were positive to PKU testing and had phenylketonuria (Benda 1960). Most children with PKU are severely retarded and not autistic, but a significant subgroup of PKU meet autistic criteria (Friedman 1969, Reiss *et al.* 1986, Fombonne and du Mazaubrun 1992).

In children with PKU, functional levels of the enzyme in the liver are inadequate to convert the first amino acid (phenylalanine) to the second one (tyrosine) in the important pathway that produces catechol amines, dopamine and norepinephrine, in the brain (see Fig. 13.2) This results in phenylalanine going into minor pathways, some of which are quite toxic to the brain. Most individuals with PKU become quite mentally retarded by this toxic assault on the brain, although very occasionally a person with PKU can be only mildly retarded.

Initiation of a low-phenylalanine diet is highly effective if started when the infant is less than 6 weeks of age (Berry *et al.* 1979). However, if infants with PKU are not started on the diet in the early weeks of life, they begin a deteriorating course which can result, among other brain abnormalities, in the development of autistic symptoms. When a child with PKU autism is identified later in life, is it of any value to start the diet? The continuing deterioration may be stopped by instituting the diet, and there is evidence of some cognitive and behavioral benefit for the older child (Lewis 1959, Lowe *et al.* 1980), although major reversal seems out of the question. Even an elderly man with PKU who had never been treated had improvement of social skills and improvement of leg tremor and spasm when placed on the diet (Williams 1998).

PKU autism should become a disease of the past since it is now possible to detect the disease *in utero* and by neonatal screening. Unfortunately, cases with PKU autism have continued to appear in the literature – three children detected in the Yale program for autism in the USA (Lowe *et al.* 1980), a 12-year-old from China (Chen and Hsiao 1989), a 3-year-old from Tunisia (Miladi *et al.* 1992), and another 12-year-old from Italy (Pavone *et al.* 1997). Both the absence of infant screening in some countries and the lack of quality control in countries where screening programs exist still leave some children at risk for PKU autism.

The Rett Complex

Autism is more common among boys, but when autistic symptoms are seen in girls the Rett complex should be included in the differential diagnosis. Autism is often the initial diagnosis in these girls, even though the autistic symptoms in classical Rett syndrome can end as early as 4 years or persist into the 7- or 8-year age group (Olsson and Rett 1987). In spite of their autistic symptoms, girls with classical Rett syndrome can be differentiated from more classical autism as described in Table 11.1. The Rett complex consists of several subgroups, many of which have symptoms of autism. The best-defined and most numerous is classical Rett syndrome; other variants have been delineated by Hagberg and Skjeldal (1994). To accurately diagnose a patient with the Rett complex, it is important to have characteristic clusters of symptoms, as seen in Tables 11.1–4, and not rely on the presence of a single symptom, such as hand-wringing.

149

TABLE 11.1
Comparison of Rett syndrome and infantile autism*

Rett syndrome	*Infantile autism*
1. Normal development to 6–18 months	1. Onset from early infancy; sometimes regression age 18–24 months
2. Progressive loss of speech and hand function	2. Loss of previously acquired skills does not occur
3. Profound mental retardation in all functional areas	3. More scatter of intellectual function. Visuospatial and manipulative skills often better than apparent verbal skills
4. Acquired microcephaly, growth retardation, decreased weight gain	4. Physical development normal in the majority
5. Stereotypic hand movements always present	5. Stereotypic behaviour is more varied in manifestation and is always more complex; midline manifestations rare
6. Progressive gait difficulties, with gait and truncal apraxia and ataxia; some may become non-ambulatory	6. Gait and other gross motor functions normal in first decade of life
7. Language always absent	7. Language sometimes absent; if present, peculiar speech patterns always present; markedly impaired non-verbal communication
8. Eye contact present, sometimes very intense	8. Eye contact with others typically avoided or inappropriate
9. Little interest in manipulating objects	9. Stereotypic ritualistic behaviour usually involves skilful but odd manipulation of objects or sensory self-stimulation
10. Seizures in at least 70% in early childhood (various seizure types)	10. Seizures (usually temporal–limbic complex partial) in 25% in late adolescence and adulthood
11. Bruxism, hyperventilation with air-swallowing and breath-holding common	11. Bruxism, hyperventilation and breath-holding not typical
12. Choreoathetoid movements and dystonia may be present	12. Dystonia and chorea not present†

* Reproduced by permission from Trevathan and Naidu (1988)
† Extrapyramidal signs may appear in some patients with autism after puberty

Rett syndrome

Rett syndrome was first described in Vienna by Andreas Rett (1966). Unaware of Rett's description, investigators from other countries – Ishikawa *et al.* (1978) in Japan, and Hagberg (1980) in Sweden – reported a similar clinical pattern in girls. The incidence of Rett syndrome may be as high as 1:15,000 live births worldwide.

The Rett Syndrome Diagnostic Criteria Work Group (1988) has established a basis for the diagnosis of Rett syndrome using necessary, supportive and exclusion criteria (see Table 11.2). Rett syndrome, in most cases, appears to be a genetic syndrome in girls that emerges during infancy with deceleration of psychomotor development and head growth, seizures, breathing irregularities and autonomic instability. One of the most striking aspects of the syndrome is that grasping and other purposeful hand movements usually disappear by the age of 3 years and are replaced by characteristic stereotyped hand-wringing movements in front of the mouth or chest. The girls have apparently normal physical and mental development until some time between the ages of 5 and 24 months, then a regression.

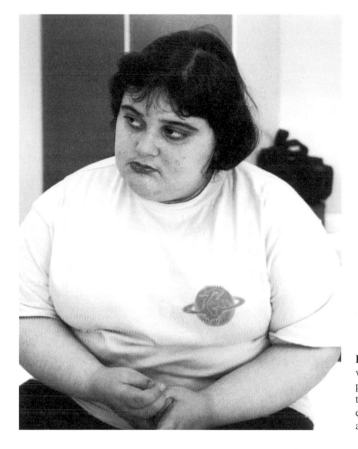

Fig. 11.1 14-year-old girl with Rett complex of the preserved speech variant type. She has short echolalic phrases in second and third person.

Although prodromal signs and symptoms are sometimes observed, which indicate a process occurring already during the first months of life, there are no predictable manifestations of this disorder until deterioration begins. Some time during the first or second year of life, the girls enter Stage I of a four-stage progression (see Table 11.3) (Hagberg and Witt-Engerström 1986). More than two-thirds eventually develop scoliosis, with a period of accelerated progression during the teenage years. Eventually one-third lose ambulation skills. As adults, there appears to be no further mental deterioration and less prominent seizures and breath-holding. There is no adequate way to test the cognitive level of these patients since they do not speak or use their hands.

In classical Rett syndrome, there is a deceleration of head growth which can be detected after age 5 months, often resulting in microcephaly. This phenomenon appears to be due to apoptosis, a biological process used by all multicellular organisms to eliminate superfluous cells, and is a prominent feature of normal neural development. Neuronal apoptosis in any young child serves to match the number of neurons to the requirements of the synaptic targets and to rid the nervous system of inappropriate or unwanted connections (Rubin *et al.* 1994, D'Mello 1998). However, it appears that in Rett syndrome

151

TABLE 11.2
Diagnostic criteria for Rett syndrome*

Necessary criteria
1. Apparently normal prenatal and perinatal period
2. Apparently normal psychomotor development through first 6 months†
3. Normal head circumference at birth
4. Deceleration of head growth between ages 5 months and 4 years
5. Loss of acquired purposeful hand skills between ages 6 and 30 months, temporally associated with communication dysfunction and social withdrawal
6. Development of severely impaired expressive and receptive language, and presence of apparent severe psychomotor retardation
7. Stereotypic hand movements such as hand-wringing/squeezing, clapping/tapping, mouthing, and 'washing'/rubbing automatisms appearing after purposeful hand skills are lost
8. Appearance of gait apraxia and truncal apraxia–ataxia between ages 1 and 4 years
9. Diagnosis tentative until 2 to 5 years of age

Supportive criteria
1. Breathing dysfunction
   a. Periodic apnoea during wakefulness
   b. Intermittent hyperventilation
   c. Breath-holding spells
   d. Forced expulsion of air or saliva
2. EEG abnormalities
   a. Slow waking background and intermittent rhythmic slowing (3–5Hz)
   b. Epileptiform discharges, with or without clinical seizures
3. Seizures
4. Spasticity often with associated development of muscle wasting and dystonia
5. Peripheral vasomotor disturbances
6. Scoliosis
7. Growth retardation
8. Hypotrophic small feet

Exclusion criteria
1. Evidence of intrauterine growth retardation
2. Organomegaly, or other signs of storage disease
3. Retinopathy or optic atrophy
4. Microcephaly at birth
5. Evidence of perinatally acquired brain damage
6. Existence of identifiable metabolic or other progressive neurological disorder
7. Acquired neurological disorders resulting from severe infections or head trauma

* Reproduced by permission from Trevathan and Naidu (1988)
† Development may appear normal until 18 months of age

the brain moves from the usual modulated apoptosis to virtual arrest of neural development, particularly seen in the prefrontal, posterior frontal and anterior temporal cortex and caudate nucleus. There is reduced neuronal cell size and increased cell-packing density extensively throughout the forebrain. As in autism, there are a reduced number of Purkinje cells in the cerebellar hemispheres, with the preservation of the neurons of the related inferior olive (Bauman 1996). There is evidence of decreased dendritic branching in the premotor frontal, motor and subicular cortex (Armstrong *et al.* 1998), raising the question of whether this is basically a disorder of developing axonodendritic connections.

TABLE 11.3
Rett syndrome: clinical characteristics and differential diagnosis by stage*

Stage	*Clinical characteristics*	*Differential diagnosis*

Stage I
Onset: 6–18mths
Duration: mths
	Developmental stagnation
	Deceleration of head/brain growth
	Lack of interest in play activity
	  and environment
	Hypotonia
	EEG background: normal or minimal
	  slowing of posterior rhythm
		Benign cogential hypotonia
		Prader–Willi syndrome
		Cerebral palsy

Stage II
Onset: 1–3yrs
Duration: wks to mths
	Rapid developmental regression
	  with irritability
	Loss of hand use
	Seizures
	Hand stereotypies: wringing,
	  clapping, tapping, mouthing
	Autistic manifestations
	Loss of expressive language
	Insomnia
	Self-abusive behaviour (e.g.
	  chewing fingers, slapping face)
	EEG: background slowing and gradual
	  loss of normal sleep activity; focal
	  or multifocal spike and wave
		Autism
		Psychosis
		Hearing or visual disturbance
		Encephalitis
		Epileptic encephalopathy
		Neurocutaneous syndromes
		Neurodegenerative disorders
		Various disorders of organic
		  acid and amino acid
		  metabolism

Stage III
Onset: 2–10yrs
Duration: mths to yrs
	Severe mental retardation/apparent dementia
	Amelioration of autistic features
	Seizures
	Typical hand sterotypies: wringing,
	  tapping, mouthing
	Prominent ataxia and apraxia
	Hyperreflexia and progressive rigidity
	Hyperventilation, breath-holding,
	  aerophagia during waking
	Weight loss with excellent appetite
	Early scoliosis
	Bruxism
	EEG: gradual disappearance of posterior
	  rhythm, generalized slowing, absent
	  vertex and spindle activity, epileptiform
	  abnormalities activated during sleep
		Spastic ataxic cerebral palsy
		Spinocerebellar degeneration
		Leukodystrophies or other
		  storage disorders
		Neuroaxonal dystrophy
		Lennox–Gastaut syndrome
		Angelman syndrome

Stage IV
Onset: 10+yrs
Duration: yrs
	Progressive scoliosis, muscle
	  wasting and rigidity
	Decreasing mobility, wheelchair-dependent
	Growth retardation
	Improved eye contact
	Virtual absence of expressive
	  and receptive language
	Trophic disturbance of feet
	Reduced seizure frequency
	EEG: poor background organization with
	  marked slowing and multifocal spikes and
	  slow spike and wave pattern activated sleep
		Unknown degenerative
		  disorder

* Reproduced by permission from Trevathan and Naidu (1988)

A neuropathological study of amino acid receptors in the frontal cortex has shown a potential neurobiological correlate (NMDA receptors) to the clinically described distinction between the active "encephalopathic" stage II/III phase and the more quiescent and less epileptic stage IV seen in older girls (Blue et al. 1999). Compared to controls, the mean density of the receptors was found to be higher in the earlier stages and lower in stage IV. This is particularly interesting because experimental data suggest that NMDA receptor activity may enhance synaptic pruning during development.

Imaging studies have demonstrated both localized (Lappalainen et al. 1997) and global (Burroni et al. 1997) hypoperfusions, depending upon the stage of the disease. MR spectroscopy studies have measured glutamate (Glu), creatinine (Cr) and N-acetyl-asparate (NA) in this patient group (Hanefeld et al. 1995, Hashimoto et al. 1998, Pan et al. in press). Again, results varied with the age of the disease. In relatively young girls, Cr/NA appears to be elevated in white matter and Glu/NA in gray matter.

Also, it has been reported that there are distention, vacuolation and membranous changes in the mitochondria in the muscles of girls with Rett syndrome (Eeg-Olofsson et al. 1988, Ruch 1989), although they are not the typical "ragged red" fibers found in mitochondrial myopathies. In children with Rett syndrome, both Complex I and combined Complex I and III oxidative phosphorylation disease entities have been identified (Shoffner, personal communication). There are strong indications that Rett syndrome is not a neuronal migration disorder and involves a postsynaptogenic developmental deficiency (Belichenko et al. 1997). The basic neuropathologic defect remains unknown; the lack of glial hyperplasia and absence of retrograde cell loss in the olive, characteristic of postnatal cerebellar insult, suggest that the pathologic process had its origin early in development.

In seven families, mutations of a gene (MECP2) on the X chromosome have been identified (Amir et al. 1999). The gene encodes X-linked methyl-CpG-binding protein 2 (MeCP2). It is an interesting, already studied gene, which regulates the expression of other genes and can actually turn off other genes – silence them – by DNA methylation. It has been reported that this gene has low expression during early organogenesis and enhanced expression in the hippocampus during the formation of the differentiated brain (Coy et al. 1999). Mutations of this gene have also been found in members of Rett families such as mothers of Rett girls and a male with congenital encephalopathy (Wan et al. 1999) as well as in three girls with the preserved speech variant (De Bona et al. 2000). A variety of cytogenetic findings have also been reported in patients with all or many Rett syndrome criteria – an inversion on chromosome 2, a duplication on the long arm of chromosome 11, deletions on chromosome 18, trisomy X, XXY, and a point mutation in mitochondrial DNA. In one girl, a tumor of the pons/midbrain was found (Vanhala et al. 1998).

A number of non-specific biochemical findings have been reported. Abnormalities in multiple neurotransmitter/receptor systems, such as the dopaminergic, cholinergic, glutamatergic and opioid pathways, emphasize the pervasive effect of the maturational arrest. Low levels of nerve-growth factor in the cerebrospinal fluid of children with Rett syndrome raise a question about the possible role of neurotrophic factors in the disease process.

Treatment in Rett syndrome remains symptomatic. Seizure control is a major challenge. Melatonin may aid the sleep disorder (McArthur and Budden 1998, Miyamoto *et al.* 1999) although long-term effects are not yet known. Appropriate orthopaedic monitoring and procedures are usually needed. Music therapy, hydrotherapy, occupational therapies and physical therapies can be helpful. In classrooms, augmentative and alternative communication can be used.

Variants

There are a number of variant forms inside the Rett complex (Hagberg and Gillberg 1993). These include the *formes frustes, the congenital variant, the late childhood variant, the preserved speech variant* (Zappella 1992b), *the male variant*, and others yet to be classified (see Table 11.4). In their paper creating the criteria for atypical cases, Hagberg and Skjeldal (1994) described 2 patients with the congenital variant, 8 *formes frustes*, and 6 with late regression.

Hagberg and Skjeldal (1994) report that the *formes frustes* variant appears to be the most prevalent atypical expression of Rett syndrome. In these girls, the supportive characteristics do not appear until late childhood. Some of these *formes frustes* girls have shown a surprisingly well-preserved, yet somewhat dyspraxic, hand function as well as the absence of the classic hand-wringing stereotypics. Also the cranial circumference curves have often remained within normal limits. Combining the *formes frustes* patients with the late childhood variant patients, the Swedish series had 155 females as of 1994.

In the preserved speech variant, Zappella *et al.* (1998) have described 30 girls and young women with this variant, all but one of whom met full symptom criteria for DSM-IV autistic disorder. They also showed many features of classical Rett syndrome. All met the required 3 out of 6 main criteria and 14 (47 per cent) met the required 5 out of 11 supportive criteria for variants (see Table 11.4). The course of this variant is more benign than classical Rett syndrome, but all the girls were severely functionally impaired. There was familial clustering in a subgroup.

There are case histories of the male variant in the literature (Coleman 1990, Topcu *et al.* 1991, Jan *et al.* 1999), as well as a description of severe encephalopathies of boys born into families with recurrent Rett syndrome (Schanen *et al.* 1998).

SMITH–MAGENIS SYNDROME (SELF-HUGGERS)

The Smith–Magenis syndrome (SMS) is more popularly known as a syndrome of self-huggers (involuntary tic-like movements of crossing both arms across the chest or clasping the hands while squeezing the arms to the sides). These unusual spasmodic "upper-body squeezes" occur in half of the patients and can be highly frequent and repetitive (up to 100 hugs per hour). The motor movements are stereotyped expressions of happiness, affection or positive excitement, most pronounced during transition periods (Finucane *et al.* 1994). They are in direct contrast to the self-abusive behaviors of these children at other times – head-banging, hand-biting, picking-off of finger or toe nails, "lick and flip" behavior, and insertion of foreign objects into body orifices. In this patient group, sleep disturbance has emerged as the strongest predictor of maladaptive behavior (Dykens and Smith 1998).

155

TABLE 11.4
Rett syndrome: A variant delineation model

Inclusion criteria: A girl of at least 10 years of age with mental retardation of unexplained origin and with at least 3 of the 6 following *primary* criteria:

A1   Loss of (partial or subtotal) acquired fine finger skill in late infancy/early childhood
A2   Loss of acquired single words/phrases/nuanced babble
A3   RS hand stereotypies, hands together or apart
A4   Early deviant communicative ability
A5   Deceleration of head growth of 2 S.D. (even when still within normal limits)
A6   The RS disease profile: A regression period (stage II) followed by a certain recovery of contact and communication (stage III) in contrast to slow neuromotor regression through school age and adolescence

and, in addition, at least 5 of the following 11 RS *supportive* manifestations:

B1   Breathing irregularities (hyperventilation and/or breath-holding)
B2   Bloating/marked air swallowing
B3   Characteristic RS teeth grinding
B4   Gait dyspraxia
B5   Neurogenic scoliosis or high kyphosis (ambulant girls)
B6   Development of lower limb neurologic abnormalities
B7   Small blue/cold impaired feet, autonomic/trophic dysfunction
B8   Characteristic RS electroencephalographic development
B9   Unprompted sudden laughing/screaming spells
B10   Impaired/delayed nociception
B11   Intensive eye communication – "eye pointing"

Exclusion criteria according to the Diagnostic Criteria Work Group [4]

Abbreviation:
RS – Rett syndrome

These children have brachycephaly, a flat midface with broad nasal bridge, brachydactyly and short stature. More variable physical features include ocular pathology, prominent jaw, down-turned mouth, ear abnormalities, congenital cardiac defects, and scoliosis. They may exhibit peripheral neuropathies (pes cavus/planus, decreased or absent deep-tendon reflexes, and insensitivity to pain). Infants present with hypotonia, lethargy and oromotor dysfunction; they develop sleep and behavioral difficulties by the third year of life. About one-quarter have abnormal EEGs and seizures. Imaging studies have shown that some of the patients have enlarged ventricles or enlarged posterior fossae. The syndrome has a prevalence estimate of approximately 1 in 25,000 births (Greenberg *et al.* 1991).

The Smith–Magenis syndrome is associated with interstitial chromosomal deletions at 17p11.2 (Smith *et al.* 1986). There is a patient in the literature whose initial diagnosis was autism at the age of 3 years; at the age of 9 years he was found to have an interstitial deletion of chromosome 17p11.2 as well as a replication, inversion and deletion on chromosome 3 (Mariner *et al.* 1986). Parental chromosomes were normal; the boy had hypertelorism and polydactyly in addition to symptoms compatible with the Smith–Magenis syndrome. There is a description of a 14-year-old boy who met DSM-III-R criteria for autistic disorder and had a deletion of 17p11.2 (Vostanis *et al.* 1994). Two further cases with Smith–Magenis syndrome have been reported to demonstrate some autistic behavior (Smith *et al.* 1986, Lockwood *et al.* 1988). The majority of children are not accurately diagnosed until they are 5 to 8 years of age, when school difficulties may lead to a diagnosis of autism or PDD (Gropman *et al.* 1998).

SOTOS SYNDROME (CEREBRAL GIGANTISM) AND MACROCRANIA

Cerebral gigantism (Sotos syndrome) is a non-progressive clinical syndrome with characteristic facies, pre- and postnatal overgrowth, advanced bone age, and developmental delay as its main features. The cranium has a circumference above two standard deviations and is dolichocephalic; the face is flat, the eyes hyperteloric and the jaw prominent. The children tend to be clumsy. Growth hormone levels are normal. Imaging studies may reveal some dilatation of the ventricular system and abnormal EEGs are common.

Some children with Sotos syndrome have been described as having autism (Morrow *et al.* 1990, Zappella 1990) and Asperger syndrome (Tantam *et al.* 1990). Andermann (1995) discussed four young people who had autism, macrocrania and epilepsy, with normal imaging studies and without an obvious family history; he raised the question about whether these patients formed a syndrome separate from the Sotos syndrome. Orstavik *et al.* (1997) also raised this question about two sisters with autism and epilepsy who had the same pattern of postnatal macrocrania as seen in Sotos syndrome but lacked the overgrowth and increased height described in that syndrome.

Macrocrania has been found in many other individuals with autism who do not meet the criteria of Sotos syndrome. Macrocephaly does not define a homogeneous grouping of autistic individuals according to clinical features (Lainhart *et al.* 1997). Besides the unknown mechanism causing macrocrania in Sotos syndrome, there are two other patterns shown to result in macrocrania in the autistic syndrome – arrested hydrocephalus and non-specific megalencephaly (an enlarged brain) (see discussion in Chapter 14).

STEINERT'S MYOTONIC DYSTROPHY

Myotonic dystrophy is one of the trinucleotide repeat diseases with the phenomenon of anticipation. When it develops at a very young age, it can present with ptosis, tenting of the upper lip and facial diplegia. Weakness may develop in the proximal hip muscles which results in difficulties with the gait. The facial diplegia may be diagnosed erroneously as Moebius syndrome, another syndrome which has a subgroup of patients within the autistic syndrome. Most patients with myotonic dystrophy have excessive CTG trinucleotide repeats on the 19th chromosome (see Chapter 15).

A girl with congenital myotonic dystrophy and infantile autism has been reported (Yoshimura *et al.* 1989). There are two case reports of patients who had both Asperger syndrome and Steinert's myotonic dystrophy (Blondis *et al.* 1996, Paul and Allington-Smith 1997). In the case of the 10-year-old girl described by Blondis *et al.* (1996), the child had the largest trinucleotide repeat expansion within her pedigree of family members with myotonic dystrophy.

157

TOURETTE SYNDROME

The Tourette syndrome is a relatively common neurological disease characterized by involuntary movements (motor tics) and vocalizations (phonic or vocal tics). In addition, patients may have obsessions, compulsions, the attentional deficit syndrome and other psychiatric symptoms. The disorder generally begins in childhood. The prevalence of Tourette syndrome in autism exceeds that expected by chance (Baron-Cohen *et al.* 1999b).

Tourette syndrome is related to autism in two ways. First, a number of children have been described with the initial diagnosis of infantile autism followed by the later development of Tourette syndrome (Realmuto and Main 1982, Barabas and Mathews 1983, Burd *et al.* 1987, Ritvo *et al.* 1990, Comings and Comings 1991, Sverd *et al.* 1993, Stern and Robertson 1997, Baron-Cohen *et al.* 1999a). The case reported by Nelson and Pribor (1993) was also a calendar savant (as was a Tourette case without autism (Moriarty *et al.* 1993)). There are also case reports of Tourette syndrome and Asperger syndrome (Berthier *et al.* 1993, Ehlers and Gillberg 1993, Kerbeshian and Burd 1996, Nass and Gutman 1997). In the study by Burd *et al.* (1987), involving 12 children with autism and Tourette syndrome, this particular subgroup scored higher on IQ tests and had better expressive language skills than children with autism in the same cohort who did not develop Tourette syndrome. However, in a study by Berthier *et al.* (1993) of seven males with the double syndrome of Asperger syndrome/Tourette syndrome compared with age-matched controls having Tourette only, individuals with the double syndrome had more psychiatric hospitalizations, poorer academic achievement, more neurological soft signs and more structural brain abnormalities by MRI. Kerbeshian and Burd (1996) have described four patients who had *three* syndromes concurrently; they were the autistic syndrome, then Tourette syndrome, then bipolar disorder. At least in North Dakota (USA), where the study was done, these three syndromes co-occur at a greater than chance expectation based on a population-based prevalence study. A chromosomal aberration has been found in one patient with both autism and Tourette syndrome; he was a boy with an IQ of about 80 with a partial trisomy of chromosome 16p, with the breakpoint at 16p13.1 (Hebebrand *et al.* 1994).

The second way in which Tourette syndrome is linked to autism is that Tourette syndrome has been reported in patients with autism who were receiving long-term neuroleptic medicine (Perry *et al.* 1989). Stahl (1980) coined the term "tardive Tourette syndrome" to describe patients whose neuroleptic withdrawal takes the form of the Tourette syndrome. In such cases, it may be hard to be sure exactly what is happening – the re-emergence of pre-existing stereotypies or the emergence of new ones, the appearance of Tourette syndrome at this age or Tourette-like withdrawal dyskinesias. Careful review of past examinations and family history, plus detailed monitoring of the future course, can help distinguish between these various possibilities.

Clonidine, an alpha2-adrenergic receptor partial agonist, is effective in reducing tics as well as symptoms of hyperactivity, impulsivity and inattention in Tourette's disorder (Leckman *et al.* 1991). (See Chapter 17 for more on clonidine.) Neuroleptics and clomipramine also can be helpful.

Recently, in a case reported from the National Institute of Mental Health in the USA, a Group A beta-hemolytic streptococcal throat infection was associated with an acute exacerbation of obsessive-compulsive disorder and tics in a 12-year-old boy. Treatment with plasmapheresis was associated with decreases in the size of the child's basal ganglia ranging from 12 per cent to 28 per cent. Fluctuations in the size of the basal ganglia correlated with the severity of symptoms (Giedd *et al.* 1996). Evaluation by history of a larger group of children suggested that about 10 per cent of tic patients report symptoms consistent with an exacerbation following a strep infection (Garvey *et al.* 1998). They appear to have the new syndrome PANDAS (pediatric autoimmune neuropsychiatric disorders associated with streptococcus). The relevance of this to patients with autism both with and without tics is currently under study. There is early evidence that both intravenous immunoglobulin and plasma exchange may be effective in lessening symptom severity (Perlmutter *et al.* 1999).

TUBEROUS SCLEROSIS COMPLEX
Another of the neurocutaneous syndromes (or phakomatoses) that can present with autism is tuberous sclerosis. The tuberous sclerosis complex, which has a prevalence of 1 in 10,000 (Franz 1998), is an autosomal dominant disorder characterized by benign tumors (hamartomas) called tubers, and malformations of one or more body systems including the central nervous system and the skin. Mental retardation is present in about half of the patients; 84 per cent have seizures. The primary diagnostic criteria are facial angiofibromas, multiple ungual fibromas, cortical tubers, subependymal nodule or giant cell astrocytoma, multiple calcified subependymal nodules protruding into the ventricle, and multiple retinal astrocytomas (Franz 1998).

The cutaneous manifestations of this disease are:

- angiofibromas called adenoma sebaceum (small, smooth, acne-like lesions usually on the face);
- ashleaf spots (hypopigmented lesions resembling a leaf);
- shagreen patches (leathery, scaly lesions);
- periungual fibromas on the hands and feet.

Tuberous sclerosis is a classic neurocutaneous syndrome, where the lesions are predominant in both the skin and the brain. In the central nervous system, the first sign of tuberous sclerosis may be the development of infantile spasms, a seizure disorder of very young babies. In a follow-up study of 214 children with infantile spasms, Riikonen and Amnell (1981) found that 25 per cent of the children who had the combination of infantile spasms, infantile autism and normal levels of motor activity also had tuberous sclerosis. Infants with the tuberous sclerosis/infantile spasms syndrome may respond to treatment by ACTH, including in the non-depot form (Kussse *et al.* 1993).

Autism and pervasive developmental disorders are common in tuberous sclerosis, according to Smalley (1998); the frequency of autism is about 25 per cent. However many of the children with autistic symptoms fail to be diagnosed with tuberous sclerosis during the early years of life; they are simply called "autistic" (Reich *et al.* 1997). After five years, if a characteristic skin lesion (adenoma sebaceum) appears on the face, the underlying disease entity is revealed. Such children will, of course, be diagnosed earlier if they have an appropriate work-up for autism (see Chapter 16). Smalley *et al.* (1992) report that in published series of tuberous sclerosis patients, in whom behavioral manifestations have been studied, autistic features have been described in from 17 to 58 per cent of the subjects. The latter figure of 58 per cent was reported by Corbett and Hunt (1988) in a series of 88 children in England. In one population-based study of 28 patients with tuberous sclerosis, 17 met DSM-III-R criteria for autistic disorder (Gillberg *et al.* 1994). Conversely, looking at the problem from the point of view of the autistic syndromes, 1–4 per cent of autistic patients have tuberous sclerosis, with a higher percentage among those with a seizure disorder (Smalley 1998). The male predominance seen in other forms of autism does not occur in the cases of autism within the tuberous sclerosis complex (Franz 1998).

What determines whether a patient with tuberous sclerosis presents with autistic symptoms? Although not fully understood, the evidence suggests that, to become autistic, the child is most likely to have a location of subependymal calcifications and cortical tubers which includes the frontal and/or temporoparietal lobes (Calderon Gonzalez *et al.* 1994). Jambaqué *et al.* (1991) noted that posterior lesions, in addition to frontal-lobe dysfunction, were observed in children with autism; their cases had bilateral lesions. Bolton and Griffiths (1997) found a strong association between tubers in the temporal lobe and autism in individuals with tuberous sclerosis. Gutierrez *et al.* (1998) noted rates of social phobia and substance abuse elevated among first-degree relatives of tuberous sclerosis probands with autism, compared to first-degree relatives of those without autism.

Patients with tuberous sclerosis often have epilepsy, ranging from mild febrile seizures (Ritvo *et al.* 1990) to a major disabling form of epilepsy. Not all of the tubers in the brain of a child with tuberous sclerosis and seizures are epileptogenic; a new method has recently been developed to determine which of the tubers are the actual source of epileptogenic foci (Chugani *et al.* 1998).

Tuberous sclerosis is a genetically heterogeneous disorder with a high mutation rate. Approximately 40 per cent of cases are related to mutations in the TSC1 gene on chromosome 9 (9q34), and most of the remaining cases are associated with alteration of the TSC2 gene on chromosome 16 (16p13.3). Both of these genes have been cloned. The TSC1 gene encodes the protein tuberin, which appears to function as a growth suppressor. The TSC2 gene codes for hamartin, whose cellular function has not yet been described although its protein product may also function as a growth suppressor (Smalley 1998). Families segregating to TSC1 and TSC2 look clinically similar and it appears that the genes may interact or play a role in a common biochemical pathway involved in cell growth and/or differentiation, with autism a common behavioral feature of both mutations. A third locus for the disorder, suggested by a child with autism and tuberous sclerosis who had a *de novo* 3;12 translocation in the presence of parents with normal karyotypes (Fahsold *et al.* 1991) remains to be understood.

The function of the gene products encoded by these genes appears to contribute to tumorigenesis only when both alleles have been inactivated. In families with tuberous sclerosis where the pattern of inheritance appears to be dominant, the inactivation of only one of the alleles through inheritance is not sufficient to cause clinical symptoms. A "second hit" (somatic mutation), inactivating the other allele, is required (Millichap 1997).

Both type 1 and type 2 forms of tuberous sclerosis are classified in the Malformations of Cortical Development scheme as a malformation due to abnormal neuronal and glial proliferation I.B.3.a.1 (see Chapter 14).

UNILATERAL CEREBELLAR HYPOPLASIA SYNDROME

Cerebellar hypoplasia is found in some patients with autism but is usually bilateral. However there is a report of two unrelated male patients who had severe psychomotor retardation with autistic features and unilateral cerebellar hypoplasia (Ramaekers *et al.* 1997). They also both had microcephaly and ipsilateral choroideo-retinal coloboma.

VELOCARDIOFACIAL SYNDROME (VCFS) – "CATCH 22"

The velocardiofacial syndrome was described in 1978 by Shprintzen *et al.* It is also referred to as "CATCH 22" syndrome (cardiac anomalies, abnormal face, thymusaplasia, cleft palate, hypocalcemia and abnormality on chromosome 22). The major clinical features of this syndrome are cleft palate or velopharnygeal insufficiency, cardiac defects and a characteristic facial appearance (a long face, a prominent nose with a bulbous nasal tip and narrow alar base, almond-shaped or narrow palpebral fissures, malar flattening, recessed chin and malformed ears). However, these features are not always apparent during infancy and childhood. The patients usually have learning disabilities or mental retardation (IQs tend to range from 30–100, mostly 50–80) and problems with speech and language, particularly articulation problems characterized by retrograde air passage through the nose.

Neurobehavioral involvement is a major feature of velocardiofacial syndrome (VCFS) (Eliez *et al.* in press). Children tend to have a bland affect with little facial expression; their social interaction seems to be different in terms of quantity and quality (Golding-Kusher *et al.* 1985). Two cases of VCFS were identified in residential homes for people with autism (Swillen *et al.* 1996). A girl with autism and profound mental retardation has been described who has VCFS (Kozma 1998). A small, but important minority of all children with the CATCH-22 syndrome have autism or autistic-like conditions (Niklasson *et al.* 2000). A lack of "drive" and energy plus features of attention-deficit/hyperactivity disorder (mainly inattention) are typical of most affected children. A survey of 91 children who met DSM-III-R criteria for PDD identified one case of VCFS (Chudley *et al.* 1998). When individuals with VCFS reach late adolescence or early adulthood, they are also at risk for schizophrenia or psychosis; the current prevalence rate for schizophrenia in this patient group has been reported to be at least 20 per cent (Coleman and Gillberg 1996).

VCFS is reported to overlap with the DiGeorge syndrome on chromosomal analysis. Both syndromes have a majority of patients with microdeletions at the 22q11.21 locus. Deletions in the long arm of the 22nd chromosome are described in a number of patients with autism (see Chapter 15). The deleted region presumably contains numerous genes and it is unlikely that all of the genes play a major role in the development of the phenotypes associated with these disorders.

Individuals with Williams syndrome, also known as the elfin-face syndrome, usually appear to have a problem exactly the opposite of autism: over-friendliness. Yet this patient group does have several problems seen in autism, such as hyperacusis, social isolation and distractibility. They also have a tendency to talk repetitively about topics that focus their attention. Individuals with Williams syndrome have been reported to have autistic behavior (Gosch and Pankau 1994). Two children with Williams syndrome and classical autistic features have been described by Reiss *et al.* (1985) and several further by Gillberg and Rasmussen (1994); these children had elevation of whole blood serotonin levels. On the other hand, two children with Williams syndrome but no autism had normal levels of whole blood serotonin (August and Realmuto 1989).

Endocrine syndromes

HYPOTHYROIDISM

Infant hypothyroidism occurs in one out of every 639 live births. The autistic syndrome has been seen in babies with congenital hypothyroidism who have been diagnosed as autistic when as young as 6 to 9 months (Ritvo *et al.* 1990, Coleman, personal communication). Older children who meet the criteria of autism or Asperger syndrome are also reported in the literature (I.C. Gillberg *et al.* 1992, Barton and Volkmar 1998). Because of the relatively high prevalence of congenital hypothyroidism, it is hard to know in any individual case of the double syndrome whether or not it is coincidental.

However, hypothyroidism is tied to the autistic syndrome in another way. The parents of autistic children are more prone to hypothyroidism – a comparison of parents of 78 autistic children with the parents of age- and sex-matched controls showed a statistically significant increase in hypothyroidism in preconception history (Weidel and Coleman 1976). Another study has confirmed that there is a high incidence among families with children who have autism and Asperger syndrome (I.C. Gillberg *et al.* 1992). Hypothyroidism found in families of patients with autism adds to the debate about the putative relationship of autoimmunity and autism (see Chapter 13).

PITUITARY DEFICIENCY

Pituitary deficiency has been reported in two cases of autism to date. Ritvo *et al.* (1990) reported a case of pituitary deficiency diagnosed shortly after birth in a boy with autism. However, since he also had septal dysplasia, which caused a lack of development of the optic nerve with resulting blindness, this complicates the interpretation of his autistic symptoms. A 9-year-old boy who fulfilled all the criteria for the ICD-10 diagnosis of autism was found to have multiple pituitary deficiency (Gingell *et al.* 1996). There is a general study of hypothalamo-pituitary function in children with autism in the medical literature (Hoshino *et al.* 1984).

There is a case of a boy born with congenital adrenal hyperplasia and XYY chromosomal karyotype who was described as autistic (Mallin and Walker 1972).

Infectious syndromes

There is evidence that infectious diseases may injure the human brain both prenatally and after birth. Prenatal infections are a difficult area to evaluate. Often the damage done to the fetus bears no relation to the severity of the disease in the mother; sometimes a pregnant woman who has no obvious infection at all may still give birth to a child severely damaged by an infection. Because of the immaturity of the brain and its protective systems, fetuses and infants up to 1 year of age are at special risk for infections, particularly viral damage. Also, infectious etiologies, although rare, are candidates to consider in the differential diagnosis of autistic symptoms starting after 30 months of age, as will be seen from information available on rubella and herpes simplex encephalitis.

The role of prenatal infections in the etiology of psychiatric disease has been studied extensively. Although there is evidence that up to 4 per cent of individuals with schizophrenia may have been exposed *in utero* to influenza (at least in Denmark – for a full discussion see Coleman and Gillberg 1996), a similarly large study of exposure to influenza during gestation for patients with autism was negative (Dassa *et al.* 1995). To study the possibility of a number of different infectious etiologies in autism, Deykin and MacMahon (1979) performed a retrospective epidemiological study of 163 individuals with autism and 355 unaffected siblings, and found a statistically significant difference between "partially autistic" patients and siblings in prenatal exposure to, or clinical illness of the mother with, rubella. Barak *et al.* (1998) have published a study of the comorbidity of epilepsy in 290 children with autism; their annual birth pattern was interpreted to support the viral hypothesis because it fitted the seasonality of viral meningitis.

Studies of seasonal variation have turned up March as the month in which the incidence of births of children with autism is highest; the finding is consistent in different climates from North Carolina to Sweden (Gillberg 1990). In Israel, at yet a different latitude, an excess of March and August births was found in autistic patients in one study (Barak *et al.* 1995) while another study found no significant seasonal effects (Landau *et al.* 1999). One 35-year study from Denmark matched 328 children with childhood psychoses with controls born at the same time (Mouridsen *et al.* 1994). In this large study, an excess of March births for boys with infantile autism was found for the years 1951–6, 1963–8 and 1976–80. These studies raise the question of whether some environmental pathogen is operating only during certain periods of the year. In schizophrenia, February and March are high-risk months for births (Mortensen *et al.* 1999). Viral infections, which tend to occur in epidemics, are a major candidate. Could viral pandemics in those falls and winters prior to the March birthdays of children with autism affect susceptible fetuses?

RUBELLA

Rubella embryopathy is a disease on the run. Since rubella vaccination programs were begun in the USA in 1968, they have expanded to include many countries. When young girls receive the inoculation prior to childbearing age, the possibility of prenatal infection by rubella of their future fetuses is eliminated. Thus the epidemics of rubella that left behind disabled children, including children with autistic traits, should become a thing of the past. The last epidemic documented as causing a number of cases of full or partial autism (Chess *et al.* 1971) occurred in 1964. Unfortunately, children with autism and congenital rubella continue to appear in the medical literature (Fombonne *et al.* 1997, Barton and Volkmar 1998).

Several important observations came out of the study of the 1964 epidemic. One was that one-third of the children who met autistic criteria at 3 years of age had *recovered* by 7 years of age; they tended to be the least retarded ones (Chess *et al.* 1971). On the other hand, there was also the finding that four new cases of autism were identified after 3 years of age in this cohort, suggesting the chronic underlying presence of the infectious agent.

HERPES SIMPLEX VIRUS ENCEPHALITIS (HSV ENCEPHALITIS)

Herpes simplex virus encephalitis is the most frequent cause of fatal endemic or sporadic encephalitis occurring in humans (Johnson 1998). Most cases are due to herpes simplex virus type 1; a small number of cases are caused by herpes simplex virus type 2, especially in neonates and immunocompromised individuals. When the virus infects the brain, it has a predilection for the orbito-frontal and temporal lobes.

There are case reports of HSV encephalitis occurring during the neonatal period of patients with a later-diagnosed autistic syndrome (Ritvo *et al.* 1990, Ghaziuddin *et al.* 1991, Ghaziuddin *et al.* 1992a). Such children could have been infected during gestation, at birth passing through an infected birth canal, or in the immediate postnatal period. In the Ritvo *et al.* (1990) series, one of the patients had psychomotor seizures, severe hearing loss and scarring of the retina, and had a twin who died at 12 days of age from congenital herpes. In an extensive study of 78 older autistic children and matched controls, 25 per cent of the children with autism tested positive for HSV type 1 antibodies, compared to 13 per cent of their matched controls, a finding of unknown relevance (Peterson and Torrey 1976). Also in that same study, there were two boys, aged 4 and 8 years, who tested positive for antibodies to HSV type 2; their mothers also carried these antibodies; no controls had HSV type 2 antibodies.

There are several reports of healthy individuals who developed autistic symptoms during a herpes simplex encephalitis occurring after infancy. In 1981, Delong *et al.* described three children, aged between 5 and 11 years, who developed an acute encephalitis accompanied by autistic features which resolved after clinical recovery. One of the patients had a high serum herpes simplex titer with lesions of the temporal lobes as defined by CT; in the other two patients, no etiological agent was found. Gillberg (1986) has described a case of a girl of 14 years who developed an autistic syndrome following an attack of herpes encephalitis. The autistic symptoms persisted after the acute symptoms of the encephalitis subsided. Eight years later, a CT showed widespread bilateral destruction of brain parenchyma and the temporal lobes, with some medial involvement of the lower parts of the parietal lobes. There is also a report in the literature of a previously healthy man who contracted herpes encephalitis at the age of 31 years and over the following months developed all the symptoms considered diagnostic of autism (Gillberg 1991). These cases of HSV encephalitis are particularly interesting from a theoretical point of view because they met all the criteria for an autistic syndrome apart from the age criterion.

One other human herpes virus (no. 6) has had its antibody studied in a population of children with autism. Serum samples were provided nationwide by parents of autistic children in the USA. A high proportion (78 per cent) of the general population has positive titers of HHV-6 antibodies; the 48 children with autism under 12 years of age also had a high proportion (76 per cent), as did 34 normal controls (61 per cent) in this study (Singh *et al.* 1998).

CYTOMEGALOVIRUS (CMV)
It is not definitely established that CMV infections are an etiological agent in autism. The high frequency of CMV in newborns (up to 1 per cent) makes it more difficult to prove causality in any particular case. Congenital CMV infections have been reported in children with autism by several investigators (Markowitz 1983, Ritvo *et al.* 1990, Fattal-Valevski *et al.* 1999). A case was detected in a prospective study of congenital CMV infection in which 72 infants were followed for more than three years (Ahlfors *et al.* 1984). In another case, there was documentation of the maternal infection which suggested a primary infection shortly before the twentieth week of gestation (Ivarsson *et al.* 1990). There has been an attempt to treat one of these children with transfer factor immunotherapy (Stubbs *et al.* 1980). In many of the identified cases of congenital CMV infection and autism, there were also concomitant neurological disorders such as seizures or spasticity.

OTHER INFECTIOUS AGENTS
There are no other infections with enough cases to definitely establish other infectious etiologies for the autistic syndromes. However, since relatively few patients with autism have received detailed medical work-ups, it is premature to rule out any infectious agent. There are limited case reports of other infectious agents that have been associated with autism. Evidence for infections that are likely to be prenatal has been found in the cases of *Treponema pallidum* (syphilis) (Rutter and Bartak 1971, Knobloch and Pasamanick 1975), rubeola virus (Deykin and MacMahon 1979), *Toxoplasma gondii* (Rutter and Bartak 1971), varicella-zoster virus (Knobloch and Pasamanick 1975), parvovirus B19 (Anlar *et al.* 1994) and human immunodeficiency virus (Pizzo *et al.* 1991, Schmitt *et al.* 1991). A postnatal *Hemophilis influenzae* meningitis was reported by Knobloch and Pasamanick (1975), and in two children by Ritvo *et al.* (1990), and epiglotitis with this agent was found in an infant who developed autistic symptoms in the month following the infection (Gillberg *et al.* 1990).

Toxic syndromes
What is the role, if any, of toxic factors in the etiology of autism? There is a discussion of possible xenobiotic factors in autism in Chapter 13. In this section, the information on possible teratogens in autism will be reviewed.

FETAL ALCOHOL SYNDROME (FAS)

Intrauterine exposure to alcohol can have dramatic teratogenic effects. The mothers of the patients are older – average age 33 years. The hallmarks of the syndrome are pre- and postnatal growth retardation, characteristic facial dysmorphology and central nervous system dysfunction. In non-retarded adolescents with fetal alcohol syndrome (FAS), there are selective problems with social competence, behavior problems and school performance, compared to controls (Olson *et al*. 1998). In the brain, alcohol can interfere with the laying down of cerebral circuits, causing abnormal neuronal migration patterns in a number of brain regions, including the prefrontal cortex (Kopera-Frye *et al*. 1996). The fetal alcohol syndrome (FAS) is classified in the Malformations of Cortical Development scheme as malformations due to abnormal neuronal migration II.B.2.e.i (see Chapter 14).

Autism and autistic-like behaviors have been reported in children with FAS (Elia *et al*. 1990, Nanson 1992, Barton and Volkmar 1998). The children with autism are usually moderately or severely retarded. These reports of FAS/autism comprise all age ranges, including children as young as 25–36 months of age (Harris *et al*. 1995). Two children with FAS and Asperger syndrome have been described; in these cases, there was a clear correlation between the occurrence and severity of the neuropsychiatric disorder and the degree of alcohol exposure *in utero* (Aronson *et al*. 1997).

Because of the unfortunate fact that FAS is a relatively common problem, with frequencies of close to 1 in 500 live births in some countries, it is hard to know if the dual diagnosis in any particular child is coincidence or not. However, because alcohol does affect neuronal migration patterns in the fetus, and that neurodevelopmental anomaly is seen in some subgroups of autism (see Chapter 14), it is possible that, in some cases, FAS predisposes a fetus to autism.

FETAL COCAINE EXPOSURE

Based on a mouse model of transplacental cocaine exposure, there is evidence that gestational cocaine exposure disrupts neocortical cytoarchitecture in animals, persisting throughout their lifespan (Ren *et al*. 1998). The pattern of brain malformations following prenatal cocaine exposure may also involved the midline of the brainstem (Leong and Ashwell 1997) if cocaine is ingested during the sixth or seventh week of fetal development.

There has been controversy about whether fetal cocaine exposure causes autism and, if so, what percentage of children are affected. The reason for this debate is that in some studies the ingested dose of cocaine varied greatly, making the amount difficult to pinpoint, and the mothers had often taken multiple drugs, making it hard to implicate a single drug as the teratogen. The debate has not been fully resolved. However, a detailed study published in the *Journal of the National Medical Association* has shown that a high level of autism (11.2 per cent) was reported in a series of 70 inner-city children after fetal exposure to cocaine (Davis *et al.* 1992). The authors raise a question about whether cocaine has specific effects different from alcohol or opiates.

FETAL VALPROATE EXPOSURE

Koch *et al.* (1996) studied the relationship between valproic acid during pregnancy and outcome of the fetuses in later life. They reported that the degree of neonatal hyper-excitability and neurological dysfunction, found at a six-year follow-up, correlated with the valproate concentrations at birth. These authors suggest that valproic acid-induced malformations and neurobehavioral and late neurological side-effects may be related to unexpectedly high levels of the drug and its active metabolites during both gestation and the perinatal period.

Cases have been reported in the literature of children with autism who were exposed *in utero* to valproic acid (Christianson *et al.* 1994, Williams and Hersh 1997).

LEAD POISONING

Lead poisoning has been described in a number of children with autism (Cohen *et al.* 1976, Accardo *et al.* 1988, Barton and Volkmar 1998). Since some of these children suffer from pica, it is often impossible to untangle information about whether the autism or the lead poisoning occurred first. There is one case in the literature in which a child with an elevated blood lead level appeared to have improvement of his repetitive behaviors and hyperactivity during the period when he received the chelating agent succimer during an on-again, off-again trial of this agent (Eppright *et al.* 1996). Unfortunately, in most cases, the brain damage from lead is already irreversible by the time it is detected.

Of great worry is the fact that children with the autistic syndromes are at increased risk of repeated lead poisonings. A study of re-exposure to lead poisoning in 17 children with PDD, including autism, found a much higher percentage of them were re-exposed compared to non-PDD children (Shannon and Graef 1996).

THALIDOMIDE EMBRYOPATHY

In a study of 100 cases of thalidomide embryopathy in Sweden, four cases met the full criteria for DSM-III-R autistic disorder and ICD-10 childhood autism (Stromland *et al.* 1994). It was estimated that the toxicity occurred 20 to 24 days after conception in the four individuals who were autistic.

Syndromes with multiple etiologies

Some non-specific syndromes are based on final-common-pathway injuries in the central nervous system of the fetus or young infant. The visual system, the auditory system or the motor system of the child may be damaged. Many of these patients with non-specific syndromes are complex etiological puzzles. Patients with autism are found among them. Visual and hearing deficits may be common in autism; actual blindness and deafness are much rarer (Steffenburg 1991).

BLINDNESS AND OTHER VISUAL PROBLEMS

Ocular problems that affect vision are often found in children with autism. In a population-based survey by Steffenburg (1991), 50 per cent of children with autism or autistic-like disorders whose vision could be properly evaluated had a refraction error – mostly hypermetropia, but myopia and astigmatism were also found. Many abnormalities of visual function have been recorded in a sample of children with autism – saccadic fixations, abnormal saccadic eye movements (Kemner *et al.* 1998), atypical optokinetic nystagmus, absent voluntary pursuit movements, etc. (Scharre and Creedon 1992).

A variety of eye disorders have been recorded in children with an autistic syndrome – septo-optic dysplasia (Ritvo *et al.* 1990), atrophy of the optic nerve (Ritvo *et al.* 1990), retinitis pigmentosa (Ritvo *et al.* 1990) and retinal degeneration/mottled retina (Cohen syndrome – see above). One study of retinal pathology, as detected by electroretinogram, showed a remarkably high number of patients with autism – 13 out of 27 – who had subnormal b-wave amplitudes (Ritvo *et al.* 1988).

A small percentage of totally blind children also suffer from an autistic syndrome (Fombonne *et al.* 1997). One form of blindness associated with autism is Leber's congenital amaurosis. It is a clinically and genetically heterogeneous autosomal recessive retinal dystrophy and the most common genetic cause of congenital visual impairment. The behavioral characteristics of five preschool boys with Leber congenital amaurosis were compared with those of five preschool boys who had been blind from birth from other causes (Rogers and Newhart-Larson 1989). The boys with Leber congenital amaurosis met criteria for infantile autism. Defects in cerebellar structure have been reported in some Leber patients (Yano *et al.* 1998). For those children who are autistic, they are reported to be more disabled by their autism – difficulties with social relatedness – than by their blindness (Boye *et al.* 1999). A case of morning glory syndrome has been reported in an autistic child (Nawratzki *et al.* 1985).

Congenitally blind children, especially with the retinopathy of prematurity (ROP), have been described as having a higher incidence of autistic symptoms such as unresponsivity and stereotypic object manipulation, which emerge between 12 and 30 months (Janson 1993, Goodman and Minne 1995). One controlled population-based study confirmed increased autism in ROP (Ek *et al.* 1998). Another study comparing congenitally blind non-autistic children and autistic children found substantial overlap in their clinical presentations (Brown *et al.* 1997).

Hobson *et al.* (1999) recently compared nine congenitally blind children, with a clinical picture that resembled the syndrome of autism, to a group of sighted autistic children. They concluded that, on the one hand, the study established that there is indeed a syndrome closely akin to (and perhaps identical with) that of early childhood autism in congenitally blind children, and that it is not confined to specific medical diagnoses. On the other hand, the findings left open the possibility that, at least in a proportion of the blind children, there might be a qualitative difference in the nature of the children's "autism," perhaps especially in the social-affective and pretend-play domains.

Deafness and Other Auditory Problems
In any non-speaking child with an autistic syndrome, part of the most basic work-up is to rule out deafness (see Chapter 16).

Auditory impairment at various levels is often a real problem in a child with autism. In a population-based survey by Steffenburg (1991), 24 per cent of children with autism or autistic-like disorders had a hearing deficit of more than 25dB. Although many of the auditory processing problems in autism are thought to be central in origin, a review of 11 auditory brainstem response studies in autism have revealed the presence of peripheral hearing impairment in a non-negligible number of individuals with autism (Klin 1993). Otitis media may be a contributory factor in such cases (Konstantareas and Homatidis 1987).

Major problems with auditory processing exist in most children with autism. One interesting study evaluating the theory-of-mind hypothesis raised the question of whether poor auditory processing, auditory inattention or actual lack of exposure to adequate conversation underlies the failure of autistic children in theory-of-mind studies. It was found that 65 per cent of a group of 26 signing, prelingually-deaf children of normal social and cognitive intelligence, aged 8 to 13 years, failed a simple test of false belief which normal preschoolers and mentally retarded children (apart from children with autism) routinely pass at a mental age of 4–5 years (Peterson and Siegal 1995).

Co-occurrence of full deafness and infantile autism has been reported (Ritvo *et al.* 1990, Gordon 1991, Fombonne *et al.* 1997). Congenital rubella infection is one etiology of a deaf child with autism (Chess *et al.* 1971). These dually disabled children are the ultimate challenge to their teachers.

CEREBRAL PALSY

Cerebral palsy is a motor impairment resulting from brain pathology that is non-progressive and is manifested in early childhood. The exact etiology of cerebral palsy is not known in many patients. Factors that appear to be involved in this syndrome include gestational infections, gestational coagulation disorders and birth asphyxia. In one epidemiological survey, 9 out of 831 children (1 per cent) with cerebral palsy were found to have classic autistic symptoms (Fombonne *et al.* 1997). However, in another study of the prevalence of the more inclusive autism spectrum disorders, 10.5 per cent of the children with cerebral palsy were found to have autistic-like symptoms (Nordin and Gillberg 1996).

There is a case in the medical literature of a child with spasticity and choreoathetosis who was described as having "social contact practically absent." The child also had self-mutilation and increased excretion of uric acid at 35 to 45 mg/kg/24 hours. A low purine diet (see Chapter 17) was said to result in "an undeniable improvement in the child's condition . . . whereas she had previously taken no interest in the outside world, she now even smiled at her parents" (Hooft *et al.* 1968).

Some children with hemiplegic cerebral palsy show marked social interaction problems, and, depending on the side of the brain lesion, a "non-verbal learning disability" or "right hemisphere syndrome," clinically similar to Asperger syndrome (Gillberg, unpublished data, 2000). Another subgroup of children with "cerebral palsy," clinically characterized by ataxia, often show marked autistic features (Gillberg and Åhsgren, unpublished data).

169

Single case reports

Aarskog syndrome – autism has been described in the facio-digito-genital syndrome of Aarskog (Assumpcao *et al.* 1999).

Achondroplasia – a child with achondroplasia and concurrent autistic symptoms has been observed by one of us (CG).

Adrenomyeloneuropathy (AMN) – a clinical subgroup of adrenoleukodystrophy-X-linked is called adrenomyeloneuropathy (AMN). It is a severely disabling disease usually with symptoms that resemble schizophrenia or dementia combined with spasticity and ataxia (Coleman and Gillberg 1996). A patient placed in a residential home because of an autistic syndrome was found to have AMN (Swillen *et al.* 1996).

Basal cell nevus syndrome – the gene responsible for this syndrome has been found to be involved in the development of primitive neuroectodermal tumors of the central nervous system (Wolter *et al.* 1997). An individual placed in a residential home because of an autistic syndrome was diagnosed as having basal cell nevus syndrome (Swillen *et al.* 1996).

Biedl–Bardet syndrome – classical autistic symptoms have been described in a case with the Biedl–Bardet syndrome (Gillberg and Wahlström 1985).

Ceroid storage disease – a patient placed in a residential home because of an autistic syndrome has been diagnosed with ceroid storage disease (Swillen *et al.* 1996).

Congenital muscular dystrophy – a case report of a 12-year-old child with early infantile autism and congenital muscular dystrophy (subtype IV, Fukuyama classification) is reported in the literature (Saccomani *et al.* 1992).

Coffin–Lowry syndrome – Coffin–Lowry syndrome (CLS) is an X-linked disorder characterized by facial dysmorphisms, mild to severe cognitive impairment and skeletal anomalies. The gene located at Xp22.2 is mutated in this syndrome (Trivier *et al.* 1996). Recent studies have shown that the gene (Rsk-2) encodes a growth-factor-regulated protein – CREB (cyclic adenosine monophosphate response element binding protein) kinase (Harum *et al.* 1998). There is a case of comorbidity with autism (Bryson *et al.* 1988).

Coffin–Siris syndrome – a girl with the Coffin–Siris syndrome has been reported to have autistic behavior (Hersh *et al.* 1982).

Neurogenic diabetes insipidus – a 33-year-old man with Asperger syndrome was found to have neurogenic diabetes insipidus associated with a primary empty sella (meaning that his pituitary gland was flattened). His response to vasopressin treatment suggested a concomitant presence of primary polydipsia (Raja *et al.* 1998).

Duchenne muscular dystrophy – a child with Duchenne muscular dystrophy was reported to have autistic symptoms (Komoto *et al.* 1984).

Laurence–Moon–Biedl syndrome – the Lawrence–Moon–Biedl syndrome has been described in a patient who met DSM-III-R criteria for autism (Steffenburg 1991).

Oculocutaneous albinism – a 4-year-old boy with oculocutaneous albinism and autism has been described by Orntiz *et al.* (1977).

Peters' plus syndrome – an individual who was placed in a residential home because of an autistic syndrome has been found to have Peters' plus syndrome (Swillen *et al.* 1996).

Prader Willi syndrome – in a girl with the Prader Willi syndrome and autism, the karyotype showed 45,XX and had a balanced Robertsonian translocation t(15q22) (Arrieta *et al.* 1994). The same translocation was present in her healthy relatives – mother, maternal grandfather, sister and a brother. No cytogenetic deletions of the paternal chromosome 15 could be identified. The relationship between the long arm of the 15th chromosome and autism is a story in itself (see Chapter 15).

Spina bifida occulta – a female with autism and an IQ of 77 was reported by Ritvo *et al.* (1990) to have a congenital skeletal anomaly, spina bifida occulta.

Trichothiodystrophy – there is a single case report of a patient with both tricho-thiodystrophy, a brittle hair syndrome, and autism. The patient also had mental retardation and seizures. Frontal and occipital hair was affected (Schepis *et al.* 1997).

Xeroderma pigmentosa – A boy of 4 years of Korean ancestry had xeroderma pigmentosa and multiple cutaneous neoplasms including melanoma (Khan *et al.* 1998). He also had autistic features and hyperactivity without typical xeroderma pigmentosa neurologic abnormalities. The boy suffered from hypoglycinemia. A molecular biological study revealed a complementation group C slice mutation. (The most important diagnostic assay for xeroderma pigmentosa is the unscheduled DNA synthesis (UDS) test. Comple-mentation group C includes patients who are moderately to severely sun-sensitive.)

Conclusion

The double syndromes vividly demonstrate the complexity of accurate diagnosis, which is the first step in preparing an educational/therapeutic stratagem for a child with autism. The double syndromes also help to illustrate some of the neuropathological hypotheses that may apply in the autistic syndromes. Examples of factors that may be more likely to be associated with autism are:

- *Full expression of the genetic defect* – fragile X cases with full expression are more likely to be autistic than those with mosaicism.
- *Full expression of the clinical phenotype* – patients with Tourette/Asperger syndromes have a more involved form of the Tourette syndrome by history, physical and laboratory criteria.
- *Lesions are often bilateral* – the anatomic location of tubers in tuberous sclerosis demonstrate bilaterality in patients who are also autistic.
- *Immaturity or actual abnormal development of cranial nerve nuclei during the first trimester may be a factor in mutism* – this possibility may be relevant to Moebius syndrome, Smith–Magenis syndrome and thalidomide babies who are autistic.
- *Malformations of cortical development* (formerly listed as neuronal migration

patterns) *that occur during the second trimester can be found in autistic subgroups –* this possibility occurs in the fetal alcohol syndrome and possibly in other toxic syndromes.

REFERENCES

Abitbol, M., Menini, C., Delezoide, A.L., Rhymer, T., Vekemans, M., Mallet, J. (1993) 'Nucleus basalis magnocellularis and hippocampus are the major sites of FMR-1 expression in the human fetal brain.' *Nature Genetics*, **4**, 147–153.

Accardo, P., Whitman, B., Caul, J., Rolfe, U. (1988) 'Autism and plumbism.' *Clinical Pediatrics*, **27**, 41–44.

Ahlfors, K., Ivarsson, S.A., Harris, S., Svanberg, L., Holmqvist, R., Lernmark, B., Theander, G. (1984) Congenital cytomegalovirus infection and disease in Sweden and the relative importance of primary and secondary infections. *Scandinavian Journal of Infectious Diseases*, **16**, 129–137.

Åkefeldt, A., Gillberg, C. (1991) 'Hypomelanosis of Ito in three cases with autism and autistic-like conditions.' *Developmental Medicine and Child Neurology*, **33**, 737–743.

Akesson, H.O. (1997) 'Rett syndrome: the Swedish Genealogic Research Project, new data and present position.' *European Child and Adolescent Psychiatry*, **6**(Suppl. 1): 96–98.

American Psychiatric Association. (1987) *Diagnostic and Statistical Manual of Mental Disorders. 3rd Edn (Revised).* Washington, DC: APA.

Amir, R.E., Van den Veyver, I.B., Wan, M., Tran, C.Q., Francke, U., Zoghbi, H.Y. (1999) 'Rett syndrome is caused by mutations in X-linked MECP2, encoding methyl-CpG-binding protein 2.' *Nature Genetics* **23**, 1185–1188.

Andermann, F. (1995) 'Autism, macrocrania and epilepsy: a syndrome?' *Brain Development*, **17**, 362.

Anlar, B., Oktem, F., Torak, T. (1994) 'Human parvovirus B19 antibodies in infantile autism.' *Journal of Child Neurology*, **9**, 104–105.

Armstrong, D.D., Dunn, K., Antalffy, B. (1998) 'Decreased dendritic branching in frontal, motor and limbic cortex in Rett syndrome compared with trisomy 21.' *Journal of Neuropathology and Experimental Neurology*, **57**, 1013–1017.

Aronson, M., Hagberg, B., Gillberg, C. (1997) 'Attention deficits and autistic spectrum problems in children exposed to alcohol during gestation: a follow-up study.' *Developmental Medicine and Child Neurology*, **39**, 583–587.

Arrieta, I., Lobato, M.N., Martinez, B., Criado, B. (1994) 'Parental origin of Robertsonian translocation (15q22) and Prader Willi associated with autism.' *Psychiatric Genetics*, **4**, 63–65.

Asarnow, J.R., Ben-Meir, S. (1988) 'Children with schizophrenia spectrum and depressive disorders: a comparative study of premorbid adjustment, onset, pattern and severity of impairment.' *Journal of Child Psychology and Psychiatry*, **29**, 477–488.

Assumpcao, F., Santos, R.C., Rosario, M., Mercadante, M. (1999) 'Brief report: Autism and Aarskog syndrome.' *Journal of Autism and Developmental Disorders*, **29**, 179–181.

August, G.J., Realmuto, G.M. (1989) 'Williams syndrome: serotonin's association with developmental disabilities.' *Journal of Autism and Developmental Disorders*, **19**, 137–141.

Bailey, A., Luthert, P., Bolton, P, Le Couteur, A., Rutter, M., Harding, B. (1993) 'Autism and megalencephaly.' *Lancet*, **341**, 1225–1226.

Bailey, A., Le Couteur, A., Gottesman, I., Bolton, P., Simonoff, E., Yudza, E., Rutter, M. (1995) Autism as a strongly genetic disorder: evidence from a British twin study. *Psychological Medicine*, **25**, 63–77.

Barabas, G., Mathews, W.S. (1983) 'Coincident infantile autism and Tourette syndrome: a case study.' *Journal of Developmental and Behavioral Pediatrics*, **4**, 280–282.

Barak, Y., Ring, A., Sulkes, J., Gabbay, U., Elizur, A. (1995) 'Season of birth and autistic disorder in Israel.' *American Journal of Psychiatry*, **152**, 798–800.

Barak, Y., Kimhi, R., Stein, D., Gutman, J., Weizman, A. (1998) 'Autistic subjects with comorbid epilepsy: a possible association with viral infections.' *Child Psychiatry and Human Development*, **29**, 245–251.

Baron-Cohen, S., Mortimore, C., Moriarty, J., Izaguirre, J., Robertson, M. (1999a) 'The prevalence of Gilles de la Tourette's syndrome in children and adolescents with autism.' *Journal of Child and Adolescent Psychiatry*, **40**, 213–218.

172

Baron-Cohen, S., Scahill, V.L., Izaguirre, J., Hornsey, H., Robertson, M.M. (1999b) 'The prevalence of Gilles de la Tourette syndrome in children and adolescents with autism: a large scale study.' *Psychological Medicine*, **29**, 1151–1159.

Barton, M., Volkmar, F. (1998) 'How commonly are known medical conditions associated with autism?' *Journal of Autism and Developmental Disorders*, **28**, 273–278.

Bauman, M.L. (1996) 'Brief report: Neuroanatomic observations of the brain in pervasive developmental disorders.' *Journal of Autism and Developmental Disorders*, **26**, 199–203.

Baumgartner, M.R., Poll-The, B.T., Verhoeven, N.M., Jakobs, C., Espeel, M., Roels, F., Rabier, D., Levade, T., Rolland, M.O., Mortinez, M., Wanders, R.J., Sandubray, J.M. (1998) Clinical approach to inherited peroxisomal disorders: a series of 27 patients. *Annals of Neurology*, **44**, 720–730.

Bay, C., Mauk, J., Radcliffe, J., Kaplan, P. (1993) 'Mild Brachmann–de Lange syndrome. Delineation of the clinical phenotype and characteristic behaviors in a six-year-old boy.' *American Journal of Medical Genetics*, **47**, 965–968.

Belichenko, P.V., Hagberg, B., Dahlstrom, A. (1997) 'Morphological study of neocortical areas in Rett syndrome.' *Acta Neuropathica (Berl)*, **93**, 50–61.

Benda, C.E. (1960) 'Childhood schizophrenia, autism and Heller's disease.' *In: Proceedings of the First International Metabolic Conference, Portland ME*. New York: Grune & Stratton.

Berry, H.K., O'Grady, D.J., Perlmutter, L.J., Bofinger, M.K. (1979) 'Intellectual development and academic achievement of children treated early for phenylketonuria.' *Developmental Medicine and Child Neurology*, **21**, 311–320.

Berthier, M.L., Santamaria, J., Encabo, H., Tolosa, E.S. (1992) 'Recurrent hypersomnia in two adolescent males with Asperger's syndrome.' *Journal of the American Academy of Child and Adolescent Psychiatry*, **31**, 735–736.

Berthier. M.L., Bayes, A., Tolosa, E.S. (1993) 'Magnetic resonance imaging in patients with concurrent Tourette's disorder and Asperger's syndrome.' *Journal of the American Academy of Child and Adolescent Psychiatry*, **32**, 633–639.

Blaser, M.E., Mautner, V.F., Ragge, N.K., Nechiporkuk, A., Riccardi, V.M., Klein, J., Sainz, J. (1996) Presymptomatic diagnosis of neurofibromatosis 2 using linked genetic markers, neuroimaging and ocular examinations. *Neurology*, **47**, 1269–1277.

Blondis, T.A., Cook, E. Jr., Koza-Taylor, P., Finn, T. (1996) 'Asperger syndrome associated with Steinert's myotonic dystrophy.' *Developmental Medicine and Child Neurology*, **38**, 840–847.

Blue, M.E., Naidu, S., Johnstone, M.V. (1999) 'Development of amino acid receptors in frontal cortex from girls with Rett syndrome.' *Annals of Neurology*, **45**, 541–545.

Bolton, P.F., Griffiths, P.D. (1997) 'Association of tuberous sclerosis of temporal lobes with autism and atypical autism.' *Lancet*, **349**, 392–395.

Bolton, M., Volmar, F. (1998) 'How commonly are known medical conditions associated with autism?' *Journal of Autism and Developmental Disorders*, **28**, 273–278.

Boye, H., Etting, A.M., Jorgensen, O.S. (1999) 'Comorbidity of infantile autism and blindness.' (In Danish) *Ugeskrift for Laeger*, **161**, 800–801.

Bregman, J.D., Volkmar, F.R. (1988) 'Autistic social dysfunction and Down syndrome.' *Journal of the American Academy of Child and Adolescent Psychiatry*, **27**, 440–441.

Brown, M.D., Voljavec, A.S., Lott, M.T., MacDonald, I., Wallace, D.C. (1992) Leber's hereditary optic neuropathy: a model for mitochondrial neurodegenerative diseases. *Federation of American Societies for Experimental Biology (FASEB) Journal*, **6**, 2791–2799.

Brown, R., Hobson, R.P., Lee, A., Stevenson, J. (1997) 'Are there "autistic-like" features in congenitally blind children?' *Journal of Child Psychology and Psychiatry*, **38**, 693–703.

Bryson, S.E., Clark, B.S., Smith, I.M. (1988) 'First report of a Canadian epidemiologic study of autistic syndromes.' *Journal of Child Psychology and Psychiatry*, **29**, 433–445.

Burd, L., Fisher, W.W., Kerbeshian, J., Arnold, M.E. (1987) 'Is the development of Tourette disorder a marker for improvement in patients with autism and other pervasive developmental disorders?' *Journal of the American Academy of Child and Adolescent Psychiatry*, **26**, 162–165.

Burroni, L., Aucone, A.M., Volterrani, D., Hayek, Y., Bertelli, P., Vella, A., Zapella, M., Vattimo, A. (1997) 'Brain perfusion abnormalities in Rett syndrome: a qualitative and quantitative SPET study with 99Tc(m)-ECD.' *Nuclear Medicine Communications*, **18**, 527–534.

Calderon Gonzalez, R., Trevion Welsh, J., Calderon Sepulveda, A. (1994) 'Autism in tuberous sclerosis.' (In Spanish) *Gaceta Medica de Mexico*, **130**, 374–349.

Campbell, M., Hardesty, A.S., Burdock, E.I. (1978) 'Demographic and perinatal profile of 105 autistic children: a preliminary report.' *Psychopharmacology Bulletin*, **14**, 36–39.

Capone, G.T., Lee, R.R. (1999) 'Children with Down syndrome and autistic features: MRI and neurologic findings.' Personal communication.

Chen, C.H., Hsiao, K.J. (1989) 'A Chinese classic phenylketonuria manifested as autism.' *British Journal of Psychiatry*, **155**, 251–253.

Chess, S. (1977) 'Follow–up report on autism in congenital rubella.' *Journal of Autism and Childhood Schizophrenia*, **7**, 68–81.

Chess, S., Korn, S.J., Fernandez, P.B. (1971) *Psychiatric Disorders of Children with Congenital Rubella.* New York: Bruner Mazel.

Christianson, A.L., Chesler, N., Kromberg, J.G. (1994) 'Fetal valproate syndrome. Clinical and neurodevelopmental features in two sibling pairs.' *Developmental Medicine and Child Neurology*, **36**, 357–369.

Chudley, A.E., Gutierrez, E., Jocelyn, L.J., Chodirker, B.N. (1998) 'Outcomes of genetic evaluation in children with pervasive developmental disorder.' *Journal of Developmental and Behavioral Pediatrics*, **19**, 321–325.

Chugani, D.C., Chugani, H.T., Muzik, O., Shah, J.R., Shah, A.K., Canady, A., Mangner, T.J., Chakraborty, P.K. (1998) 'Imaging epileptic tubers in children with tuberous sclerosis using α-[^{11}C]methyl-L-tryptophan positron emission tomography.' *Annals of Neurology*, **44**, 858–866.

Cohen, D.J., Johnson, W.T., Caparulo, B.K. (1976) 'Pica and elevated blood lead levels in autistic and atypical children.' *American Journal of the Diseases of Children*, **130**, 47–48.

Cohen, I.L., Sudhalter, V., Pfadt, A., Jenkins, E.C., Brown, W.T., Vietze, P.M. (1991) 'Why are autism and the fragile X syndrome associated? Conceptual and methodological issues. *American Journal of Human Genetics*, **48**, 195–202.

Cohen, I.L., Nolin, S.L., Sudhalter, V., Ding, X.H, Dobkin, C.S., Brown, W.T. (1996) 'Mosaicism for the FMR1 gene influences adaptive skills development in fragile X-affected males.' *American Journal of Medical Genetics*, **64**, 365–369.

Cohen, M.M., Rollnick, B.R., Kaye, C.I. (1989) 'Oculo-auriculovertebral spectrum: an update critique.' *Cleft Palate Journal*, **26**, 276–286.

Coleman, M. (Ed.) (1976) *The Autistic Syndromes.* Amsterdam: North-Holland and New York: Elsevier.

—— (1986) 'Down's syndrome children with autistic features.' *Down's Syndrome: Papers and Abstracts for Professionals*, **9**, 1–2.

—— (1990) 'Is classical Rett syndrome ever present in males?' *Brain and Development*, **12**, 31–32.

Coleman, M., Abassi, V. (1984) 'Down's syndrome and hypothyroidism: coincidence or consequence.' *Lancet*, **i**, 569.

Coleman, M., Gillberg, C. (1996) *The Schizophrenias.* New York: Springer.

Collacott, R.A., Cooper, S.-A., McGrother, C. (1992) 'Differential rates of psychiatric disorders in adults with Down's syndrome compared to other mentally handicapped adults.' *British Journal of Psychiatry*, **161**, 671–674.

Comings, D.E., Comings, B.G. (1991) 'Clinical and genetic relationships between autism-pervasive developmental disorder and Tourette syndrome: a study of 19 cases.' *American Journal of American Genetics*, **39**, 180–191.

Corbett, J., Hunt, A. (1988) 'Recent research on tuberous sclerosis.' *Journal of the Royal Society of Medicine*, **81**, 481–482.

Cox, J.F., Sedlacek, Z., Bachner, D., Delius, H., Poustka, A. (1999) 'A complex pattern of evolutionary conservation and alternative polyadenylation within the long 3′-untranslated region of the methyl-CpG-binding protein 2 gene (MeCP2) suggests a regulatory role in gene expression.' *Human Molecular Genetics*, **8**, 1253–1262.

Coy, I.F., Sedlacek, Z., Bachner, D., Delius, H., Poustka, A. (1999) 'A complex pattern of evolutionary conservation and alternative polyadenylation within the 3′-untranslated region of the methyl-CpG-binding protein 2 gene (MeCP2) suggests a regulatory role in gene expression.' *Human Molecular Genetics*, **8**, 1253–1262.

Dassa, D., Takei, N., Sham, P.C., Murray, R.M. (1995) 'No association between prenatal exposure to influenza and autism.' *Acta Psychiatrica Scandinavica*, **92**, 145–149.

Davidovitch, M., Patterson, B., Gartside, P. (1996) 'Head circumference measurements in children with autism.' *Journal of Child Neurology*, **11**, 398–393.

174

Davis, E., Fennoy, I., Laraque, D., Kanem, N., Brown, G., Mitchell, J. (1992) 'Autism and developmental abnormalities in children with perinatal cocaine exposure.' *Journal of the National Medical Association*, **84**, 315–319.

Deb, S., Bramble, D., Drybabla, G., Boyle, A., Bruce, J. (1994) 'Polydipsia amongst adults with learning disability in an institution.' *Journal of Intellectual Disability Research*, **38**, 359–367.

De Bona, C., Zappella, M., Hayek, G., Meloni, I., Vitelli, F., Bruttini, M., Cusano, R., Loffredo, P., Longo, I., Renieri, A. (in press) 'Preserved speech variant is allelic of classic Rett syndrome.' *European Journal of Human Genetics.*

DeLong, G.R., Bean, S.C., Brown, F.R. (1981) 'Acquired reversible autistic syndrome in acute encephalopathic illness in children.' *Archives of Neurology*, **38**, 191–194.

Deykin, E.Y., MacMahon, G. (1979) 'Viral exposure and autism.' *American Journal of Epidemiology*, **109**, 628–638.

D'Mello, S.R. (1998) 'Molecular regulation of neuronal apoptosis.' *Current Topics in Developmental Biology*, **39**, 187–213.

Dykens, E.M., Smith, A.C. (1998) 'Distinctiveness and correlates of maladaptive behavior in children and adolescents with Smith–Magenis syndrome.' *Journal of Intellectual Disability Research*, **42**, 481–489.

Dykens, E.M., Volkmar, F.R. (1997) 'Medical conditions associated with autism.' *In:* Cohen, D.J., Volkmar, F.R. (Eds) *Handbook of Autism and Pervasive Developmental Disorders. 2nd Edn.* New York: Wiley, pp. 388–410.

Eeg-Olofsson, O., al-Zuhair, A.G., Teebi, A.S., al-Essa, M.M. (1988) 'Abnormal mitochondria in the Rett syndrome.' *Brain Development*, **10**, 260–262.

Ehlers, S., Gillberg, C. (1993) 'The epidemiology of Asperger syndrome. A total population study.' *Journal of Child Psychology and Psychiatry*, **34**, 1327–1350.

Ek, U., Fernell, E., Jacobson, L., Gillberg, C. (1998) 'Relation between blindness due to retinopathy of prematurity and autistic spectrum disorders: a population based study.' *Developmental Medicine and Child Neurology*, **40**, 297–301.

Elia, M., Bergonzi, P., Ferri, R., Musumeci, S.A., Paladino, A., Panerai, S., Ragusa, R.M. (1990) 'The etiology of autism in a group of mentally retarded subjects.' *Brain Dysfunction*, **3**, 228–240.

Eliez, S., Palacio-Espasa, F., Spira, A., Lacroix, M., Pont, C., Luthi, F., Robert-Tissot, C., Feinstein, C., Antonarakis, S.E., Cramer, B. (in press) 'Young children with Velo-Cardio-Facial syndrome. Psychological and language phenotypes.' *European Child and Adolescent Psychiatry.*

Eppright, T.D., Sanfacon, J.A., Horwitz, E.A. (1996) 'Attention deficit hyperactivity disorder, infantile autism and elevated blood-lead levels: a possible relationship.' *Molecular Medicine*, **93**, 136–138.

Fahsold, R., Rott, H.D., Claussen, U., Schmalenberger, B. (1991) 'Tuberous sclerosis in a child with de novo translocation t(3:12)(p26.3)(p23.3).' *Clinical Genetics*, **40**, 326–328.

Failla, P., Romano, C., Schepis, C. (1997) 'Hypomelanosis of Ito: a syndrome requiring a multisystem approach.' *Australia's Journal of Dermatology*, **38**, 65–70.

Fattal-Valevski, A., Kramer, U., Leitner, Y., Nevo, Y., Greenstein, Y., Harel, S. (1999) 'Characterization and comparison of autistic subgroups: 10 years' experience with autistic children.' *Developmental Medicine and Child Neurology*, **41**, 21–25.

Fehlow, P., Bernstein, K., Tennstedt, A., Walther, F. (1993) 'Early infantile autism and excessive aerophagy with symptomatic megacolon and ileus in a case of Ehlers–Danlos syndrome.' (In German) *Padiatrie und Grenzgebiete*, **31**, 259–267.

Feinstein, C., Reiss, A.L. (1998) 'Autism: the point of view from fragile X studies.' *Journal of Autism and Developmental Disorders*, **28**, 393–405.

Fernell, E., Olsson, V.A., Karlgren-Leitner, C., Norlin, B., Hagberg, B., Gillberg, C. (1999) 'Autistic disorders in children with CHARGE association.' *Developmental Medicine and Child Neurology*, **41**, 270–272.

Finucane, B.M., Konor, D., Haas-Givler, B., Kurtz, M.B., Scott, C.I. Jr. (1994) 'The spasmodic upper-body squeeze: a characteristic behavior in the Smith–Magenis syndrome.' *Developmental Medicine and Child Neurology*, **36**, 70–83.

Fisman, S., Steele, M., Short, J., Byrne, T., Lavallee, C. (1996) 'Case study: anorexia nervosa and autistic disorder in an adolescent girl.' *Journal of the American Academy of Child and Adolescent Psychiatry*, **35**, 937–940.

Fombonne, E., du Mazaubrun, C. (1992) 'Prevalence of infantile autism in four French regions.' *Soc Psychiatr Epidemiol*, **27**, 203–210.

Fombonne, E., du Mazaubrun, C., Cans, C., Grandjean, H. (1997) 'Autism and associated medical disorders in a French epidemiological survey.' *Journal of the American Academy of Child and Adolescent Psychiatry*, **36**, 1561–1569.

Franz, D.N. (1998) 'Diagnosis and management of tuberous sclerosis complex.' *Seminars in Pediatric Neurology*, **5**, 253–268.

Friedman, E. (1969) 'The autistic syndrome and phenylketonuria.' *Schizophrenia*, **1**, 249–261.

Frith, C.D., Frith, U. (1991) 'Elective affinities in autism and schizophrenia.' *In:* Bebbington, P. (Ed.) *Social Psychiatry, Theory, Methodology and Practice.* New Brunswick, NJ: Transaction Books, pp. 65–88.

Fryns, J.P., Buttiens, M. (1987) 'X-linked mental retardation with marfanoid habitus.' *American Journal of Medical Genetics*, **28**, 267–274.

Fryns, J.P., Legius, E., Devriendt, K., Meire, F., Standaert, L., Baten, E., van den Berghe, H. (1996) 'Cohen syndrome: the clinical symptoms and stigmata at a young age.' *Clinical Genetics*, **49**, 237–241.

Gaffney, G.R., Kuperman, S., Tsai, L.Y., Minchin, S. (1988) 'Morphological evidence of brainstem involvement in infantile autism.' *Biological Psychiatry*, **24**, 578–586.

Garvey, M.A., Giedd, J., Swedo, S.E. (1998) 'PANDAS: the search for environmental triggers of pediatric neuropsychiatric disorders. Lessons from rheumatic fever.' *Journal of Child Neurology*, **13**, 413–423.

Gath, A., Gumley, D. (1986) 'Behavior problems in retarded children with special reference to Down's syndrome.' *British Journal of Psychiatry*, **149**, 156–161.

Ghaziuddin, M. (1997) 'Autism in Down syndrome: family history correlates.' *Journal of Intellectual Disability Research*, **41**, 87–91.

Ghaziuddin, M., Tsai, L. (1991) 'Depression in autistic disorder.' *British Journal of Psychiatry*, **159**, 721–723.

Ghaziuddin, M., Tsai, L.Y., Ghaziuddin, N. (1991) 'Brief report: Haloperidol treatment of trichotillomania in a boy with autism and mental retardation.' *Journal of Autism and Developmental Disorders*, **21**, 365–371.

Ghaziuddin, M., Tsai, L.Y., Eilers, L., Ghaziuddin, N. (1992a) 'Brief report: Autism and herpes simplex encephalitis.' *Journal of Autism and Developmental Disorders*, **22**, 107–113.

Ghaziuddin, M., Tsai, L.Y., Ghaziuddin, N. (1992b) 'Autism in Down syndrome: presentation and diagnosis.' *Journal of Intellectual Disability Research*, **36**, 449–456.

Ghaziuddin, M., Bolyard, B., Alessi, N. (1994) 'Autistic disorder in Noonan syndrome.' *Journal of Intellectual and Disability Research*, **38**, 67–72.

Giedd, J.N., Rapoport, J.L., Leonard, H.L., Richter, D., Swedo, S.E. (1996) 'Case study: acute basal ganglia enlargement and obsessive-compulsive symptoms in an adolescent boy.' *Journal of the American Academy of Child and Adolescent Psychiatry*, **35**, 913–915.

Gillberg, C. (1986) 'Brief report: Onset at age 14 of a typical autistic syndrome. A case report of a girl with herpes simplex encephalitis.' *Journal of Autism and Developmental Disorders*, **16**, 369–375.

—— (1990) 'Do children with autism have March birthdays?' *Acta Psychiatrica Scandinavica*, **82**, 152–156.

—— (1991) 'Outcome in autism and autistic-like conditions.' *Journal of the American Academy of Child and Adolescent Psychiatry*, **30**, 375–382.

—— (1998) 'Chromosomal disorders and autism.' *Journal of Autism and Developmental Disorders*, **28**, 415–424.

Gillberg, C., Coleman, M. (1996) 'Autism and medical disorders: a review of the literature.' *Developmental Medicine and Child Neurology*, **38**, 191–202.

Gillberg, C., Forsell, C. (1984) 'Childhood psychosis and neurofibromatosis – more than a coincidence?' *Journal of Autism and Developmental Disorders*, **14**, 1–8.

Gillberg, C., Rasmussen, P. (1994) 'Brief report: Four case histories and a literature review of Williams syndrome and autistic behavior.' *Journal of Autism and Developmental Disorders*, **24**, 381–393.

Gillberg, C., Steffenburg, S. (1987) 'Autistic behavior in Moebius syndrome.' *Acta Paediatrica Scandinavica*, **78**, 314–316.

Gillberg, C., Wahlström, J. (1985) 'Chromosome abnormalities in infantile autism and other childhood psychoses: a population study of 66 cases.' *Developmental Medicine and Child Neurology*, **27**, 293–304.

Gillberg, C., Winnergard, I. (1984) 'Childhood psychosis in a case of Moebius syndrome.' *Neuropediatrics*, **15**, 147–149.

Gillberg, C., Ehlers, S., Schaumann, H., Jakobsson, G., Dahlgren, S.O, Lindblom, R., Bagenholm, A., Tjuus, T., Blidner, E., (1990) 'Autism under age 3 years: a clinical study of 28 patients referred for autistic symptoms in infancy.' *Journal of Child Psychology and Psychiatry*, **31**, 921–934.

Gillberg, I.C., Gillberg, C., Ahlsen, C. (1994) 'Autistic behavior and attention deficits in tuberous sclerosis: a population-based study.' *Developmental Medicine and Child Neurology*, **36**, 50–56.

Gillberg, I.C. (1991) 'Autistic syndrome with onset at age 31 years: herpes encephalitis as a possible model for childhood autism.' *Developmental Medicine and Child Neurology*, **33**, 920–924.

Gillberg, I.C., Gillberg, C., Koop, S., Svenny, C. (1992) 'Hypothyroidism and autism spectrum disorders.' *Journal of Child and Adolescent Psychiatry*, **33**, 531–542.

Gillberg, I.C., Gillberg, C., Ratsam, M., Johansson, M. (1996) 'The cognitive profile of anorexia nervosa: a comparative study including a community-based sample.' *Comparative Psychiatry*, **37**, 23–30.

Gingell, K., Parmar, R., Sungum-Paliwal, S. (1996) 'Autism and multiple pituitary deficiency.' *Developmental Medicine and Child Neurology*, **38**, 545–549.

Goldfischer, S., Moore, C.L., Johnson, A.B., Spiro, A.J., Valsamis, M.P., Wisniewski, H.K., Ritch, R.H., Norto, W.T., Rapin, I., Gartner, L.M. (1973) 'Peroxismal and mitochondrial defects in cerebro-hepato-renal syndrome.' *Science*, **183**, 62–64.

Golding-Kushner, K.J., Weller, G., Shprintzen, R.J. (1985) 'Velo-cardio-facial syndrome: language and psychological profiles.' *Journal of Craniofacial Genetics*, **51**, 259–266.

Goodman, R., Minne, C. (1995) 'Questionnaire screening for comorbid pervasive developmental disorders in congenitally blind children: a pilot study.' *Journal of Autism and Developmental Disorders*, **25**, 195–203.

Gordon, A.G. (1991) 'Co occurrence of deafness and infantile autism.' *American Journal of Psychiatry*, **148**, 1615.

Gosch, A., Pankau, R. (1994) ' "Autistic" behavior in two children with Williams–Beuren syndrome.' (Letter) *American Journal of Medical Genetics*, **53**, 83–84.

Greenberg, F., Guzzetta, V., de Oca-Luna, R.M., Magenis, R.E., Smith, A.M., Richter, S., Kondo, I., Dobyns, W.B, Patel, P.I., Lupski, J.R. (1991) 'Molecular analysis of the Smith–Magenis Syndrome: a possible contiguous-gene syndrome associated with del(17)(p11.2).' *American Journal of Human Genetics*, **49**, 1207–1218.

Griebel, V., Krageloh-Mann, I., Michaelis, R. (1989) 'Hypomelanosis of Ito – report of four cases and survey of the literature.' *Neuropediatrics*, **20**, 234–237.

Gropman, A., Smith, A.C.M., Greenberg, F. (1998) 'Neurological aspects of the Smith Magenis syndrome.' (Abstract) *Annals of Neurology*, **44**, 542.

Guerrieri, F., Neri, G. (1991) 'A girl with Lujan–Fryns syndrome.' *American Journal of Medical Genetics*, **38**, 290–291.

Gurling, H.M., Bolton, P.F., Vincent, J., Melmer, G., Rutter, M. (1997) 'Molecular and cytogenetic investigations of the fragile X region including the Frag A and Fra E CGG trinucleotide repeat sequences in families multiplex for autism and related phenotypes.' *Human Heredity*, **47**, 254–262.

Gutierrez, G.C., Smalley, S.L., Tanguay, P.E. (1998) 'Autism in tuberous sclerosis complex.' *Journal of Autism and Developmental Disorders*, **28**, 97–103.

Hagberg, B. (1980) 'Infantile autism, dementia and loss of hand use: a report of 16 Swedish girl patients.' Paper presented at the Research Session of the European Federation of Child Neurology Societies, Manchester, England.

Hagberg, B., Gillberg, C. (1993) 'Rett variants Rettoid phenotypes.' *In:* Hagberg, B. (Ed.) *Rett Syndrome – Clinical and Biological Aspects.* Clinics in Developmental Medicine No. 127. London: Mac Keith Press, pp. 40–60.

Hagberg, B.A., Skjeldal, O.H. (1994) 'Rett variants: a suggested model for inclusion criteria.' *Pediatric Neurology*, **11**, 5–11.

Hagberg, B., Witt-Engerström, I. (1986) 'Rett syndrome: a suggested staging system for describing impairment profile with increasing age toward adolescence.' *American Journal of Medical Genetics*, **24**, 47–59.

Hagerman, R.J., Cronister, A.J. (Eds) (1991) 'Epidemiology.' *Fragile X Syndrome.* Baltimore: Johns Hopkins University Press.

Hanefeld, F., Christen, H.-J., Holzbach, U., Kruse, B., Frahm, J., Hanicke, W. (1995) 'Cerebral proton magnetic resonance spectroscopy in Rett syndrome.' *Neuropediatrics*, **26**, 126–127.

Harding, A.E., Sweeny, M.G., Govan, G.G., Riodan-Eva, P. (1995) 'Pedigree analysis in Leber hereditary optic neuropathy families with a pathogenic mtDNA mutation.' *American Journal of Human Genetics*, **57**, 77–86.

Harris, S.R., MacKay, L.L., Osborn, J.A. (1995) 'Autistic behaviors in offspring of mothers abusing alcohol and other drugs.' *Alcoholism Clinical and Experimental Research*, **19**, 660–665.

Harum, K.H., Ahn, S., Johnstone, M.V., Ginty, D.D. (1998) 'Defective growth factor to transcription factor signaling in Coffin–Lowry syndrome.' (Abstract) *Annals of Neurology*, **44**, 562.

Hashimoto, T., Kawano, N., Fukuda, K., Endo, S., Mori, K., Yoneda, Y., Yamaue, T., Harada, M., Miyoshi, K. (1998) '1H MR spectroscopy of the brain in three cases of Rett syndrome: comparison with autism and normal controls.' *Acta Neurologica Scandinavica*, **98**, 8–14.

Hebebrand, R.J., Martin, M., Korner, J., Roitzheim, B., de Braganca, K., Werner, W., Remschmidt, H. (1994) 'Partial trisomy 16p in an adolescent with autistic disorder and Tourette's syndrome.' *American Journal of Medical Genetics*, **54**, 268–270.

Hermida, A., Eiris, J., Alvarez-Moreno, A., Alonso-Martin, A., Barreiro, J., Castro-Gago, M. (1997) Hypomelanosis of Ito: autism, segmental dilatation of colon and unusual neuroimaging findings. (In Spanish) *Review Neurologique*, **25**, 71–74.

Hersh, J.H., Bloom, A.S., Weisskopf, B. (1982) 'Childhood autism in a female with Coffin–Siris syndrome.' *Journal of Developmental and Behavioral Pediatrics*, **3**, 249–251.

Herzberg, B. (1976) 'The families of autistic children.' *In:* Coleman, M. (Ed.) *The Autistic Syndromes.* Amsterdam: North-Holland.

Hinds, H.L., Ashley, C.T., Sutcliffe, J.S., Nelson, D.L., Warren, S.T., Housman, D.E., Schalling, M. (1993) 'Tissue specific expression of FMR-1 provides evidence for a functional role in fragile X syndrome.' *Nature Genetics*, **3**, 36–43.

Hobson, R.P., Lee, A., Brown, R. (1999) 'Autism and congenital blindness.' *Journal of Autism and Developmental Disorders*, **29**, 45–56.

Holroyd, S., Reiss, A.L. (1993) 'Cognitive development and behavior in Joubert syndrome. Response.' *Biological Psychiatry*, **33**, 855.

Holroyd, S., Reiss, A.L., Bryan, R.N. (1991) 'Autistic features in Joubert syndrome: a genetic disorder with agenesis of the cerebellar vermis.' *Biological Psychiatry*, **29**, 287–294.

Hooft, C., van Nevel, C., Schaepdryver, A.F. (1968) 'Hyperuricosuric encephalopathy without hyperuricaemia.' *Archives of Disease in Childhood*, **43**, 734–737.

Hoshino, Y., Watanabe, M., Tachibana, R., Kaneko, M., Kumashiro, H. (1984) 'The hypothalamo-pituitary function in autistic children.' *Neurosciences*, **10**, 285–291.

Howlin, P., Wing, L., Gould, J. (1995) 'The recognition of autism in children with Down's syndrome: Implications for intervention.' *Developmental Medicine and Child Neurology*, **37**, 406–414.

Ishikawa, A., Goto, T., Narasaki, M., Wokochi, K., Kitahara, H., Fukuyama, Y. (1978) 'A new syndrome (?) of progressive psychomotor deterioration with peculiar stereotyped movement and autistic tendency: a report of three cases.' *Brain and Development*, **3**, 258.

Ivarsson, S.A., Bjerre, I., Vegfors, P., Ahlfors, K. (1990) 'Autism as one of several disabilities in two children with congenital cytomegalovirus infection.' *Neuropediatrics*, **21**, 102–103.

Jacobsen, J., King, B.H., Leventhal, B.L., Christian, S.L., Ledbetter, D.H., Cook, E.H., Jr. (1998) 'Molecular screening for proximal 15q abnormalities in a mentally retarded population.' *Journal of Medical Genetics*, **35**, 534–538.

Jambaqué, I., Cusmai, R., Curatolo, P., Cortesi, F., Perrot, C., Dulac, O. (1991) 'Neuropsychological aspects of tuberous sclerosis in relation to epilepsy and MRI findings.' *Developmental Medicine and Child Neurology*, **33**, 698–705.

Jan, M.M., Dooley, J.M., Gordon, K.E. (1999) 'Male Rett syndrome variant: application of diagnostic criteria.' *Pediatric Neurology*, **20**, 238–240.

Janson, U. (1993) 'Normal and deviant behavior in blind children with ROP.' *Acta Ophthalmologica Supplement*, **210**, 20–26.

Jenkins, E.C., Brown, W.T., Brooks, J., Duncan, C.J., Rudellii, R.D., Wisniewski, H.M. (1984) 'Experience with prenatal fragile X detection.' *American Journal of Medical Genetics*, **17**, 215–239.

Johns, D.R. (1998) 'Genetic basis of mitochondrial disease.' *In:* Jameson, J.L. (Ed.) *Principles of Molecular Medicine.* Totowa, NJ: Humana Press, pp. 941–947.

Johnson, H.G., Ekman, P., Friesen, W. (1976) 'A behavior phenotype in the de Lange syndrome.' *Pediatric Research*, **10**, 843–850.

Johnson, R.T. (1998) *Viral Infections of the Nervous System. 2nd Edn.* Philadelphia: Lippincott-Raven.

Jones, K.L. (1997) *Smith's Recognizable Patterns of Human Malformation. 5th Edn.* Philadelphia: Saunders.

Julu, P.O., Kerr, A.M., Hansen, S., Apartopoulos, F., Jamal, G.A. (1997) 'Functional evidence of brain stem immaturity in Rett syndrome.' *European Child and Adolescent Psychiatry*, **6**(Suppl. 1): 47–54.

178

Kemner, C., Verbaten, M.N., Cuperus, J.M., Camfferman, G., van Engeland, H. (1998) 'Abnormal saccadic eye movements in autistic children.' *Journal of Autism and Developmental Disorder*, **28**, 61–67.

Kent, D.M., Hayward, R. (1998) 'Treating unrelated disorders in patients with chronic disease.' *New England Journal of Medicine*, **339**, 926.

Kerbeshian, J., Burd, L. (1996) 'Case study: comorbidity among Tourette's syndrome, autistic disorder, and bipolar disorder.' *Journal of the American Academy of Child and Adolescent Psychiatry*, **35**, 681–685.

Khan, S.G., Levy, H.L., Legerski, R., Quackenbush, E., Readon, J.T., Emmert, S., Sancar, A., Li, L., Schneider, T.D., Cleaver, J.E., Kraemer, K.H. (1998) 'Xeroderma pigmentosa Goup C slice mutation associated with autism and hypoglycinemia.' *Journal of Investigative Dermatology*, **111**, 791–796.

Klin, A. (1993) 'Auditory brainstem responses in autism: brainstem dysfunction or peripheral hearing loss?' *Journal of Autism and Developmental Disorders*, **23**, 15–35.

Knobloch, H., Pasamanick B. (1975) 'Some etiologic and prognostic factors in early infantile autism and psychosis.' *Journal of Pediatrics*, **55**, 182–191.

Koch, S., Jager-Roman, E., Losche, C., Nau, H., Rateng, D., Helge, H. (1996) 'Antiepileptic drug treatment in pregnancy: drug side effects in the neonate and neurological outcome.' *Acta Paediatrica*, **16**, 739–746.

Komoto, J., Usni, S., Otsuki, S., Terao, A. (1984) 'Infantile autism and Duchenne muscular dystrophy.' *Journal of Autism and Developmental Disorders*, **14**, 191–195.

Konstantareas, M.M., Homatidis, S. (1987) 'Brief report: Ear infections in autistic children.' *Journal of Autism and Developmental Disorders*, **17**, 585–594.

Kopera-Frye, K., Dehaene, S., Streissguth, A.P. (1996) 'Impairment of number processing induced by prenatal alcohol exposure.' *Neuropsychologia*, **34**, 1187–1196.

Kozma, C. (1998) 'On cognitive variability in velocardiofacial syndrome: profound mental retardation and autism.' *American Journal of Medical Genetics*, **81**, 269–270.

Kusse, M.C., van Nieuwenhuizen, O., van Huffelen, A.L., van der Mey, W., Thijssen, J.H., van Ree, J.M. (1993) 'The effect on non-depot ACTH on infantile spasms.' *Developmental Medicine and Child Neurology*, **35**, 1067–1073.

Lainhart, J.E., Piven, J., Wzorck, M., Landa, R., Santangelo, S.L., Coon, H., Folstein, S.E. (1997) 'Macrocephaly in children and adults with autism.' *Journal of American Academy of Child and Adolescent Psychiatry*, **36**, 282–290.

Lalande, M., Minossian, B.A., DeLorey, T.M., Olsen, R.W. (1999) 'Parental imprinting and Angelman syndrome.' *Advances in Neurology*, **79**, 421–429.

Landau, E.C., Cicchetti, D.V., Klin, A., Volkmar, F.R. (1999) 'Season of birth in autism: a fiction revisited.' *Journal of Autism and Developmental Disorders*, **29**, 385–393.

Landgren, M., Gillberg, C., Stromland, K. (1992) 'Goldenhar syndrome and autistic behavior.' *Developmental Medicine and Child Neurology*, **34**, 999–1005.

Lappalainen, R., Liewendahl, K., Sainio, K., Nikkinen, P., Riikonen, R.S. (1997) 'Brain perfusion SPECT and EEG findings in Rett syndrome.' *Acta Neurologica Scandinavica*, **95**, 44–50.

Leckman, J.F., Hardin, M.T., Riddle, M.A., Stevenson, J., Ort, S., Cohen, D.J. (1991) 'Clonidine treatment of Gilles de la Tourette's syndrome.' *Archives of General Psychiatry*, **48**, 324–328.

Leong, S., Ashwell, K.W. (1997) 'Is there a zone of vascular vulnerability in the fetal brain stem?' *Neurotoxicology and Teratology*, **19**, 265–275.

Lewis, E. (1959) 'The development of concepts in a girl with dietary treatment for phenylketonuria.' *British Journal of Medical Psychology*, **32**, 282–287.

Lewis, K.E., Lubetsky, M.J., Wegner, S.L., Steele, M.W. (1995) 'Chromosomal abnormalities in a psychiatric population.' *American Journal of Medical Genetics*, **60**, 53–54.

Li, S.Y., Chen, Y.C., Lai, T.J., Hsu, C.Y., Wang, Y.C. (1993) 'Molecular and cytogenetic analyses of autism in Taiwan.' *Human Genetics*, **92**, 441–445.

Lockwood, D., Hecht, F., Dowman, C., Hecht, B.K., Rizkallah, T.H., Goodwin, T.M., Allanson, J. (1988) 'Chromsome subband 17p11.2 deletion: a minute deletion syndrome.' *Journal of Medical Genetics*, **25**, 732–737.

Lowe, T.L., Tanaka, K., Seashore, M.R., Young, J.G., Cohen, D.J. (1980) 'Detection of pheylketonuria in autistic and psychotic children.' *Journal of the American Medical Association*, **243**, 126–128.

Lubs, H.A. (1969) 'A marker X-chromosome. *American Journal of Human Genetics*, **21**, 231–244.

Lujan, J.E., Carlin, M.E., Lubs, H.A. (1984) 'A form of X-linked mental retardation with marfanoid habitus.' *American Journal of Medical Genetics*, **17**, 311–322.

Lund, J. (1988) 'Psychiatric aspects of Down syndrome.' *Acta Psychiatrica Scandinavica*, **78**, 364–374.

McArthur, A.J., Budden, S.S. (1998) 'Sleep dysfunction in Rett syndrome: a trial of exogenous melatonin treatment.' *Developmental Medicine and Child Neurology*, **40**, 186–192.

Mallin, S.R., Walker, F.A. (1972) 'Effects of the XYY karyotype in one of two brothers with congenital adrenal hyperplasia.' *Clinical Genetics*, **3**, 490–494.

Maria, B.L., Drane, W.B., Quisling, R.J., Hoaug, K.B. (1997) 'Correlation between gadolinium-diethylenetriaminepentaacetic acid contrast enchancement and thallium 201 chloride uptake in brainstem glioma.' *Journal of Child Neurology*, **12**, 341–348.

Mariner, R., Jackson, A.W., Levitas, A., Hagerman, R.J., Braden, M., McBogg, P.M., Berry, R., Smith, A.C.M. (1986) 'Autism, mental retardation and chromosomal abnormalities.' *Journal of Autism and Developmental Disorders*, **16**, 425–440.

Markowitz, P.I. (1983) 'Autism in a child with congenital cytomegalovirus infection.' *Journal of Autism and Developmental Disorders*, **13**, 249–253.

Mazzocco, M.M., Pennington, B.F., Hagerman, R.J. (1993) 'The neurocognitive phenotype of female carriers of fragile X: additional evidence for specificity.' *Journal of Developmental and Behavioral Pediatrics*, **14**, 328–335.

Mazzocco, M.M., Kates, W.R., Baumgardner, T.L., Freund, L.S., Reiss, A.L. (1997) 'Autistic behaviors among girls with fragile X syndrome.' *Journal of Autism and Developmental Disorders*, **27**, 415–435.

Meyer, G.A., Blum, N.J., Hitchcock, W., Fortina, P. (1998) 'Absence of fragile X CGG trinucleotide repeat expansion in girls diagnosed with a pervasive developmental disorder.' *Journal of Pediatrics*, **133**, 363–365.

Miladi, N., Larnaout, A., Kaabachi, N., Helayem, M., Ben Hamida, M. (1992) 'Phenylketonuria: an underlying etiology of autistic syndrome. A case report.' *Journal of Child Neurology*, **7**, 22–23.

Miller, M.T., Stromland, K., Gillberg, C., Johansson, M., Nilsson, E.W. (1998) 'The puzzle of autism: an ophthalmologic contribution.' *Transactions of the American Ophthalmologic Society*, **96**, 369–385.

Millichap, J.G. (1997) Neurocutaneous syndromes; Infantile spasms and neurofibromatosis 1. *In:* Millichap, J.G. (Ed.) (1997) *Progress in Pediatric Neurology III*. Chicago: PNB Publishers, pp. 435–437; 41–42.

Miyamoto, A., Oki, J. Takahashi, S., Okuno, A. (1999) 'Serum melatonin kinetics and long-term melatonin treatment for sleep disorders in Rett syndrome.' *Brain Development*, **21**, 59–62.

Moebius, P.J. (1888) 'Uber angeborene doppelseitige Abducens-Facialis-Lähmung.' *Münchener Medizinische Wochenschrift*, **35**, 91–94.

Moncla, A., Malzac, P., Voelckel, M.A., Auguier, P. Girardot, L., Mattei, M.G.N., Mattei, J.F., Lalande, M., Livet, M.O. (1999) 'Phenotype–genotype correlation in 20 deletion and 20 non-deletion Angelman syndrome patients.' *European Journal of Human Genetics*, **7**, 131–139.

Moriarty, J., Ring, H.A., Robertson, M.M. (1993) 'An idiot savant calendrical calculator with Gilles de la Tourette syndrome: implications for an understanding of the savant syndrome.' *Psychological Medicine*, **23**, 1019–1021.

Morrow, J.D., Whitman, B.Y., Accardo, P.J. (1990) 'Autistic disorder in Sotos syndrome: a case report.' *European Journal of Pediatrics*, **149**, 567–569.

Mortensen, P.B., Pedersen, C.B., Westergaard, T., Wohlfahrt, J., Ewald, H., Mors, O., Andersen, P.K., Melbye, M. (1999) 'Effects of family history and place and season of birth on the risk of schizophrenia.' *New England Journal of Medicine*, **340**, 603–608.

Moser, A.B., Kreiter, N., Bezman, L., Lu, S., Raymond, G.V., Naidu, S., Moser, H.W. (1999) 'Plasma very long chain fatty acids in 3,000 peroxisome disease patients and 29,000 controls.' *Annals of Neurology*, **45**, 100–110.

Moser, H.W., Raymond, G.V. (1998) 'Genetic peroxismal disorders: why when and how to test.' *Annals of Neurology*, **44**, 713–714.

Mouridsen, S.E., Andersen, L.B., Sorensen, S.A., Rich, B., Isager, T. (1992) 'Neurofibromatosis in infantile autism and other types of childhood psychoses.' *Acta Paedopsychiatrica*, **55**, 15–18.

Mouridsen, S.E., Nielsen, S., Rich, B., Isager, T. (1994) 'Season of birth in infantile autism and other types of childhood psychoses.' *Child Psychiatry and Human Development*, **25**, 31–43.

Nanson, J.L. (1992) 'Autism in fetal alcohol syndrome: a report of six cases.' *Alcoholism Clinical and Experimental Research*, **16**, 558–565.

Nass, R., Gutman, C. (1997) 'Boys with Asperger's disorder, exceptional verbal intelligence, tics, and clumsiness.' *Developmental Medicine and Child Neurology*, **39**, 691–695.

Nawratzki, I., Schwartzenberg, T., Zaubermann, H., Yanko, L. (1985) 'Bilateral morning glory syndrome with midline brain lesion in an autistic child.' *Metabolic, Pediatric and Systemic Ophthalmology*, **8**, 35–36.

Nelson, E.C., Pribor, E.F. (1993) 'A calendar savant with autism and Tourette syndrome. Response to treatment and thoughts on the interrelationships of these conditions.' *Annals of Clinical Psychiatry*, **5**, 135–140.

Niklasson, L., Rasmussen, P., Oskarsdottir, S., Gillberg, C. (2000) 'Neuropsychiatric problems in individuals with the CATCH-22 syndrome' (submitted).

Nilsson, E.W., Gillberg, C., Gillberg, I.C., Rastam, M. (1999) 'Ten-year follow-up of adolescent-onset anorexia nervosa: personality disorders.' *Journal of the Amercian Academy of Child and Adolescent Psychiatry*, **38**, 1389–1395.

Nordin, V. (1997) Autism spectrum disorder in children with mental and physical disability. Ph.D. thesis. Göteborg University.

Nordin, V., Gillberg, C. (1996) 'Autism spectrum disorders in children with physical or mental disability or both. I: Clinical and epidemiological aspects.' *Developmental Medicine and Child Neurology*, **38**, 297–313.

North, K.N. (1998) 'Neurofibromatosis 1 in childhood.' *Seminars in Pediatric Neurology*, **5**, 231–242.

Okuno, T., Matsuo, M., Higa, T., Hattori, H. (1997) 'Neuroimagings in neuronal migration disorders.' (In Japanese) *No To Hattatsu*, **29**, 123–128.

Olson, H.C., Feldman, J.J., Streissguth, A.P., Sampson, P.D., Bookstein, F.L. (1998) 'Neuropsychological deficits in adolescents with fetal alcohol syndrome: clinical findings.' *Alcoholism Clinical and Experimental Research*, **22**, 1998–2012.

Olsson, B., Rett, A. (1987) 'Autism and Rett syndrome: behavioral investigations and differential diagnosis.' *Developmental Medicine and Child Neurology*, **29**, 429–441.

Ornitz, E.M., Guthrie, D., Farley, A.H. (1977) 'The early development of autistic children.' *Journal of Autism and Childhood Schizophrenia*, **7**, 207–229.

Orstavik, K.H., Stromme, P., Ek, J., Torvik, A., Skjeldal, O.H. (1997) 'Macrocephaly, epilepsy, autism, dysmorphic features, and mental retardation in two sisters: a new autosomal recessive syndrome?' *Journal of Medical Genetics*, **34**, 849–851.

Ozonoff, S., Williams, B.J., Gale, S., Miller, J.N. (1999) 'Autism and autistic behavior in Joubert syndrome.' *Journal of Child Neurology*, **14**, 636–641.

Pan, J.W., Lane, J.B., Hetherington, H., Percy, A.K. (in press) 'Rett syndrome: 1H spectroscopic imaging at 4.1T.' *Journal of Child Neurology*.

Pascual-Castroviejo, I., Roche, C., Martinez-Bermejo, A., Arcas, J., Lopez-Martin, V., Tendero, A., Esquiroz, J.L., Pascual-Pascual, S.I. (1998) Hypomelanosis of Ito. A study of 76 infantile cases. *Brain Development*, **20**, 36–43.

Pastuszak, A.L., Schuler, L., Speck-Martins, C.E., Coelho, K.E., Cordello, S.M., Vargas, F., Brunoni, D., Schwarz, I.V., Larrandaburu, M., Safattle, H., Meloni, V.F., Koren, G. (1998) 'Use of misoprostol during pregnancy and Mobius' syndrome in infants.' *New England Journal of Medicine*, **338**, 1991–1885.

Paul, M., Allington-Smith, P. (1997) 'Asperger's syndrome associated with Steinert's myotonic dystrophy.' *Developmental Medicine and Child Neurology*, **39**, 280–281.

Paul, R., Cohen, D.J., Volkmar, F.R. (1983) 'Autistic behaviors in a boy with Noonan syndrome.' (Letter) *Journal of Autism and Developmental Disorders*, **13**, 433–434.

Pavone, L., Fiumara, A., Bottaro, G., Mazzone, D., Coleman, M. (1997) 'Autism and celiac disease: failure to validate the hypothesis that a link might exist.' *Biological Psychiatry*, **42**, 72–75.

Perlmutter, S.J., Leitman, S.F., Garvey, M.A., Hamburger, S., Feldman, E., Leonard, H.L., Swedo, S.E. (1999) 'Therapeutic plasma exchange and intravenous immunoglobulin for obsessive-compulsive disorder and tic disorders in childhood.' *Lancet*, **354**, 1153–1158.

Perry, R., Nobler, M.S., Campbell, M. (1989) 'Tourette-like symptoms associated with neuroleptic therapy in an autistic child.' *Journal of the American Academy of Child and Adolescent Psychiatry*, **28**, 93–96.

Peterson, C.C., Siegal, M. (1995) 'Deafness, conversation and theory of mind.' *Journal of Child Psychology and Psychiatry*, **36**, 459–474.

Peterson, M.R., Torrey, E.F. (1976) 'Viruses and other infectious agents as behavioral teratogens.' *In:* Coleman, M. (Ed.) *The Autistic Syndromes.* Amsterdam: North-Holland, pp. 23–42.

Pizzo, R.G., Albizzati, A., Cervini, R., Grioni, A., Musetti, L., Saccani, M., Rossetti, M., Guareschi, A., Cazzullo, A. (1991) 'Autistic symptoms in 5 sero-reverted HIV+ children.' *Brain Dysfunction.*

Raja, M., Azzoni, A., Giammarco, V. (1998) 'Diabetes insipidus and polydipsia in a patient with Asperger's disorder and an empty sella: a case report.' *Journal of Autism and Developmental Disorders*, **28**, 235–239.

Ramaekers, V.Th., Heimann, G., Reul, J., Thron, A., Jaeken, J. (1997) 'Genetic abnormalities and cerebellar structural abnormalities in childhood.' *Brain*, **120**, 1739–1751.

Realmuto, G.M., Main, B. (1982) 'Coincidence of Tourette disorder and infantile autism.' *Journal of Autism and Developmental Disorders*, **12**, 367–372.

Reich, M., Lenoir, P., Malvy, J., Perrot, A., Sauvage, D. (1997) 'Bourneville's tuberous sclerosis and autism.' (In French) *Archives de Pediatre*, **4**, 170–175.

Reiss, A.L., Feinstein, C., Rosenbaum, K.N., Borengasser-Caruso, M.A. (1985) 'Autism associated with Williams syndrome.' *Journal of Pediatrics*, **106**, 247–249.

Reiss, A.L., Feinstein, C., Rosenbaum, K.N. (1986) 'Autism in genetic disorders.' *Schizophrenia Bulletin*, **12**, 724–738.

Reiss, A.L., Lee, J., Freund, L. (1994) 'Neuroanatomy of fragile X syndrome: the temporal lobe.' *Neurology*, **44**, 1317–1324.

Ren, J.O., Tabit, E., Kosofsy, B.E. (1998) 'Dose-related alterations in neocortical cytoarchitecture following prenatal cocaine exposure.' (Abstract) *Annals of Neurology*, **44**, 563.

Rett, A. (1966) *Uber ein cerebral-atrophisches Syndrome bei Hyperammonämie.* Vienna: Hollinek.

Rett Syndrome Diagnostic Criteria Work Group (1988) 'Diagnostic criteria for Rett syndrome.' *Annals of Neurology*, **23**, 425–428.

Riikonen, R., Amnell, G. (1981) 'Psychiatric disorders in children with earlier infantile spasms.' *Developmental Medicine and Child Neurology*, **23**, 747–760.

Ritvo, E.R., Creel, D., Realmuto, G., Crandall, A.S., Freeman, B.J., Bateman, B., Barr, R., Pingree, C., Coleman, M. (1988) 'Electroretinograms in autism: a pilot study of b-wave amplitudes.' *American Journal of Psychiatry*, **147**, 1614–1621.

Ritvo, E.R., Mason-Brothers, A., Freeman, B.J., Pingree, C., Jenson, W.R., McMahon, W.M., Petersen, C.B., Jorde, L.B., Mo, A., Ritvo, A. (1990) 'The UCLA–University of Utah Epidemiologic Survey of Autism: the etiologic role of rare diseases.' *American Journal of Psychiatry*, **147**, 1614–1621.

Rogers, P.T., Coleman, M. (1992) *Medical Care in Down Syndrome: A Preventive Medicine Approach.* New York: Marcel Dekker.

Rogers, S.J., Newhart-Larson, S. (1989) 'Characteristics of infantile autism in five children with Leber's congenital amaurosis.' *Developmental Medicine and Child Neurology*, **31**, 598–608.

Rubin, L.L., Gatchalian, C.L., Rimon, G., Brooks, S.F. (1994) 'The molecular mechanisms of neuronal apoptosis.' *Current Opinion in Neurobiology*, **4**, 696–702.

Ruch, A. (1989) 'Mitochondrial alterations in Rett syndrome.' *Pediatric Neurology*, **5**, 320–323.

Rutter, M., Bartak, L. (1971) 'Causes of infantile autism: some considerations from recent research.' *Journal of Autism and Childhood Schizophrenia*, **1**, 20–32.

Rutter, M., Bailey, A., Bolton, P., Le Couteur, A. (1994) 'Autism and known medical conditions: myth and substance.' *Journal of Child Psychology and Psychiatry*, **35**, 311–322.

Saccomani, L., Veneselli, E., Di Stefano, S., Celle, M.E., De Negri, M. (1992) 'Early autism and congenital muscular dystrophy: a clinical case.' (In Italian) *Pediatria Medica e Chirargica*, **14**, 231–233.

Schanen, N.C., Kurczynski, T.W., Brunelle, D., Woodcock, M.M., Dure, L.S. 4th, Percy, A.K. (1998) 'Neonatal encephalopathy in two boys in families with recurrent Rett syndrome.' *Journal of Child Neurology*, **13**, 229–231.

Scharre, J.E., Creedon, M.P. (1992) 'Assessment of visual function in autistic children.' *Optometry and Vision Science*, **69**, 433–439.

Schepis, C., Elia, M., Siragusa, M., Barbareschi, M. (1997) 'A new case of trichothiodystrophy associated with autism, seizures and mental retardation.' *Pediatric Dermatology*, **14**, 125–128.

Schmitt, B., Seeger, J., Kreuz, W., Eneukel, S., Jacobi, G. (1991) 'Central nervous system involvement of children with HIV infection.' *Developmental Medicine and Child Neurology*, **33**, 535–540.

Shannon, M., Graef, J.W. (1996) 'Lead intoxication in children with pervasive developmental disorders.' *Journal of Toxicology and Clinical Toxicology*, **34**, 177–181.

Shprintzen, R.J., Goldberg, R.B., Lewin, M.L., Sidoti, E.J., Berkman, V., Arggmeso, R.V., Young, D. (1978)

'A new syndrome involving palate, cardiac anomalies, typical facies and learning disabilities: the velo-cardio-facial syndrome.' *Cleft Palate Journal*, **15**, 56–62.

Sieg, K.G. (1992) 'Autism and Ehlers–Danlos syndrome.' *Journal of the American Academy of Child and Adolescent Psychiatry*, **31**, 173.

Silva, M.I., Cieuta, C., Guerrini, R., Plouin, P., Livet, M.O., Dulac, O. (1996) 'Early clinical and EEG features of infantile spasms in Down syndrome.' *Epilepsia*, **37**, 977–982.

Singh, V.K., Lin, S.X., Yang, V.C. (1998) 'Rapid communication: serological association of measles virus and human herpesvirus-6 with brain autoantibodies in autism.' *Clinical Immunology and Immuno-pathology*, **89**, 105–108.

Smalley, S.L. (1998) 'Autism and tuberous sclerosis.' *Journal of Autism and Developmental Disorders*, **28**, 407–414.

Smalley, S.L., Tanguay, P.E., Smith, M., Gutierrez, G. (1992) 'Autism and tuberous sclerosis.' *Journal of Autism and Developmental Disorders*, **22**, 339–355.

Smith, A.C.M., McGavran, L., Robinson, J., Waldstein, G., Macfarlane, J., Zonona, J., Reiss, J., Lahr, M., Allen, L. Magenis, E. (1986) 'Interstitial deletion of (17)(p11.2p11.2) in nine patients.' *American Journal of Medical Genetics*, **24**, 393–414.

Smith, P.R, Cooper, J.M., Govan,, G.G., Riordan-Eva, P., Harding, A.E., Schapira, A.H. (1995) 'Antibodies to human optic nerve in Leber's hereditary optic neuropathy.' *Journal of Neurological Science*, **30**, 134–138.

Stahl, S.M. (1980) 'Tardive Tourette syndrome in an autistic patient after long-term neuroleptic administration.' *American Journal of Psychiatry*, **137**, 1267–1269.

Steffenburg, S. (1991) 'Neuropsychiatric assessment of children with autism: a population-based study.' *Developmental Medicine and Child Neurology*, **33**, 495–511.

Steffenburg, S., Gillberg, C., Steffenburg, U., Kyllerman, M. (1996) 'Autism in Angelman syndrome: a population-based study.' *Pediatric Neurology*, **14**, 131–136.

Steiner, J., Adamsbaum, C., Desguerres, I., Lalande, G., Raynaud, F., Ponsot, G., Kalifa, G. (1996) 'Hypomelanosis of Ito and brain abnormalities: MRI findings and literature review.' *Pediatric Radiology*, **26**, 763–768.

Stern, J.S., Robertson, M.M. (1997) 'Tics associated with autistic and pervasive developmental disorders.' *Neurological Clinics*, **15**, 345–355.

Stromland, K., Nordin, V., Miller, M., Akerstrom, B., Gillberg, C. (1994) 'Autism in thalidomide embryopathy: a population study.' *Developmental Medicine and Child Neurology*, **36**, 351–356.

Stubbs, E.G., Budden, S.S., Burger, D.R., Vanderbark, A.A. (1980) 'Transfer factor immunotherapy of an autistic child with congenital cytomegalovirus.' *Journal of Autism and Developmental Disorders*, **10**, 451–458.

Sverd, J., Montero, G., Gurevich, N. (1993) 'Brief report: Cases for an association between Tourette syndrome, autistic disorder and schizophrenia-like syndrome.' *Journal of Autism and Developmental Disorder*, **23**, 407–413.

Swillen, A., Hellemans, H., Steyaert, J., Fryns, J.-P. (1996) 'Autism and genetics: high incidence of specific genetic syndromes in 21 autistic adolescents and adults living in two residential homes in Belgium.' *American Journal of Medical Genetics (Neuropsychiatric Genetics)*, **67**, 315–316.

Tantam, D., Evered, C., Hersov, L. (1990) 'Asperger's syndrome and ligamentous laxity.' *Journal of The American Academy of Child and Adolescent Psychiatry*, **29**, 892–896.

Tevathan, E., Naidu, S. (1988) 'The clinical recognition and differential diagnosis of Rett syndrome.' *Journal of Child Neurology*, **3**(Suppl.): S6–S16.

Topcu, M., Topaloglu, H., Renda, Y., Berker, M., Turanli, G. (1991) 'The Rett syndrome in males.' (Letter) *Brain and Development*, **13**, 62.

Trivier, E., De Cesare, D., Jacquot, S., Pannetier, S., Zackai, E., Young, I., Mandel, J.L., Sassone-Corsi, P., Hanauer, A.V. (1996) 'Mutations in the kinase Rsk-2 associated with Coffin–Lowry syndrome.' *Nature*, **384**, 567–570.

Vanhala, R., Gaily, E., Paetau, A., Riikonen, R. (1998) 'Pons tumour behind a phenotypic Rett syndrome presentation.' *Developmental Medicine and Child Neurology*, **40**, 836–839.

Van Steensel, M.A., Steijlen, P.M. (1998) 'Hypomelanosis of Ito: a symptom, not a syndrome.' *American Journal of Medical Genetics*, **80**, 435.

Veenstra-VanderWeele, J., Gonen, D., Leventhal, B.L., Cook, E.H. Jr. (1999) 'Mutation screening of the UBE3A/E6-AP in autistic disorder.' *Molecular Psychiatry*, **4**, 64–67.

183

Von Aster, M., Zachmann, M., Brandeis, D., Wohlrab, G., Richner, M., Steinhausen, H.C. (1997) 'Psychiatric, neuropediatric and neuropsychological symptoms in a case of hypomelanosis of Ito.' *European Child and Adolescent Psychiatry*, **6**, 227–233.

Vostanis, P., Harrington, R., Prendergast, M., Farndon, P. (1994) 'Case reports of autism with interstitial deletion of chromosome 17 (p11.2p11.2) and monosomy of chromosome 5 (5pter→5p15.3).' *Psychiatric Genetics*, **4**, 109–111.

Wakabayashi, S. (1979) 'A case of infantile autism associated with Down syndrome.' *Journal of Autism and Developmental Disorders*, **9**, 31–36.

Wan, M., Lee, S.S., Zhang, X., Houwink-Manville, I., Song, H.R., Amir, R.E., Budden, S., Naidu, S., Pereira, J.L., Lo, I.F., Zoghbi, H.Y., Schanen, N.C., Francke, U. (1999) 'Rett syndrome and beyond: recurrent spontaneous and familial MECP2 mutations at CpG hotspots.' *American Journal of Human Genetics*, **65**, 1520–1529.

Weidel, L., Coleman, M. (1976) 'The autistic and control population of this study.' *In:* Coleman, M. (Ed.) *The Autistic Syndromes*. New York: Elsevier.

Wentz, E. (2000) *Ten-Year Outcome of Anorexia Nervosa with Teenage Onset*. Göteborg, Sweden: Kompendiet-Göteborg.

Wentz-Nilsson, E., Gillberg, C., Gillberg, I.C., Råstam, M. (1999) 'Anorexia nervosa 10 years after onset. Personality disorders.' Submitted.

Williams, K. (1998) 'Benefits of normalizing plasma phenylalanine: impact on behaviour and health. A case report.' *Journal of Inherited Metabolic Diseases*, **21**, 785–790.

Williams, P.G., Hersh, J.H. (1997) 'A male with fetal valproate syndrome and autism.' *Developmental Medicine and Child Neurology*, **39**, 632–634.

—— (1998) 'Brief report: The association of neurofibromatosis 1 and autism.' *Journal of Autism and Developmental Disorders*, **28**, 567–571.

Wing, L., Gould, J. (1979) 'Severe impairments of social interaction and associated abnormalities in children: epidemiology and classification.' *Journal of Autism and Developmental Disorders*, **9**, 11–29.

Wolff, S. (1992) 'Psychiatric morbidity and criminality in "schizoid" children grown-up: a record survey.' *European Child and Adolescent Psychiatry*, vol. 1.

Wolter, M., Reifenberger, J., Sommer, C., Ruzicka, T., Reifenberger, G. (1997) 'Mutations in the human homologue of the Drosophila segment polarity gene patched (PTCH) in sporadic basal cell carcinoma of the skin and primitive neuroectodermal tumors of the central nervous system.' *Cancer Research*, **57**, 2581–2585.

Yano, S., Oda, K., Watanabe, Y., Watanabe, S., Matsuishi, T., Kojima, K., Abe, T., Kato, H. (1998) 'Two sib cases of Leber congenital amaurosis with cerebellar vermis hypoplasia and multiple systemic anomalies.' *American Journal of Medical Genetics*, **78**, 429–432.

Yoshimura, I., Sasaki, A., Alimoto, H., Yoshimura, N. (1989) 'A case of congenital myotonic dystrophy with autism.' (In Japanese) *No To Hattatsu*, **24**, 379–384.

Zappella, M. (1990) 'Autistic features in children affected by cerebral gigantism.' *Brain Dysfunction*, **3**, 241–244.

—— (1992a) 'Hypomelanosis of Ito is frequently associated with autism.' *European Child and Adolescent Psychiatry*, **1**, 170–173.

—— (1992b) 'The Rett girls with preserved speech.' *Brain and Development*, **14**, 98–101.

—— (1993) 'Autism and hypomelanosis of Ito in twins.' *Developmental Medicine and Child Neurology*, **35**, 826–832.

Zappella, M., Gillberg, C., Ehlers, S. (1998) 'The preserved speech variant: a subgroup of the Rett complex: a clinical report of 30 cases.' *Journal of Autism and Developmental Disorder*, **28**, 510–526.

12
EPILEPSY AND ELECTROPHYSIOLOGY

In 1943, Kanner described eleven children with his then new "autistic disturbances of affective contact." One of these eleven suffered from epilepsy. In 1971, Kanner reported on a follow-up of the eleven patients; by then, two patients – 18 per cent of his original series of eleven children – were suffering from epilepsy. Thus, in this seminal report which defined autism, the patients already formed a clinically heterogeneous group – those with and those without seizures. What has become clear over the years since Kanner's discovery is that patients with autism are, in fact, at greater risk of seizures than they are of many other types of developmental problems, such as developmental dysphasia or Down syndrome (Wong 1993). The frequency of epilepsy in autism, regardless of IQ, is higher than in 'non autistic' severe mental retardation (Gillberg *et al.* 1986), even though a population of individuals with severe mental retardation is likely to include a fraction with double syndromes.

The higher prevalence of epilepsy in a group of individuals with the autistic syndrome is best explained by the fact that we are dealing with a syndrome – a collection of different diseases which share a distinctive pattern of behavior. Some disease entities within the autistic syndrome are seizure-free; in others, many, but not all, individuals suffer from epilepsy (see Chapters 10 and 11). In Table 12.1, those disease entities containing a number of patients with a seizure disorder are listed. Both patients with classical autism and those with double syndromes may suffer from epilepsy. So, if one looks at studies of autistic individuals, the percentage of those with epilepsy varies greatly. The prevalence of epilepsy in the general population is 0.5 per cent; the published figures on epilepsy in autism range from 4 per cent to 47 per cent (Carod *et al.* 1995). Besides the fact that each group of autistic patients contains a different mixture of disease entities, some of which have seizures and some of which do not, there is another factor to consider. The frequency of epilepsy varies with the length of the follow-up period, rising as the follow-up period lengthens. Although epilepsy in children with autism often appears during the first three years of life (Ritvo *et al.* 1990), there appears to be another spurt around the time of puberty (Rutter 1970, Gillberg and Steffenburg 1987), as is seen in other affected populations.

New details about epilepsy in autism are available from recent studies. In a large American series of 302 children with autism, Tuchman *et al.* (1991) reported that epilepsy occurred in 14 per cent. In this series, girls were affected more frequently than boys (24 per cent vs. 11 per cent). When cognitive and motor disabilities were excluded, the risk of epilepsy in children with autism was only 6 per cent. Elia *et al.* (1995) also found females more frequently affected by seizures than males in an Italian series of subjects with autism and mental retardation. An epidemiological study of infantile autism conducted in a

TABLE 12.1
Underlying disease entities in the autistic syndrome that may have seizures

Infants

Infantile spasms
Cytochrome c oxidase deficiency
Malformations of cortical development
Tuberous sclerosis

Children and adolescents

Classic autism
Purine autism

Double syndromes
Angelman syndrome
Fragile X syndrome
Phenylketonuria
Rett syndrome
Sanfilippo's syndrome, type A
Tuberous sclerosis

county in Norway found that 9 out of 28 persons (32 per cent) with autism had epilepsy (Herder 1993). In a Spanish series of 62 children with autism (Carod *et al.* 1995), 47 per cent had some kind of epileptic syndrome, including two children with brain tumors – which is an unusual finding in any autism series.

Standard EEGs are helpful when they reveal frankly epileptiform activity (Rapin 1997). Based on a review of the medical literature up to the time of their study, Tsai *et al.* (1985) reported that the majority of children with autism have shown some kind of EEG abnormality whether they had seizures or not. However, if the abnormal EEG readings are limited to epileptiform findings, this figure declines. Rossi *et al.* (1995) examined 106 patients with autism and found that 23.6 per cent had paroxysmal EEG abnormalities compared to 18.9 per cent with actual clinical seizures.

Looking at the picture the other way around, there is also the question of how much autism itself contributes to the population of those with epilepsy and mental retardation. A population-based study of 6- to 13-year-olds, which identified 98 children with active epilepsy and mental retardation, reported that an autistic disorder was present in 27 per cent and an autistic-like disorder in 11 per cent of these children (Steffenburg *et al.* 1995).

Autistic regression and epilepsy
A subgroup, possibly a third, of autistic toddlers regress in language, sociability, play and often cognition (Rapin 1995). Fluctuation in language or behavior raises the suspicion of epilepsy. Epilepsy or a paroxysmal EEG may occasionally be associated with autistic regression. However, in the experience of an outstanding clinician, I. Rapin, epilepsy probably plays a relatively minor, although non-negligible, pathogenetic role in autistic regression (Rapin 1995). Nevertheless, a prolonged sleep EEG that includes study of stage

III and stage IV sleep is recommended for children without seizures who have regressed or who have fluctuating deficits, and for mute and poorly intelligible children who may have verbal auditory agnosia (Tuchman and Rapin 1997). In the medical literature, there is a rare subgroup of children with chronic motor tics who have both autistic regression and seizures, as described by Nass *et al.* (1998). Seizures consisted of absence or myoclonic patterns, usually resistant to antiepileptic drugs. The patients had a specific pattern of occipital spiking on EEG.

After language is developed and after 2 years of age, a few children may undergo a rapid regression in language, sociability, play and apparent cognition. This has been called childhood disintegrative disorder and is thought to be a separate disorder from an autistic syndrome (see Chapter 10).

Bilateral hippocampal sclerosis

Severe epilepsy with episodes of status epilepticus is found in children with early-life bilateral hippocampal sclerosis, as reported by DeLong and Heinz (1997). These children had a profound failure of learning of both complex social and adaptive skills. They all failed to attain language or lost what little they had. These losses persisted in spite of adequate motor and sensory function and even after epilepsy was controlled. MRI imaging showed bilateral hippocampal sclerosis, while PET scans demonstrated isolated bilateral anterior temporal lobe hypometabolism. The authors noted that these children had the cognitive deficits seen in severe infantile autism.

Landau–Kleffner (acquired epileptic aphasia) syndrome

Landau–Kleffner syndrome is an acquired epileptic aphasia or verbal auditory agnosia affecting children between 2 and 5 years of age who have already developed speech. There are seizures and/or often a bilateral paroxysmal EEG pattern. In the classical Landau–Kleffner syndrome, aphasia is acquired and other higher cortical functions usually do not deteriorate. In a variation of the syndrome called "epilepsy with continuous spike-waves during slow wave speech," speech is disturbed in 50 per cent of cases, and intellectual deterioration occurs, with psychiatric symptoms, often reminiscent of autism, developing. According to Hirsch *et al.* (1990), they are probably variations of a single syndrome. Corticosteroids are usually tried in this patient group and may have a temporary beneficial effect. There is also an experimental surgical therapy called subpial intracortical transection (Morrell *et al.* 1995).

Types of seizures

Many patterns of seizures are seen in patients with autism – infantile spasms, atonic seizures, myoclonic seizures, atypical absence, complex partial seizures, and generalized tonic–clonic seizures. Most known EEG patterns are also found in this patient group, including the continuous spike-waves variant (electrical status epilepticus in slow wave sleep – ESES), mentioned above.

Infantile Spasms and Hypsarrhythmia (West Syndrome)

Infantile spasms begin in early infancy with multiple myoclonic jerks, jackknife seizures or salaam attacks. The EEG changes have a characteristic picture of abundant spikes and polyspikes along with high voltage slowing. The association of infantile spasms with the EEG picture of hypsarrhythmia has become known as the West syndrome, referring to the physician who first described the features in his own son.

After the infantile spasms have subsided, the child is sometimes left with the development of autistic symptoms. Taft and Cohen (1971) first noted the relationship between hypsarrhythmia and infantile spasms with autism. The percentage of patients with infantile spasms who later become autistic varies in different studies, from 2 per cent (Prats *et al.* 1991) to 16 per cent (Riikonen and Amnell 1981). Millichap (1997) estimates that the percentage averages around 10 per cent. Looking at the problem from a different perspective, one could ask what percentage of autistic patients with all forms of epilepsy have infantile spasms? In the large series of 302 autistic patients studied by Tuchman *et al.* (1991), infantile spasms occurred in 12 per cent of the autistic patients with epilepsy.

It is known that patients with malformations of cortical development typically present with infantile spasms. Patients with infantile spasms who later develop an autistic syndrome may have one of a number of different disease entities, placing these patients in the category of one of the double syndromes. Those disease entities that may have infantile spasms in early infancy include tuberous sclerosis, neurofibromatosis 1, Down syndrome, phenylketonuria and minor hydrocephalus. Tuberous sclerosis is one of the more common double syndromes underlying autism. In a study of 38 patients with tuberous sclerosis and epilepsy, 17 had infantile spasms (Ohtsuka *et al.* 1998). A number of patients with neurofibromatosis 1 have also been reported with infantile spasms (Millichap 1997). (For more details on these double syndromes, see Chapters 11 and 14.)

One study suggests that both temporal lobes often appear to be involved in those patients with infantile spasms who will later develop autism (Chugani *et al.* 1996). This was a follow-up study of 14 babies with infantile spasms and a PET study showing bitemporal hypometablism; 10 of them later became autistic.

Infantile Convulsions Not Meeting Criteria of Infantile Spasms

In the first few weeks of life, infantile spasms are, by far, the most likely seizure pattern to be associated with later development of autistic symptoms. However, there are other rare possibilities. A patient with adenylosuccinase deficiency, a purine disorder some-times associated with autistic features, has presented with epilepsy in early infancy (Maaswinkel-Mooij *et al.* 1997). There is a case in the literature of an infant with EEG and clinical symptoms that met the criteria of benign familial neonatal convulsions who later became autistic (Alfonso *et al.* 1997).

Atonic Seizures

Atonic seizures refer to generalized seizures in which the dominant motor manifestation is loss of postural tone, associated with loss of consciousness, usually for several minutes. They are simply *grand mal* seizures with limpness – rather than stiffness and repetitive jerking. Such cases have been reported in children with autism in the Tuchman *et al.* (1991) series.

MYOCLONIC EPILEPSIES OF EARLY CHILDHOOD (MINOR MOTOR SEIZURES)

Myoclonic seizures refer to single or multiple, brief, shocklike jerking movements of the head, trunk or extremities. The infant form of these epilepsies begins in infancy or the preschool years and is often seen in combination with tonic–clonic patterns. It may be associated with a burst of slow 1- to 2.5-per-second spike-and-wave complexes on EEG.

Myoclonic seizures are seen in patients with autism but it is unusual to find them as an isolated seizure type. Most often they are found in combination with other seizure patterns, particularly tonic–clonic, and are classified as the myoclonic epilepsies (Gillberg and Steffenburg 1987, Olsson *et al.* 1988). As the exception to the rule, there are several cases in the medical literature of solitary myoclonic seizures and autism (Boyer *et al.* 1981, Gillberg 1984). The Gillberg (1984) case involved a boy with classical autism and myoclonic seizures who became seizure-free on valproic acid, and thereafter quickly improved in regard to both his severe behavioral symptoms and his language disturbances.

ABSENCE EPILEPSY (*PETIT MAL*)

Absence seizures refer to staring spells, usually less than 20 seconds in duration, sometimes with slight flickering of the eyes. There are associated bilateral 2–4 Hz spike-and-slow wave (spike-and-dome) complexes on EEG. EEGs are indicated for children in whom epilepsy is suspected, but it should be kept in mind that non-epileptic staring spells are much more common than absence seizures (Rapin 1997).

There are a few studies which have found absence seizures in patients with autism (Ritvo *et al.* 1990, Tuchman *et al.* 1991). The absence seizures may be described as atypical. There is a case in the literature of an 8-year-old boy in whom absence seizures were reported to "masquerade" as autism. He had almost continuous bilateral synchronous 3 Hz spike-and-slow wave complexes on EEG and improved dramatically – both psychiatrically and neurologically – with ethosuximide monotherapy (Gillberg and Schaumann 1983).

COMPLEX PARTIAL SEIZURES (PSYCHOMOTOR EPILEPSY)

If a child blanks out or stares, there are two possible seizure types to consider. One is absence seizures, as described above. The other is complex partial seizures, which usually last between 30 seconds and 2 minutes and are accompanied by a variety of automatisms, such as lip-smacking, hand-wringing or plucking at clothes. Other signs of a partial complex seizure might be a temporary "dreamy state" or impaired consciousness with an affective disturbance such as fear or anger. The EEG may show either a unilateral or bilateral focus, usually frontal or temporal.

It is easy to see how such seizure activity might be hard to pick out in a child with autism. Corbett (1982) raised the question of how likely it was that such seizure activity might be under-reported in non-verbal children with autism. A population-based study of epilepsy in prepubertal children with autism or autistic-like conditions found that complex partial seizures were present in 71 per cent of those who had an onset of seizures in early childhood (Olsson *et al.* 1988). In another study of young people with autism, aged 16 to 23 years, Gillberg and Steffenburg (1987) found that the majority of those with epilepsy and a prepubertal onset had complex partial seizures.

GENERALIZED TONIC–CLONIC SEIZURES (*GRAND MAL*)
In seizure parlance, the word "tonic" refers to a stiffening of the body with rigid extension of the trunk and extremities. The word "clonic" refers to generalized seizures with repetitive bilateral clonic jerking of the extremities. In tonic–clonic (*grand mal*) seizures, there is typically alternate stiffening and jerking associated with loss of consciousness.

Generalized tonic–clonic seizures are the most frequent form of epilepsy in the general population. They are relatively common in children and adolescents with autism (Olsson *et al.* 1988, Tuchman *et al.* 1991, Carod *et al.* 1995). In autism, tonic–clonic seizures may be associated with other types of seizures, either as a sequela after infantile spasms, or immediately following complex partial seizures (Gillberg and Steffenburg 1987, Olsson *et al.* 1988).

Medical work-up

Medical work-up is indicated for diagnostic purposes for all patients with an autistic syndrome (see Chapter 16). A complete work-up is particularly important before starting anticonvulsants in patients with autism and epilepsy, to rule out the possibility of an underlying metabolic disease which might be adversely affected by a specific anticonvulsant. Examples relating to valproic acid demonstrate this. A test for lactate/pyruvate levels is needed in children with suspected mitochondrial disorders before valproate treatment is employed, in order to prevent potential fatalities (Chabrol *et al.* 1994). Also, 24-hour urinary calcium needs to be studied before giving valproic acid, a drug that itself predisposes to osteoporotic fractures. Since children with autism are often low in serum magnesium (see Chapter 13), this test has particular relevance to any child with a seizure disorder. Recurrent epileptic attacks occurring to an autistic person in an institution may signal that the patient is suffering from intermittent water intoxication due to compulsive water drinking and episodic release of antidiuretic hormone (Hiratani *et al.* 1997).

Antiepileptic therapies in autism

Ideal therapies against epilepsy are tailored to the specifics of the individual patient's etiology of the seizure disorder. At present few such therapies exist. A disease entity within the autistic syndrome that includes many children with epilepsy is purine autism (see Chapter 10). When patients with purine autism have a seizure disorder, one of the choices for an anticonvulsant is a specific drug – allopurinol – which directly affects purine metabolism (Coleman *et al.* 1986).

Non-specific anticonvulsant therapies in patients with autism and epilepsy include valproic acid, carbamazepine, and steroids, as well as new drugs being developed. The need for new drugs exists because seizure control cannot be obtained in all patients. Some of the best antiepileptic drugs (phenytoin, phenobarbitone and the benzodiazepines) are of limited value in autism, since they may be detrimental to the behavioral status of particular children with both autism and epilepsy. In a few patients, seizure control by successful antiepileptics is accompanied by an improved psychiatric status. If an individual with autism and epilepsy needs to be placed on a class of drugs other than anticonvulsants, *e.g.* drugs such as neuroleptics, caution is indicated in the selection of the additional drugs to ensure that the drugs used for behavior do not affect the seizure disorder.

Valproic acid is a standard antiepileptic monotherapy for autism or potential autism, and it has been reported to be effective in children with autism with a variety of different seizure presentations. It has been used in *infantile spasms* at doses as high as 100 to 300 mg/kg/day, with control of the hypsarrhythmic EEG pattern achieved within two weeks for over three-quarters of the children (Prats *et al.* 1991). Gillberg and Schaumann (1983) described a boy with autism and frequent *myoclonic seizures* who became seizure-free on valproic acid, and thereafter rapidly improved in regard to his behavioral and language disabilities. There is a report of a dramatically accelerated rate of acquisition of both language and social skills, concomitant with control of *absence seizures*, in twin boys with autism begun on valproic acid at 3 years of age (Childs and Blair 1997). A girl with autism and *complex partial seizures* had improvement in her EEG and a suppression of her staring spells on valproic acid (Gillberg and Schaumann 1983). However, like all drugs, valproic acid has side-effects. Occasionally valproate causes a serious or fatal hepatotoxicity, particularly in young children under 2 years of age. Early symptoms are exacerbation of seizures, drowsiness, nausea and anorexia, vomiting, jaundice, infections with fever, apathy and coma (Bryant and Dreifuss 1996). Longer-term concerns are problems with weight gain and the effect of the drug on calcium metabolism which can be at risk in patients with autism (see Chapter 13). Valproate may be associated with decreased mineralization of bone which may predispose to osteoporotic fractures (Sheth *et al.* 1995). In girls, there is also a concern regarding the effect of long-term use on reproductive endocrine disorders (Vainionpää *et al.* 1999).

Carbamazepine, also used in monotherapy for patients with autism and epilepsy, has its share of side-effects and is contraindicated in combination with liquid neuroleptics. Its efficacy as a drug to suppress behavioral symptoms in autism is not well established (Smith and Perry 1992).

Steroid therapy has been a standard for the treatment of infantile spasms. In infantile spasms, ACTH or prednisolone is begun as soon as possible after the onset of the first seizure. Steroid therapy is also being tried experimentally for seizure disorders in young children with autism. A combination therapy of valproic acid plus a weekly bolus of 10 mg/kg prednisone or methylprednisolone was reported to improve speech in 36 out of 44 young children with language regression and an abnormal sleep Digitrace 24 EEG (Chez *et al.* 1998). No side-effects of cushingoid features were detected after 18 months. In addition to standard steroids, a group in the Netherlands has reported using a synthetic analog of adrenocorticotrophic hormone(4-9) in autism. In a double-blind, placebo-crossover trial, this synthetic analog, called ORG 2766, has been reported to show benefit to the behavioral component in children with autism (Buitelaar *et al.* 1992, 1996), including an improved quality of their social interaction. In evaluation of steroid therapy, it must be remembered that steroids themselves can produce mood-altering symptoms – euphoria being a common one.

A small fraction of children with autism and epilepsy do not become seizure-free on standard monotherapy. Development of new anticonvulsant drugs is a priority in neurology. One of the relatively new drugs currently being tried is lamotrigine. In a study by Uvebrant and Bauziene (1994), 13 children with autism and intractable epilepsy were treated with lamotrigine as an anticonvulsant. In an interesting development, eight of the children had a decrease of behavioral autistic symptoms during the lamotrigine therapy, including several with an unchanged seizure situation. Other new drugs being investigated for use in autism are vigabatrin, gabapentin, clobazam and topiramate.

Antiepileptic neurosurgery may be a final option for refractory patients. Two boys who had brain surgery for their epilepsy initially improved dramatically regarding their autistic symptoms; however one subsequently relapsed (Gillberg *et al.* 1996). Surgery is also being tried in some forms of autistic regression associated with abnormal EEGs. It has been reported that seven children with autistic epileptiform regression had improvement of seizure control after multiple subpial regression (Nass *et al.* 1999). A great deal more research is necessary to evaluate this new approach; the cases where the surgery fails may tend not to be published.

Electrophysiology

One of the most difficult things to understand in the field of autism is the many papers describing brainstem auditory evoked potentials, cortical evoked potentials and event-related potentials in this patient group. The difficulty arises because the studies done by outstanding investigators have been found to contradict each other. The studies are remarkable in their lack of a coherent answer to specific questions. Even studies with a large number of patients – 109 children in the Wong and Wong (1991) study – are contradicted by other studies (Klin 1993). The inconsistent literature is particularly disappointing because of the greater consistency of results of evoked potential studies in other developmental syndromes, which have more specifically defined etiologies, such as Down syndrome.

A glimpse of what might underlie this confusing literature is provided by the electrophysiological studies performed by the Lelord group in France (Martineau *et al.* 1992a, 1992b, Lelord *et al.* 1993). Their studies agree that the cognitive deficit in the ability to maintain cross-modal associations is preceded by a more elementary perceptive abnormality in children with autism. What is illuminating is that they interpret their results as allowing the separation of autistic children into three subgroups which present different patterns of ability to form cross-modal associations. The three subgroups present different clinical profiles regarding attention, intention, motility, association, contact and communication.

Another possible explanation for the inconsistent results is the chance that calcium levels in the brain might vary from patient to patient. A subgroup of children with autism (not negligible in size) have abnormal calcium levels in the urine (see Chapter 13). It has been shown in the medical literature on dialysis that the lower the calcium level, the greater the BAER absolute latency and interpeak latency values (Pratt *et al.* 1986). Thivièrge *et al.* (1990) in their BAER study of 20 children with autism did not attempt to measure calcium levels, but they were puzzled by the contradictory results in the literature and came up with the suggestion that calcium levels in the brainstem might help explain the incompatible reports from excellent centers.

Thus there is the possibility that a population of autistic children, even though they are carefully diagnosed, is not homogeneous regarding many electrophysiological phenomena, to say nothing of their underlying diagnosis. When scientists start experiments with mixed populations, there is inevitable variability in the results – no matter how carefully a study is performed, how brilliant the investigator, or how sophisticated the equipment. The older literature on this subject, including ERG and sleep studies, is summarized in Chapter 12 of the second edition of this textbook. This literature is based on the assumption that autism is one specific entity that can be studied as a whole. In the future, when electrophsyiological studies are performed on specific disease entities within the autistic syndrome (see Chapters 10 and 11 of this edition), data that will survive the test of time is likely to emerge.

In the last decade, new variations of electrophysiological studies have been introduced into the field, still based on studying all patients with autism mixed together as one whole group. Midlatency auditory evoked reponses (P1), measuring the ascending reticular activating system and their thalamic target cells, have been reported as abnormal in children with autism (Buchwald *et al.* 1992). Studies from the Netherlands have shown that the occipital event-related potential P3 waves are smaller in children with autism compared to controls (Verbaten *et al.* 1991). In 1994, Kemner *et al.* compared autistic children with three control groups (normal, attention-deficit, dyslexic) and found that the children with autism differed from controls with respect to visual and somatosensory event-related potential P2N2 and the visual event-related potential P3. These authors also found that children with autism show abnormalities of processing of both proximal (somatosensory) and distal (visual) stimuli. The studies raise the question of under-stimulation of the occipital lobe by visual stimuli in autism (Kemner *et al.* 1995). A reassuring study, evaluating speech prosody, indicated "remarkably normal P3 and behavioral processing of prosodic stimuli by high functioning adults" with autism (Erwin *et al.* 1991).

Summary

Individuals with an autistic syndrome are more likely to have a seizure disorder than most categories of individuals with mental retardation. Some disease entities within the autistic syndrome have patients with epilepsy; others do not. Individual diagnosis and treatment are the best approach to epilepsy in autism. Electrophysiological studies that treat patients with autism as a single diagnostic group are often not replicated. In the future, electro-physiological studies limited to individual disease entities within the autistic syndrome should prove to be more consistent and revealing.

REFERENCES

Alfonso, I., Hahn, J.S., Papazian, O., Martinez, Y.L., Reyes, M.A., Aicardi, J. (1997) 'Bilateral tonic–clonic epileptic seizures in non-benign familial neonatal convulsions.' *Pediatric Neurology*, **16**, 249–251.

Boyer, J.-P., Deschatrette, A., Delwarde, M. (1981) 'Autism convulsif?' (In French) *Pédiatrie*, **5**, 353–368.

Bryant, A.E. III, Dreifuss, F.E. (1996) 'Valproic hepatic fatalities. III. US experience since 1986.' *Neurology*, **46**, 465–469.

Buchwald, J.S., Erwin, R., van Lancker, D., Guthrie, D., Schwafel, J., Tanguay, P. (1992) 'Midlatency auditory evoked responses: P1 abnormalities in adult autistic subjects.' *Electroencephalography and Clinical Neurophysiology*, **84**, 164–171.

Buitelaar, J.K., van Engeland, H., de Kogel, K.H., de Vries, H., van Hoof, J.A., van Ree, J.M. (1992) 'The use of adrenocorticotrophic hormone (4-9) analog ORG 2766 in autistic children: effects on organization of behavior.' *Biological Psychiatry*, **31**, 1119–1129.

Buitelaar, J.K., Dekker, M.E., van Ree, J.M, van Engeland, H. (1996) 'A controlled trial with ORG 2766, an ACTH-(4-9) analog, in 50 relatively able children with autism.' *European Neuropsychopharmacology*, **6**, 13–19.

Carod, F.J., Prats, J.M., Garaizar, C., Zuazo, E. (1995) 'Clinical-radiological evaluation of infantile autism and epileptic syndromes associated with autism.' (In Spanish) *Review Neurologique*, **23**, 1203–1207.

Chabrol, B., Mancini, J., Chretien, D., Rustin, P., Munnich, A., Pinsard, N. (1994) 'Valproate-induced hepatic failure in a case of cytochrome C oxidase deficiency.' *European Journal of Pediatrics*, **153**, 133–135.

Chez, M.G., Loeffel, M., Buchanan, C.P., Field-Chez, M. (1998) 'Pulse high-dose steroids as combination therapy with valproic acid in epileptic aphasia patients with pervasive developmental delay or autism.' (Abstract) *Annals of Neurology*, **44**, 539.

Childs, J.A., Blair, J.L. (1997) 'Valproic acid treatment of epilepsy in autistic twins.' *Journal of Neuroscience Nursing*, **29**, 244–248.

Chugani, H.T., Da Silva, E., Chugani, D.C. (1996) 'Prognostic implications of bitemporal hypometabolism on positron emission tomography.' *Annals of Neurology*, **39**, 643–649.

Coleman, M., Landgrebe, M., Landgrebe, A. (1986) 'Purine seizure disorders.' *Epilepsia*, **23**, 263–269.

Corbett, J. (1982) 'Epilepsy and the electroencephalogram in early childhood psychosis.' *In:* Wing, J.K., Wing, L. (Eds) *Handbook of Psychiatry. Vol. 3*. London: Cambridge University Press, pp.198–202.

DeLong, G.R., Heinz, E.R. (1997) 'The clinical syndrome of early-life bilateral hippocampal sclerosis.' *Annals of Neurology*, **42**, 11–17.

Elia, M., Musumeci, S.A., Ferri, R., Bergonzi, P. (1995) 'Clinical and neurophysiological aspects of epilepsy in subjects with autism and mental retardation.' *American Journal of Mental Retardation*, **100**, 6–16.

Erwin, R., van Lancker, D., Guthrie, D., Schwafel, J., Tanguay, P., Buchwald, J.S. (1991) 'P3 responses to prosodic stimuli in adult autistic patients.' *Electroencephalography and Clinical Neurophysiology*, **80**, 561–571.

Gillberg, C. (1984) 'Infantile autism and other childhood psychoses in a Swedish urban region. Epidemiological aspects.' *Journal of Child Psychology and Psychiatry*, **25**, 35–43.

Gillberg, C., Schaumann, H. (1983) 'Epilepsy presenting as infantile autism? Two case studies.' *Neuropediatrics*, **14**, 206–212.

Gillberg, C., Steffenburg, S. (1987) 'Outcome and prognostic factors in infantile autism and similar conditions: a population-based study of 46 cases followed through puberty.' *Journal of Autism and Developmental Disorders*, **17**, 273–287.

Gillberg, C., Persson, E., Grufman, M., Themnér, U. (1986) 'Psychiatric disorders in mildly and severely mentally retarded urban children and adolescents: epidemiological aspects.' *British Journal of Psychiatry*, **149**, 68–74.

Gillberg, C., Uvebrant, P., Carlsson, G., Hedstrom, A., Silfvenius, H. (1996) 'Autism and epilepsy (and tuberous sclerosis?) in two pre-adolescent boys: neuropsychiatric aspects before and after epilepsy surgery.' *Journal of Intellectual Disability Research*, **40**, 75–81.

Giovanardi Rossi, P., Parmeggiani, A., Bach, V., Santucci, M., Visconti, P. (1995) 'EEG features and epilepsy in patients with autism.' *Brain Development*, **17**, 169–174.

Herder, G.A. (1993) 'Infantile autism among children in the county of Nordland. Prevalence and etiology.' (In Norwegian) *Tidsskrift for den Norske Laegeforening*, **113**, 2247–2249.

194

Hiratani, M., Munesue, T., Terai, K., Haruki, S. (1997) 'Two cases of infantile autism with intermittent water intoxication due to compulsive water drinking and episodic release of antidiuretic hormone.' (In Japanese) *No To Hattatsu*, **29**, 367–372.

Hirsch, E., Marescaux, C., Maquet, P., Metz-Lutz, M.N., Kiesmann, M., Salmon, E., Franck, G., Kurtz, D. (1990) Landau–Kleffner syndrome: a clinical and EEG study. *Epilepsia*, **31**, 756–767.

Kanner, L. (1943) 'Autistic disturbances of affective contact.' *Nervous Child*, **2**, 217–250.

—— (1971) 'Follow-up study of eleven children originally reported in 1943.' *Journal of Autism and Childhood Schizophrenia*, **1**, 119–145.

Kemner, C., Verbaten, M.C., Cuperus, J.M., Camfferman, G., van Engeland, H. (1994) 'Visual and somatosensory event-related brain potentials in autistic children and three different control groups.' *Electroencephalography and Clinical Neurophysiology*, **92**, 225–237.

—— (1995) 'Auditory event-related brain potentials in autistic children and three different control groups.' *Biological Psychiatry*, **38**, 150–165.

Klin, A. (1993) 'Auditory brainstem responses in autism: brainstem dysfunction or peripheral hearing loss?' *Journal of Autism and Developmental Disorders*, **23**, 15–35.

Lelord, G., Herault, J., Perrot, A., Hameury, L., Lenoir, P., Adrien, J.L., Mallet, J., Muh, J.P. (1993) 'Childhood autism: a relating deficiency due to a developmental disorder of the nervous system.' (In French) *Bulletin de Academie Nationale de Medicine*, **177**, 1423–1430.

Maaswinkel-Mooij, P.D., Laan, L.A., Onkenhout, W., Brouwer, O.F., Jaeken, J., Poorthuis, B.J. (1997) 'Adenylosuccinase deficiency presenting with epilepsy in early infancy.' *Journal of Inherited Metabolic Disease*, **20**, 606–607.

Martineau, J., Roux, S., Adrien, J.L., Garreau, B., Barthelemy, C., Lelord, G. (1992a) 'Electrophysiological evidence of different abilities to form cross-modal associations in children with autistic behavior.' *Electroencephalography and Clinical Neurophysiology*, **82**, 60–66.

Martineau, J., Roux, S., Garreau, B., Adrien, J.L., Lelord, G. (1992b) 'Unimodal and crossmodal reactivity in autism: presence of auditory evoked responses and effect of the repetition of auditory stimuli.' *Biological Psychiatry*, **31**, 1190–1203.

Millichap, J.G. (1997) *Progress in Pediatric Neurology III*. Chicago: PNB Publishers, p. 41(infantile spasms and neurofibromatosis 1).

Morrell, F., Whisler, W.W., Smith, V.D.C., Hoeppner, T.J., de Toledo-Morrell, L., Pierre-Louis, S.J., Kanner, A.M., Buelow, J.M., Ristanovic, R., Bergen, D. (1995) 'Landau–Kleffner syndrome. Treatment with subpial intracortical transection.' *Brain*, **118**, 1529–1546.

Nass, R., Gross, A., Devinsky, O. (1998) 'Autism and autistic epileptiform regression with occipital spikes.' *Developmental Medicine and Child Neurology*, **40**, 453–458.

Nass, R., Gross, A., Wisoff, J., Devinsky, O. (1999) 'Outcome of multiple subpial transections for autistic epileptiform regression.' *Pediatric Neurology*, **21**, 464–470.

Ohtsuka, Y., Ohmori, I., Oka, E. (1998) 'Long-term follow-up of childhood epilepsy associated with tuberous sclerosis.' *Epilepsia*, **39**, 1158–1163.

Olsson, I., Steffenburg, S., Gillberg, C. (1988) 'Epilepsy in autism and autistic-like conditions: a population-based study.' *Archives of Neurology*, **45**, 666–668.

Prats, J.M., Garaizar, C., Rua, M.J., Garcia-Nieto, M.L., Madoz, P. (1991) 'Infantile spasms treated with high doses of sodium valproate: initial response and follow-up.' *Developmental Medicine and Child Neurology*, **33**, 617–625.

Pratt, H., Brosky, G., Goldhsher, M., Ben-David, Y., Harari, R., Podoshin, L., Eliachar, I., Gruska, E., Better, O., Garty, J. (1986) 'Auditory brain stem evoked potentials in patients undergoing dialysis.' *Electroencephalography and Clinical Neurophysiology*, **63**, 18–24.

Rapin, I. (1995) 'Autistic regression and disintegrative disorder: how important is the role of epilepsy?' *Seminars in Pediatric Neurology*, **2**, 278–285.

—— (1997) 'Autism.' *New England Journal of Medicine*, **337**, 97–104.

Riikonen, R., Amnell, G. (1981) 'Psychiatric disorders in children with earlier infantile spasms.' *Developmental Medicine and Child Neurology*, **23**, 747–760.

Ritvo, E.R., Freeman, B.J., Pingree, C., Mason-Brothers, A., Jorde, L.B., Jenson, W.R., McMahon, W.M., Petersen, P.B., Mo, A., Ritvo, A. (1990) 'The UCLA-University of Utah epidemiological survey of autism prevalence.' *American Journal of Psychiatry*, **146**, 194–199.

Rossi, P.G., Parmeggiani, A., Bach, V., Santucci, M., Visconti, P. (1995) 'EEG features and epilepsy in patients with autism.' *Brain Development*, **17**, 169–174.

Rutter, M. (1970) 'Autistic children. Infancy to adulthood.' *Seminars in Psychiatry*, **2**, 435–450.

Sheth, R.D., Wesolowshi, C.A., Jacob, J.C., Penney, S., Habbe, G.R., Riggs, J.E., Bodensteiner, J.B.(1995) 'Effect of carbamazepine and valproate on bone mineral density.' *Journal of Pediatrics*, **127**, 245–262.

Smith, D.A., Perry, P.J. (1992) 'Nonneuroleptic treatment of disruptive behavior in organic mental syndromes.' *Annals of Pharmacotherapy*, **26**, 1400–1408.

Steffenburg, U., Hagberg, G., Viggedal, G., Kyllerman, M. (1995) 'Active epilepsy in mentally retarded children. I. Prevalence and additional neuro-impairments.' *Acta Paediatrica*, **84**, 1147–1152.

Taft, L.T., Cohen, H.J. (1971) 'Hypsarrhythmia and infantile spasms: a clinical report.' *Journal of Autism and Childhood Schizophrenia*, **3**, 287.

Thivièrge, J., Bedard, C., Côté, R., Maziade, M. (1990) 'Brainstem auditory evoked response and subcortical abnormalities in autism.' *American Journal of Psychiatry*, **147**, 1609–1613.

Tsai, L.Y., Tsai, M.C., August, G.J. (1985) 'Brief report: implication of EEG diagnoses in the subclassification of infantile autism.' *Journal of Autism and Childhood Schizophrenia*, **15**, 339–344.

Tuchman, R.F., Rapin, I. (1997) 'Regression in pervasive developmental disorders: seizures and epileptiform electroencephalogram correlates.' *Pediatrics*, **99**, 560–565.

Tuchman, R.F., Rapin, I., Shinnar, S. (1991) 'Autistic and dysphasic children. II: epilepsy.' *Pediatrics*, **88**, 1219–1225.

Uvebrant, P., Bauziene, R. (1994) 'Intractable epilepsy in children. The efficacy of lamotrigine treatment.' *Neuropediatrics*, **25**, 284–289.

Vainionpää, L.K., Rättyä, J., Knip, M., Tapanainen, J.S., Pakarinen, A.J., Lanning, P., Tekay, A., Myllylä, V.V., Isojärvi, J.I.T. (1999) 'Valproate-induced hyperandrogenism during pubertal maturation in girls with epilepsy.' *Annals of Neurology*, **45**, 444–450.

Verbaten, M.N., Roelofs, J.W., van Engeland, H., Kenemans, J.K., Slagen, J.L. (1991) 'Abnormal visual event-related potentials of autistic children.' *Journal of Autism and Developmental Disorders*, **21**, 449–470.

Wong, V. (1993) 'Epilepsy in children with autistic spectrum disorder.' *Journal of Child Neurology*, **8**, 316–322.

Wong, V., Wong, S.N. (1991) 'Brainstem auditory evoked potential study in children with autistic disorder.' *Journal of Autism and Developmental Disorders*, **23**, 15–35.

13
BIOCHEMISTRY, ENDOCRINOLOGY AND IMMUNOLOGY

There are many fascinating problems under investigation regarding the biochemistry, endocrinology and immunology in children with an autistic syndrome. To take one example, recent studies have suggested that neurotransmitters themselves may also have roles as neural morphogens during brain development. Thus it is theoretically possible that early abnormalities in the stimulation of dopamine or serotonin receptor subtypes could lead to the kind of neuroanatomical changes observed in autism (Todd 1992).

In this chapter, as in Chapters 12 and 14, the work reported here was almost always performed on a group of individuals with autism, treating them as though they all had a single disease. This needs to be kept in mind when evaluating these studies.

Biochemistry

AMINO ACIDS AND ORGANIC ACIDS

Amino acid and organic acid testing in the urine are standard tests which can be useful in identifying disease entities found in children with mental retardation. However, they have usually not been productive when performed on specimens from children with autism. The exception is patients who have phenylketonuria (PKU), a disease producing abnormal levels of phenylalanine in the serum and phenylpyruvic acid in the urine (see Chapter 11).

A study by Perry *et al.* (1978) of amino acid levels in the plasma, urine and CSF of 28 children with infantile autism showed no known disease entities. In the CSF portion of that study, ethanolamine appeared to be elevated in some of the children. Another study of amino acids in the CSF of children with autism (Winsberg *et al.* 1980) reported that two children had an elevation of arginine, although most results were unremarkable. Four amino acids or their amines – aspartic acid, glutamine, glutamic acid and gamma-aminobutyric acid – have been measured inside the platelets of 18 persons with autism, and were found to be significantly decreased compared to controls (Rolf *et al.* 1993). Moreno-Fuenmayor *et al.* (1996) reported variation in levels of excitatory amino acids in the plasma of 14 children with autism.

The children in the study by Perry *et al.* (1978) also had organic acid levels in plasma, urine and CSF tested by gas chromotography. None of the known diseases of organic acid metabolism was found, although unidentified peaks were noted.

KREBS CYCLE ANALOGS

A marked increase in analogs of the Krebs cycle and arabinose was found in the urine of two brothers with autistic features (Shaw *et al.* 1995).

SEROTONIN (5-HYDROXYTRYPTAMINE; 5HT)

Serotonin is a neurotransmitter in the central nervous system that also exists in the platelets of the blood and thus is a brain amine whose levels can easily be studied in humans. It has at least 14 distinct receptor subtypes (Martin *et al.* 1998). Its metabolic pathway is seen in Fig. 13.1. Gene knockout experiments have shown that many genes play multiple roles in different tissues during development. Serotonin appears to play at least two different roles in the developing brain, first as a morphogenetic agent involved as a trophic or differentiation factor during formation of the brain *in utero*, and later as a major neurotransmitter in children and adults. Serotonin content, serotonin uptake sites and serotonin receptor binding, as measured in animal studies, are all higher in the young brain, compared with adult values, and decline before puberty. A recent study involving α-[^{11}C]-methyl-L-tryptophan and PET was interpreted to suggest that human children undergo a period of changing brain serotonin synthesis capacity with age and that this normal developmental process was disrupted in the 30 children with autism who participated in the study (Chugani *et al.* 1999). This paper even raises the question of whether fetal serotonin depletion might be a factor related to the increased neuronal cell numbers and/or macrocephaly found in some autistic brains (see Chapter 14).

The level of serotonin – as measured by whole blood, platelet or serum methods – has been found to be below normal in a number of human diseases, and above normal in a number of others. Patients with autism and an associated known medical disorder (double syndromes) fall into both categories. Those with the double syndromes of PKU autism or de Lange autism may have low serotonin levels in their blood; those with the double syndromes of congenital rubella, tuberous sclerosis, infant hypothyroidism and Williams syndrome may have high levels. In addition, there are many individuals with autism who do not have either a specific diagnosis or a known double syndrome but do have high levels of 5HT in their blood. High levels of serotonin occur much more frequently in autism than low levels. In fact, the most consistent biochemical abnormality found in autism is that over 25 per cent of the patients have an elevated 5HT level in platelets, whole blood or serum (Cook 1990). Percentages of patients with elevated serotonin as high as 70 per cent have been reported (Levy and Bicho 1997). Levels of 5HIAA, the end product of serotonin metabolism, have not been found to be elevated in most studies of the cerebrospinal fluid in children with autism (Narayan *et al.* 1993). In one study, levels

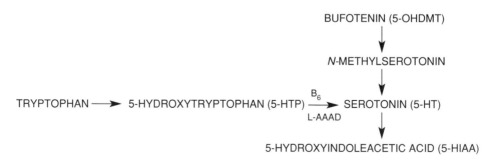

Fig. 13.1 The metabolic pathway of serotonin (5-hydroxytryptamine).

of bufotenin, a minor metabolite of this pathway, were detected in the urine of patients with autism (Himwich *et al.* 1972).

Serotonin, at least theoretically, might have a special relevance to autism and other developmental disorders because it is involved in early neurogenesis (Azmitia *et al.* 1990). However, abnormal levels of serotonin in the blood are not specific to autism. They include diseases such as sudanophilic leukodystrophy, histidinemia, Huntington disease, motor neurone disease, migraine, Raynaud's syndrome, hyperthyroidism, intestinal obstruction, carcinoid disease, asthma, cirrhosis of the liver, and many more (Coleman 1973). A number of variables such as age, drugs and levels in other family members (Leboyer *et al.* 1999) must be taken into account when evaluating whole blood or platelet serotonin in a particular patient. It is interesting that parents of autistic children who themselves have elevated levels of whole blood serotonin have been reported to have significantly higher scores of depression and obsessive-compulsive disorder than parents with normal serotonin levels (Cook *et al.* 1994).

Subjects with autism and elevated whole blood serotonin levels have been shown to have elevated 5HT transport into platelets (Cook and Leventhal 1996). However, the high levels in the platelets do not necessarily mean that this translates to high levels in the central nervous system; in fact, there is reason to think otherwise. A direct measurement was made at autopsy on a child with a leukodystrophy who had many excessively elevated 5HT levels recorded in his whole blood during his lifetime (Coleman *et al.* 1977). The brain level of 5HT was diminished compared to a control who died the same day from a total anomalous pulmonary venous return. The results were a decreased 5HT level in the basal ganglia of 36 per cent, cerebellar gray matter 30 per cent, pons 52 per cent and medulla 69 per cent.

Thus the platelet serotonin binding site, although it is clinically useful, is only a partial model of the 5HT binding site in the brain. Actually, for a partial model, it is surprisingly useful. Recently it has been determined that the human platelet serotonin uptake site and the brain serotonin transporter are both proteins encoded by the same single-copy gene (Lesch *et al.* 1993). It is rare in brain studies that one has exactly the same neurotransmitter and its binding site floating around in the blood, so easy to measure. This may help to explain why abnormal serotonin levels as measured in the blood can sometimes give an indication of the success of a therapeutic intervention in the brain. An example of a disease with high serotonin levels in the blood is seen in infant hypothyroidism, where the levels are high in whole blood (Coleman 1970). Early initiation of thyroid replacement therapy in babies with infant hypothyroidism can be of great value in ameliorating their potential mental retardation. In one such case, the serotonin level came down into the normal range seven days after thyroid therapy was started (Coleman and Hur 1973). The same principle in reverse can be seen in low serotonin patients, such as those with phenylketonuria (PKU). In one case, placement of the patient on a special low phenylalanine diet (the treatment for PKU) resulted in marked improvement of low serotonin blood level, moving it up toward the normal range (McKean 1971). Regarding future research, the improvement of serotonin levels in the blood of autistic patients who start out with abnormal levels could be used as one indirect measure of the success of any new experimental treatments.

There have been several studies related to tryptophan, the initial step of the serotonin pathway in individuals with autism (see Fig. 13.1). Because the ratio of serum tryptophan to large amino acids is thought to be a possible marker of tryptophan availability for brain serotonin synthesis, this ratio was studied in 40 children with autism (D'Eufemia *et al.* 1995). A significantly lower ratio was observed in the children with autism compared to the normal controls. In another study, tryptophan was depleted on a temporary basis causing adults with autism to have a worsening of toe-walking, whirling, flapping, pacing, banging and hitting self, and rocking (McDougle *et al.* 1996a). However, the patients appeared more anxious and no change was noted in social relatedness or repetitive thoughts and behavior. An imaging approach using α-[^{11}C]-methyl-L-tryptophan found that tryptophan metabolites were reduced in one or the other frontal cortex in seven boys with autism, but were increased in their contralateral dentate nucleus (Chugani *et al.* 1997). In this study, which inventoried the dentatothalamocortical pathway, there were statistically significant differences between the boys with autism and their non-autistic siblings. A later study showed that high-functioning girls had a pattern similar to the boys but that low-functioning girls did not (Chugani *et al.* 1998a). All of these studies are difficult to interpret since only 1 per cent of tryptophan goes down the serotonin pathway; other metabolic pathways which begin with tryptophan also include pathways where psychiatric symptoms occur, such as the one to nicotinic acid (Lishman 1987). However, in favor of the likelihood of low serotonin in the brain in some patients with autism is the observation that serotonin-reuptake inhibitor drugs (which increase the amount of 5HT at the receptor site) have improved specific symptoms in up to half the patients with autism (McDougle *et al.* 1996b) (see Chapter 17).

In patients with autism and seizures, serotonin levels may have a relationship to seizure activity. Increased serotonin content and immunoreactivity have been reported in human epileptic tissue removed for seizure control. This is the theoretical basis of the PET studies performed with the tracer α-[^{11}C]-methyl-L-tryptophan ([^{11}C]AMT) in children with tuberous sclerosis and epilepsy (Chugani *et al.* 1998b). Whereas glucose metabolism PET showed multifocal cortical hypometabolism corresponding to the locations of the tubers, [^{11}C]AMT studies showed selective increased uptake only in epileptogenic tubers, with a decrease in nonepileptogenic tubers. Such studies could lead to pinpointed surgery to control seizures.

Recently there has been a revived interest in the meaning of abnormal blood levels of serotonin in persons with autism related to the evidence of an association between autistic disorder and a variant of the promoter region of the serotonin transporter (5HTT) gene (Cook *et al.* 1997). Chugani *et al.* (1999) have postulated that expression of a polymorphism of the serotonin transporter in autism might result in altered serotonin modulation of the thalamocortical connectivity during development, possibly explaining the abnormal sensory perception of autism (O'Neill and Jones 1997). It is interesting that the polymorphism in the promoter region of the gene is also associated with measures of anxiety and depression. The drugs that affect the serotonin transporter protein are also efficacious with obsessive-compulsive disorder (McDougle *et al.* 1998). No differences in allele and genotype frequencies for the 5-HT2A receptor marker were found in one study of children with autism compared with age-matched healthy students (Hérault *et al.* 1996).

An interesting new pilot study has compared the severity of repetitive behaviors in adult autistic patients to a measure of serotonergic function (Hollander *et al.* 2000). The growth hormone response to the 5-HT 1d agonist, sumatriptan, was measured in 11 adult patients with autism or Asperger disorder. The authors report that, in their study, the severity of repetitive behaviors paralleled the sensitivity of the 5-HT 1d receptor as manifest by the sumatriptan-elicited growth hormone response.

CATECHOL AMINES

When it was discovered that a child with phenylketonuria (PKU) was clinically diagnosed as having autism (see Chapter 11), research interest in autism focused on a metabolic pathway leading from phenylalanine toward neurotransmitters of the catechol amine pathways (see Fig. 13.2) An extensive literature in autism developed, showing both normal and abnormal levels of various catechol amines, their end-products and the enzymes of their pathways (see the second edition of this book). However, since the patients tested were not screened for individual disease entities in most cases, often not even for PKU, it is hard to know if some disease entities within the autistic syndrome do or do not have catechol amine abnormalities or lags in maturation. Apparently, if patients with autism are grouped together and tested as whole, it is unlikely that there are consistent abnormalities to be found (Minderaa *et al.* 1994). One interesting recent study demonstrated low medial pre-frontal dopaminergic activity by new techniques using regional FDOPA ratios measured by PET (Ernst *et al.* 1997). The studies were based on fourteen 13-year-olds with autism, compared to controls.

Genetic studies in autism which explore genes of the catechol amine pathway are still at the early stages. In a study of 50 children with autism and age-matched controls, no difference for allele frequencies was found in the genes coding for tyrosine hydroxylase, dopamine beta hydroxylase and DRD3 (Martineau *et al.* 1994). The A1 allele of the Taq I polymorphism of the dopamine D2 receptor has been reported to have an increased

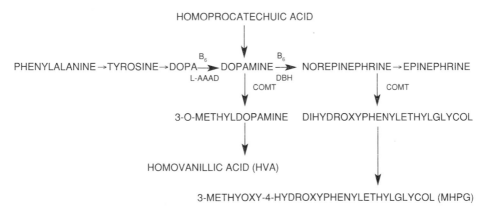

Fig. 13.2 The metabolic pathway of the catechol amines (dopamine and norepinephrine).

201

prevalence in autism (Comings *et al.* 1991). However, because increased prevalence of the A1 allele is found in a number of other behavior disorders, it is thought to act as a modifying gene rather than as the primary etiologic agent. (For more information on genetic studies in autism, see Chapter 15.)

MELATONIN
Melatonin (N-acetyl-methoxytryptamine) is involved in regulation of sleep/wake cycles. Abnormalities of circadian rhythm in autism first noticed by Yamazaki (Yamazaki *et al.* 1975) have been further documented with a study of melatonin in a group of adults with a severe autistic syndrome (Nir *et al.* 1995). Although not out of phase, the serum melatonin levels differed from normal in amplitude and mesor. The usefulness of melatonin for sleep problems in autism has been raised (Lord 1998). Because melatonin is contraindicated in individuals with autoimmune disorders (see below), this would have to be evaluated on an individual basis.

CYCLIC AMP
Cyclic AMP (adenosine monophosphate) is believed to act as the "second messenger" inside the cell for neurotransmitters such as serotonin and catecholamines. It also affects calcium release in platelets (Moos and Goldberg 1988). There have been several studies performed in autistic children (Belmaker *et al.* 1978, Hoshino *et al.* 1979, 1980, Goldberg *et al.* 1984); the studies suggest that plasma cyclic AMP may be elevated in psychiatrically disturbed children, including those with autism.

PTERINS
Pterins comprise a class of vital co-factors in brain function; tetrahydrobiopterin (THB) is essential for brain cells to make monoamine neurotransmitters. THB is synthesized directly at those sites where it is used as a co-factor, in the serotoninergic and dopaminergic synaptosomes. A derivative of THB, called 6R-BH4, has been found to directly stimulate the release of neurotransmitters such as dopamine and serotonin independently of its co-factor activity (Miwa *et al.* 1992). When plasma and urinary levels of tetrahydrobiopterin, neopterin and monapterin were assessed in 16 children with autism and 12 healthy controls, the results indicated that plasma and urinary levels of tetrahydrobiopterin were not statistically different between the two groups (Eto *et al.* 1992). Messahel *et al.* (1998) studied urinary levels of neopterin and biopterin in a group of children with autism, their siblings and age-matched control children; both urinary neopterin and biopterin were raised in the children with autism compared to controls, and their siblings showed intermediate results (Harrison and Pheasant 1995). In the Eto *et al.* (1992) study, plasma levels of neopterin and monapterin were significantly depressed. One study of 20 children with autism found these two pterin compounds significantly reduced in the cerebrospinal fluid (Tani *et al.* 1994).

In 1987, a group of investigators conducted double-blind, placebo-controlled trials of the effect of administration of THB on 84 autistic children for 12 weeks, and reported that it was of benefit with no significant side-effects (Takesada *et al.* 1987). This work needs evaluation and follow-up. Folate is a pterin (see below).

202

GANGLIOSIDES

Gangliosides are a type of glycolipids found in all cells yet especially abundant in nerve cells. They are mainly situated on outer-membrane surfaces; increased synaptic activity leads to added release of gangliosides. In one study, the four major gangliosides, GM1, GD1a, GD1b and GT1b were found to be increased in the cerebrospinal fluid of 20 children with autism compared with age-matched controls and children with non-progressive neurological disorders (Lekman *et al.* 1995). Another study of 66 children with the autistic syndrome studied all four gangliosides and found that one ganglioside, GM1, was significantly increased in their cerebrospinal fluid compared to 29 controls (Nordin *et al.* 1998).

GLIAL FIBRILLARY ACIDIC PROTEIN (GFA)

Glial fibrillary acid protein is thought to be a marker of the degree of gliosis and an indicator of neuronal density. A study of GFA in the cerebrospinal fluid of 47 children with autism found elevated levels at three times the levels of normal controls, putting this patient group into a category with other chronic neurological diseases (Rosengren *et al.* 1992, Ahlsen *et al.* 1993). These results, combined with the newer findings in gangliosides (see above), raise the question of increased synaptic activity in patients with autism.

ENDORPHINS

The endogenous opioids, or endorphins and enkephalins, constitute a chemically complex family of peptides which serve as so-called neuroregulators. In 1979, Panksepp suggested a theoretical basis for the involvement of the endogenous opioids in the development of autism. Based on his animal studies, he proposed that opiate antagonists can increase prosocial behaviors, including affiliative vocalizations, seeking of social contact and social grooming (Panksepp *et al.* 1985). There is also the suggestion that endogenous opioids play a role in self-injurious behavior (see Chapter 7) in children with various types of developmental disabilities (Aman 1993).

The endorphin, beta-endorphin, has been studied extensively in patients with autism, although the results are not always consistent. It has been observed that morning levels of plasma beta-endorphins in subjects with severe self-injury are significantly lower than those of autistic subjects without severe self-injurious behavior (Willemsen-Swinkels *et al.* 1996). In the study by Ernst *et al.* (1992), there was a strong correlation between plasma beta-endorphin levels and the severity of stereotypies in children with autism. The authors noted that their baseline levels were lower than those reported in the literature. In other studies, plasma beta-endorphin levels have been reported as lower in children with autism compared to normal controls (Weizman *et al.* 1988, Sandman *et al.* 1991). Yet Tordjman *et al.* (1997b) found plasma levels of beta-endorphin to be higher in 48 individuals with autism compared to both mentally retarded and normal controls. Leboyer *et al.* (1994) performed a detailed study measuring beta-endorphin in 17 children with autism, 67 matched controls and 22 girls with Rett syndrome. Medial C-terminal directed beta-endorphin was much higher in patients with autism (70 pg/ml) and in Rett syndrome (35 pg/ml) than in controls (8 pg/ml). In contrast, N-terminal directed beta-endorphin was lower than controls in patients with autism. Brambilla *et al.* (1997) used peripheral blood mononuclear cells to look at beta-endorphin values and found them to be significantly higher in 12 children with autism compared to 10 diagnosed as PDD and 11 healthy controls. To add to the difficulty of interpretation of a child's level of beta-endorphin, familial factors also need to be taken into account. A study has been performed of mothers of subjects with autism which reports that 53 per cent of the mothers had elevated levels of C-terminal directed beta-endorphin protein immunoreactivity (Leboyer *et al.* 1999).

Gillberg *et al.* (1985) reported elevated CSF endorphin fraction II in 20 children with autism. Eleven of these children had levels above the highest control values as well as decreased pain sensitivity. Regarding beta-endorphin in the cerebrospinal fluid, abnormally high (Ross *et al.* 1987), abnormally low (Gillberg *et al.* 1990), and normal (Nagamitsu *et al.* 1997) levels of CSF beta-endorphin have now been reported in autism.

LACTATE/PYRUVATE

A question has arisen as to whether lactic acidosis identifies a subgroup of autism, or is a non-specific finding, such as serotonin in autism. In 1985, four patients with autism were reported to have abnormally elevated levels of lactic acid and pyruvic acid in the blood (Coleman and Blass 1985); the authors estimated that these patients constituted a cohort of about 5 per cent or less of the medical practice from which they were identified. Frequency of lactic acidosis in populations of patients with autism have varied from 4 per cent (1 in 27) (Fattal-Valevski *et al.* 1999) to 43 per cent (13 out of 30) (László *et al.* 1994). In the study by László *et al.* (1994), all of the patients met DSM-III criteria, and 9 of them also had hyperpyruvatemia. In the Fattal-Valevski *et al.* (1999) study, the patient met DSM-III-R criteria. One has to be careful in evaluating elevated lactic acid levels because sometimes the result is merely related to the fact that the child was struggling too hard during the time the blood was drawn, a characteristic of many children with autism. In such situations, the test must be repeated with the child adequately restrained.

Lactic acidosis is not a specific biochemical abnormality. Rather, it indicates difficulty in the utilization of sugar, which increases the rate of lactate production relative to the rate of lactate utilization, and may be due to a decrease in gluconeogenesis. There are a number of possibilities regarding the underlying cause of a finding of lactic acidosis. An inborn error of metabolism in the family of disorders of carbohydrate metabolism can be considered. Elevated lactate levels can point to a respiratory chain defect as seen in mitochondrial disorders – a boy with autism and a mitochondrial disorder, who had a sister with lactic acidosis, is described in Chapter 15.

One of the patients in the Coleman and Blass (1985) lactic acidosis study was also a candidate for the general category of purine autism since he had hyperuricemia and hyperuricosuria (see Chapter 10). A study by Miyazaki *et al.* (1998) has demonstrated that patients with infantile spasms who showed a good initial response to ACTH treatment had a significantly higher cerebrospinal fluid level of pyruvate and a lower serum lactate:pyruvate ratio during therapy; infantile spasms can be followed by an autistic syndrome (see Chapter 12). In view of the finding of so many subgroups of autism with antenatal malformations of cortical development (see Chapter 14), it is of interest that cerebral lactic acidosis (Chow *et al.* 1987) and blood lactic acidosis (Lombes *et al.* 1996) can also be associated with those malformations. Lactic acidosis is a non-specific finding in autism which can point the examiner toward more exact testing in the evaluation of patients.

Endocrinology
THYROID STUDIES
Baseline thyroid function was extensively studied in patients with autism in the 1970s and 1980s, with minor results; most patients were euthyroid. One useful outcome of these studies was helping a few patients with delayed bone ages to improve with triiodothyronine (Campbell *et al.* 1973, 1978); the drug had to be administered with careful monitoring (Abassi *et al.* 1978). Beyond these baseline thyroid studies were the additional loading test studies of thyrotropin-releasing hormone (TRH), which measured the thyroid-stimulating hormone (TSH) response. The studies were hard to interpret since some studies found lower levels and others higher levels – in short, contradictory responses. This is a phenomenon often seen when populations of several diseases (see Chapters 10 and 11) are mixed together and studied as one disease entity called autism. Marginal changes in the diurnal rhythms of serum TSH have been reported in autistic adults (Nir *et al.* 1995). Rarely, a patient with autism is found to actually have hypothyroidism (see Chapter 11).

HUMAN GROWTH HORMONE
Human growth hormone as tested by loading with L-5HTP produced a normal response (Hoshino *et al.* 1984) while testing by insulin (Deutsch *et al.* 1985); and L-dopa (Deutsch *et al.* 1986) resulted in abnormal responses in a subgroup of children with autism. Realmuto *et al.* (1990) also found an abnormal response to L-dopa loading, while Ragusa *et al.* (1993) confirmed an abnormal response when testing with insulin in one patient.

ANDROGENS
Idiopathic precocious puberty is a syndrome that has been reported in children with autistic features (Gillberg 1984, Mouridsen 1989, Tordjman *et al.* 1997a). In the Gillberg epidemiological study, the frequency was found to be 1:2,500 for all childhood psychoses. In the girl reported by Mouridsen, extensive neuroradiological and endocrinological testing was uninformative. Tordjman *et al.* (1997a) observed precocious puberty in 33 per cent (4 out of 12) prepubertal children with autism. This led these investigators to study testosterone levels in autism; they found that high plasma testosterone concentrations were present in three subjects with autism who exhibited aggression against others, including a girl. However in a larger study of plasma levels of testosterone and adrenal androgen DHEA-S in 39 male autistic subjects, it was found that altered secretion of the androgens is not a common feature of autism (Tordjman *et al.* 1995).

CORTICOSTEROIDS
Levels of adrenocorticotropin hormone (ACTH) are a measure of hypothalamic function and an index of stress in humans. A small study by Yamazaki *et al.* (1975) was interpreted

as evidence of hypothalamic dysfunction related to basal ACTH secretion in children with autism; a normal circadian rhythm could scarcely be observed. A large study of plasma levels of ACTH in 48 individuals with autism found elevated levels compared to mentally retarded and normal controls (Tordjman *et al.* 1997b). The authors point out that the elevated mean for the whole was due to the highest results in the more severely affected individuals, suggesting that they were the most stressed. In a study primarily focused on the use of naltrexone in autism, 70 per cent of the children were found to have abnormally low levels of ACTH (Bouvard *et al.* 1995). In a small study comparing cortisol levels in institutionalized patients and normal controls, cortisol levels did not differ between the groups (Sandman *et al.* 1991).

Jensen *et al.* (1985) performed a test of dexamethasone-suppressing cortisol secretion on 13 children with autism and found it positive in 11 of them. This non-specific test is thought to indicate a dysregulation of the hypothalamic-pituitary-adrenal axis. Earlier, in 1975, Maher *et al.* had reported that 11 children with autism hypersecreted cortisol in response to insulin-induced hypoglycemia.

OXYTOCIN

Oxytocin is a neuropeptide involved in the regulation of social behavior in animals. Originally thought only to be regulatory in nursing mothers, it is now known to have unique effects on the normal expression of species-typical social behavior, communication and rituals in animals. This finding has led to speculation about the possible role of oxytocin in autism (Modahl *et al.* 1992, Panksepp 1993, Freeman 1997, Insel *et al.* 1999). A study of oxytocin levels in 29 children with autism found significantly lower plasma levels than in a normal control group (Modahl *et al.* 1998).

Immunology

Psychoneuroimmunology, a term introduced by Adler in 1981, refers to the inter-disciplinary field based on the observation that neurons and immune cells share the ability to respond to external stimuli. Problems with the patient's immunological system have been reported in many diseases of the brain, including autism. Abnormalities of the immune system in autism may parallel other cellular abnormalities in the brain, both controlled by similar genetic mechanisms. An example of this principle in autism might be seen in inherited enzyme deficiencies in purine nucleotide metabolism, which often affect both the central nervous system and the immune system (Stubbs *et al.* 1982) (see Chapter 10). Another example is the monoclonal antibody D8/17, which identifies a B lymphocyte antigen that may serve as a marker for compulsion severity in autism (Hollander *et al.* 1999); D8/17 is already known to have expanded expression in rheumatic fever, Sydenham's chorea, and subgroups of obsessive-compulsive disorder and Tourette syndrome with repetitive behaviors.

The infectious diseases identified to date in individuals with an autistic syndrome are rubella, herpes simplex encephalitis, and possibly cytomegalovirus disease (see Chapter 11). Some of these cases were part of a general epidemic (rubella) but many were sporadic. In the case of infections, it is not known whether (1) these infections occurred by chance; (2) the patients were predisposed due to an already altered immune system in themselves (and/or their mothers if the infection was prenatal); or (3) a prenatal or perinatal infection altered the later immune responses of the children with autism. In very young children, an inherited deficiency of the immune system may prevent the patient from clearing a pathogen in a timely and normal fashion, placing the child at higher risk for the pathogen to interfere with brain development and/or triggering an autoimmune response, either of which might possibly result in the symptoms of autism.

Many immunological studies in autism have found general immune function of one type or another modified, depending upon the age of the individuals with autism being studied. Such studies include abnormalities in T cells and T cell subsets (Stubbs *et al.* 1977, Warren *et al.* 1990, Yonk *et al.* 1990, Warren *et al.* 1995, Gupta *et al.* 1998), depressed responses to T cell mitogens (Stubbs *et al.* 1977, Warren *et al.* 1986), decreased natural killer cell function (Warren *et al.* 1987), a lower percentage of helper-inducer cells (Denney *et al.* 1996), elevation of interleukin-12 (Singh 1996), elevation of interferon-gamma (Singh 1996), and elevation of alpha-interferon levels (Stubbs 1995).

In one study, which focused on immunological signs of food allergy, IgA antigen-specific antibodies for casein, lactalbumin and beta-lactoglobulin, and IgG and IgM for casein were found to be higher in 36 patients with autism compared to 20 healthy controls (Lucarelli *et al.* 1995). Another study found levels of IgA to be decreased (Warren *et al.* 1997). A study of 12 children with PDD found 4 (one-third) with a low serum IgA (Wakefield *et al.* 1998). Menage *et al.* (1992) raised the question of an IgE mechanism in autistic hypersensitivity.

Warren *et al.* (1994) have reported that a major subset of patients with autism had decreased C4B complement protein levels resulting from inheritance of a null allele of the C4B gene. The C4B null allele has been associated with increased viral and bacterial infections. Another study showed that it is not specific to autism – there is also an increased amount of the C4B null allele in attention-deficit hyperactivity disorder and dyslexia (Warren *et al.* 1996).

The possibility of autoimmune problems in autism is under investigation (Singh *et al.* 1993, 1997b, van Gent *et al.* 1997). The question of autoimmunity was originally raised by the finding of an increased incidence of hypothyroid disease in the parents of children with autism compared to the parents of matched controls (Wiedel and Coleman 1976). Another study found 12.5 per cent of mothers of children with autism suffering from rheumatoid arthritis (Raiten and Massaro 1986). A family with documented autoimmune disease and autism has been described (Money *et al.* 1971). Most autoimmune disorders arise in older adults at a time when the immune system has declined in its competence. However, such disorders may arise early in life when there is an inherited deficiency of the immune system. Family and population studies indicate that several different genes can increase susceptibility to autoimmune disease (Carson 1992). An important component of the development of autoimmune disorders can be infection with a pathogen that triggers an abnormal immune response to self tissue; genetic factors may influence the immune responses to an infectious agent, which can trigger autoimmunity.

Antibodies to myelin basic protein have been found to be positive in children with autism; the results were significant at p<0.0001 compared to age-matched controls (Singh *et al.* 1993). Cell-mediated immune response to human myelin basic protein has been reported (Weizman *et al.* 1982). Also in favor of the possible involvement of cell-mediated immunity are the findings of elevated urinary neopterin and biopterin in children with autism (Messahel *et al.* 1998). (See earlier section on pterin – p. 201.) In a study of antibodies to specific viruses, Singh *et al.* (1997b) have reported that positive measles or human herpes virus 6 titers were related to autoantibodies, especially those of anti-myelin basic protein, in children with autism but not in controls. (Herpes virus 6 is the agent of roseola infantum, a very mild disease of childhood.) Circulating autoantibodies to neuronal and glial filament proteins were found to be significantly increased in autistic subjects (Singh *et al.* 1997b). Autoantibodies to nerve-growth factor have been reported in children with "active" Kanner's and Asperger's syndromes (Bashina *et al.* 1997). In some studies, the autoantibodies to serotonin receptors (5HT1A/5HT2) do not appear to be characteristic of autism (Yuwiler *et al.* 1992, Cook *et al.* 1993), while other studies report the presence of such antibodies (Singh *et al.* 1997a). This is an example of laboratories disagreeing with each other – one explanation is that each laboratory's results were technically accurate but that they were testing patients with different disease entities within the autistic syndrome.

The immunological findings in patients with autism raise the question of whether there will ever be an established immunotherapy for any group of children within the autistic syndrome, or whether immunological abnormalities in any given patient will best respond to treatment of the individual's underlying metabolic disorder. ACTH, which has been given to some patients (see Chapter 12), is an immunosuppressant (Buitelaar *et al.* 1992).

VITAMIN AND MINERAL/ION LEVELS

Vitamin levels have not been systematically studied in autism. However, an autistic child with vitamin A deficiency and xerophthalmia has been described in the literature (Steinemann and Christiansen 1998). A study of folate levels in 16 children with autism compared to 12 healthy controls showed no statistical difference between the two groups (Eto *et al.* 1992). In Rett syndrome, decreased levels of nicotinamide (vitamin B3) have been reported (Rocchigiani *et al.* 1995). Studies pertaining to vitamin B6 (pyridoxine) and vitamin C (ascorbic acid) are discussed in Chapter 17.

Regarding minerals, levels of several ions have been reported as abnormal in children with autism. The most consistent finding has been reports of lower levels of magnesium. Saladino and Sankar (1973) reported that magnesium levels were lower in erythrocytes of a group of children seen for pediatric psychiatric reasons than they were in normal controls. In a large study of 59 children with autism (Coleman *et al.* 1976), serum magnesium levels were significantly lower than in age- and sex-matched controls (p<0.001). Another study (Hayek 1991) also showed lower values of magnesium in erythrocytes in children with autism. In that same study, girls with Rett syndrome were studied separately and did not have a significantly lower value. Low levels of magnesium in humans are known to predispose to apathy, irritability and seizures. Since magnesium is lost in the processing of many modern foods, evaluation of magnesium levels is indicated in children with autism, particularly if they have seizures.

Calcium is a mimic/antagonist of magnesium. A study has been performed of serum and 24-hour urinary levels of calcium in 72 children with autism compared to age- and sex-matched controls for 67 of them (Coleman *et al.* 1976). This study found no statistically significant differences in serum or urine levels, although the urine results were highly skewed, with 22 of the patients having levels more than two standard deviations below the mean. At the time of the study, some of these low-calcium patients, who also had steatorrhea, had received the diagnosis of celiac disease from their pediatricians. Later follow-up studies indicated that these children did not have celiac disease (McCarthy and Coleman 1979).

Potassium levels have been tested in patients with autism; a depression of red blood cell potassium was reported in child psychiatry patients compared to controls (Saladino and Sankar 1973).

Serum copper levels were tested in 60 patients with autism and age-, sex-matched controls; no statistical difference was found (Mahanand *et al.* 1976). Testing zinc levels in humans is notoriously inaccurate due to technical problems; an attempt at studying zinc levels in serum in 64 children with autism and age-, sex-matched controls found an elevation in the children with autism (Mahanand *et al.* 1976).

In contrast to the other ions discussed, lead has no known enzymatic function in the human body. Xenobiotic (toxic) contamination with lead has been found in some children with autism (see Chapter 11).

XENOBIOTIC EXPOSURE

Finally, there is the controversial question of whether children with autism might have been exposed to various agents that are xenobiotic to the central nervous system, and whether they might have a decreased ability to detoxify such agents. In one study, abnormal liver detoxification profiles were reported in 20 children with autism, aged 3 to 12 years (Edelson and Cantor 1998). McFadden (1996) has raised the question of whether detoxification problems in a child, combined with exposure to food that is toxic to that child, could be an underlying factor in the unresolved concept of *diet responsive autism* (see Chapter 17).

A significant number of individuals with chronic disease have impaired sulfur-dependent detoxification of phenolic xenobiotics and amines. In a study of sulfation capacity in autism, a subgroup of children with autism were selected by investigators at the University of Birmingham if they had a family history of both migraine and allergies (Waring *et al.* 1996). Acetaminophen was used as an *in vivo* probe drug. The children selected were shown to have reduced levels of excretion of the sulfate conjugate, but not the glucuronide metabolite, compared to age-matched controls. The children also had significantly reduced levels of the enzyme *p*-sulfotransferase in platelets, and of inorganic sulfate in plasma. Alberti *et al.* (1999) also report the same detoxification problems in autism. To paraphrase Dr. Rosemary Waring, *this sulfation problem may not be the cause of autism but it certainly makes the situation much worse.*

In the first large biochemical study, which was performed on 78 children with autism in the United States, the parents of autistic children were found to have more exposure to chemicals than the parents of matched controls (Wiedel and Coleman 1976). The validity of the study can be questioned because the parents who brought their children to such a study were self-selected parents interested in the biochemistry of autism – in four of the families, both mother and father had been exposed to chemicals, mostly working as chemists. In an attempt to answer the question of self-selection by parents, another study took 20 unselected children with autism in a residential setting and compared their families to the families of 20 mentally retarded children and 20 normal children in the same town (Felicetti 1981). The preconception questionnaire showed that 21 per cent of the parents of the autistic children, compared to 10 per cent of the parents of the normal children, and 3 per cent of the parents of the mentally retarded children, had been exposed to chemicals – again a statistically significant finding, despite the relatively small number of children in the study. In this second study, five of the parents of the children with autism were found to be professional chemists.

The problem of possible xenobiotic exposure on the part of either the parents of children with autism or the children themselves *in utero* is becoming a political topic around the world, due to apparent clusters of cases in particular geographic locations. Attempts to isolate the factors causing such clusters have not been successful; possible reasons for such clusters include coincidence, a viral epidemic or toxic exposures. Prospective studies of people who work with chemicals (chemists, crop-dusters, workers in chemical factories, etc.), which follow the health of their offspring, are the best scientific way to resolve the question of chemical xenobiotic exposure in autism.

REFERENCES

Abassi, V., Linscheid, T., Coleman, M. (1978) 'Triiodothyronine (T3) concentration and therapy in autistic children.' *Journal of Autism and Childhood Schizophrenia*, **8**, 383–388.

Adler, R. (1981) *Psychoneuroimmunology*. New York: Academic Press.

Ahlsen, G., Rosengren, L., Belfrage, M., Palm, A., Haglid, K., Hamberger, A., Gillberg, C. (1993) 'Glial fibrillary acidic protein in the cerebrospinal fluid of children with autism and other neuropsychiatric disorders.' *Biological Psychiatry*, **33**, 734–743.

Alberti, A., Pirrone, P., Elia, M., Waring, R.H., Romano, C. (1999) 'Sulphation deficit in "low-functioning" autistic children: a pilot study.' *Biological Psychiatry*, **46**, 420–424.

Aman, M.G. (1993) 'Efficacy of psychotropic drugs for reducing self-injurious behavior in the developmental disabilities.' *Annals of Clinical Psychiatry*, **5**, 171–188.

Azmitia, E.C., Frankfurt, M., Davila, M., Whitaker-Azmitia, P.M., Zhou, F.C. (1990) 'Plasticity of fetal and adult CNS serotonergic neurons: role of growth-regulatory factors.' *Annals of the New York Academy of Sciences*, **600**, 343–363.

Bashina, V.M., Kozlova, I.A., Kliushnik, T.P., Simashkova, N.V., Danilovskaia, E.V., Gorbachevskaia, N.L., Turkova, I.L., Iakupova, L.P., Grachev, V.V. (1997) 'An elevation in the level of autoantibodies to nerve-growth factor in the blood serum of schizophrenic children.' (In Russian) *Zhurnal Neuropatologii Psikhiatrii Imeni S.S. Korsakova*, **97**, 47–51.

Belmaker, R.H., Hattab, J., Ebstein, R.P. (1978) 'Plasma dopamine-beta-hydroxylase in childhood psychosis.' *Journal of Autism and Childhood Schizophrenia*, **8**, 293–298.

Bouvard, M.P., Leboyer, M., Launay, J.M., Recasens, C., Plumet, M.H., Waller-Perotte, D., Tabuteau, F., Bondoux, D., Dugas, M., Lensing, P. *et al.* (1995) 'Low-dose naltrexone effects on plasma chemistries and clinical symptoms in autism: a double-blind, placebo-controlled study.' *Psychiatry Research*, **58**, 191–201.

Brambilla, F., Guareschi-Cazzullo, A., Tacchini, C., Musetti, C., Panerai, A.E., Sacerdote, P. (1997) 'Beta-endorphin and cholcystokinin 8 concentrations in peripheral blood mononuclear cells of autistic children.' *Neuropsychobiology*, **35**, 1–4.

Buitelaar, J.K., van Engeland, H., de Kogel, K.H., de Vries, H., van Hooff, J.A., van Ree, J.A. (1992) 'The use of adrenocorticotrophic hormone (4-9) analog ORG2766 in autistic children; effects on the organization of behavior.' *Biological Psychiatry*, **31**, 1119–1129.

Campbell, M., Fish, B., David, R., Shapiro, T., Collins, P., Koh, C. (1973) 'Liothyronine treatment in psychotic and nonpsychotic children under 6 years of age.' *Archives of General Psychiatry*, **29**, 602–608.

Campbell, M., Small, A.M., Hollander, C.S., Korein, J., Cohen, I.L., Kalmijn, M., Ferris, S. (1978) 'A controlled crossover study of triiodothyronine in autistic children.' *Journal of Autism and Childhood Schizophrenia*, **8**, 371–381.

Carson, D.A. (1992) 'Genetic factors in the etiology and pathogenesis of autoimmunity.' *Federation of American Societies for Experimental Biology (FASEB) Journal*, **6**, 2800–2805.

Chow, C.W., Anderson, R.M., Kenny, G.C.T. (1987) 'Neuropathology in cerebral lactic acidosis.' *Acta Neuropathologica*, **74**, 393–396.

Chugani, D.C., Muzik, O., Rothermel, R., Behen, M., Chakraborty, P., Mangner, T., da Silva, E.A., Chugani, H.T. (1997) 'Altered serotonin synthesis in the dentatothalamocortical pathway in autistic boys.' *Annals of Neurology*, **42**, 666–669.

Chugani, D.C., Behen, M.E., Muzik, O., Chugani, H.T. (1998a) 'Focal abnormalities of serotonin synthesis in autistic children.' (Abstract) *Annals of Neurology*, **44**, 555.

Chugani, D.C., Chugani, H.T., Muzik, O., Shah, J.R., Shah, A.K., Canady, A., Mangner, T.J., Chakraborty, P.K. (1998b) 'Imaging epileptogenic tubers in children with tuberous sclerosis using α-[^{11}C]]methyl-L-tryptophan positron emission tomography.' *Annals of Neurology*, **44**, 858–866.

Chugani, D.C., Muzik, O., Behen, M., Rothermel, R., Janisse, J.J., Lee, J., Chugani, H.T. (1999) 'Developmental changes in brain serotonin synthesis capacity in autistic and nonautistic children.' *Annals of Neurology*, **45**, 287–295.

Coleman, M. (1970) 'Serotonin levels in infant hypothyroidism.' (Letter) *Lancet*, **2**, 235.

—— (1973) 'Appendix IX.' *In:* Coleman, M. (Ed.) *Serotonin in Down's Syndrome.* Amsterdam: North-Holland.

Coleman, M., Blass, J.P. (1985) 'Autism and lactic acidosis.' *Journal of Autism and Developmental Disorders*, **15**, 1–8.

Coleman, M., Hur, F. (1973) 'Platelet serotonin in disturbances of the central nervous system.' *In:* Coleman, M. (Ed.) *Serotonin in Down's Syndrome.* Amsterdam: North-Holland, pp. 5–24.

Coleman, M., Landgrebe, M.A., Landgrebe, A.R. (1976) 'Celiac autism: calcium studies and their relationship to celiac disease in autistic patients.' *In:* Coleman, M. (Ed.) *The Autistic Syndromes.* New York: Elsevier, pp. 197–205.

Coleman, M., Hart, P.N., Randall, J., Lee, J., Hijada, D., Bratendahl, C.G. (1977) 'Serotonin levels in the blood and central nervous system of a patient with sudanophilic leukodystrophy.' *Neuropädiatrie*, **8**, 459–466.

Comings, D.E., Comings, B.G., Muhleman, D., Dietz, G., Shahbahrami, B., Tast, D., Knell, E., Kocsis, P., Daumgarten, R., Kovuou, B.W. *et al.* (1991) 'The dopamine D2 receptor locus as a modifying gene in neuropsychiatric disorders.' *Journal of the American Medical Association*, **266**, 1793–1800.

Cook, E.H. (1990) 'Autism: review of neurochemical investigation.' *Synapse*, **6**, 292–308.

Cook, E.H., Leventhal, B.L. (1996) 'The serotonin system in autism.' *Current Opinion in Pediatrics*, **8**, 348–354.

Cook, E.H. Jr., Perry, B.D., Dawson, G., Wainwright, M.S., Leventhal, B.L. (1993) 'Receptor inhibition by immunoglobulins: specific inhibition by autistic children, their relatives and control subjects.' *Journal of Autism and Developmental Disorders*, **23**, 67–78.

Cook, E.H. Jr., Charak, D.A., Arida, J., Spohn, J.A., Roizen, N.J., Leventhal, B.L. (1994) 'Depressive and obsessive-compulsive symptoms in hyperserotonemic parents of children with autistic disorder.' *Psychiatry Research*, **52**, 25–33.

Cook, E.H. Jr., Courchesne, R., Lord, C., Cox, N.J., Yan, S., Lincoln, A., Haas, R., Courchesne, E., Leventhal, B.L. (1997) 'Evidence of linkage between the serotonin transporter and autistic disorder.' *Molecular Psychiatry*, **2**, 247–250.

Denney, D.R., Frei, B.W., Gaffney, G.R. (1996) 'Lymphocyte subsets and interleukin-2 receptors in autistic children.' *Journal of Autism and Developmental Disorders*, **26**, 87–97.

D'Eufemia, P., Finocchiaro, R., Celli, M., Viozzi, L., Monteleone, D., Giardini, O. (1995) 'Low serum tryptophan to large neutral amino acids ratio in idiopathic infantile autism.' *Biomedical Pharmacotherapy*, **49**, 288–292.

Deutsch, S., Campbell, M., Sachar, E., Green, W.H., David, R. (1985) 'Plasma growth hormone response to oral L-DOPA in infantile autism.' *Journal of Autism and Developmental Disorders*, **15**, 205–212.

Deutsch, S., Campbell, M., Perry, R., Green, W.H., Poland, R.E., Rubin, R.T. (1986) 'Plasma growth hormone response to insulin-induced hypoglycemia in infantile autism: a pilot study.' *Journal of Autism and Developmental Disorders*, **16**, 59–68.

Edelson, S.B., Cantor, D.S. (1998) 'Autism: xenobiotic influences.' *Toxicology and Industrial Health*, **14**, 553–563.

Ernst, M., Devi, L., Silva, R.R., Gonzalez, N.M., Small, A.M., Malone, R.P., Campbell, M. (1992) 'Plasma beta-endorphin levels, naltrexone and haloperidol in autistic children.' *Psychopharmacological Bulletin*, **29**, 221–227.

Ernst, M., Zametkin, A.J., Matochik, A.J., Pascualvaca, D., Cohen, R.M. (1997) 'Low medial prefrontal dopaminergic activity in autistic children.' *Lancet*, **350**, 638.

Eto, I., Bandy, M.D., Butterworth, C.E. Jr. (1992) 'Plasma and urinary levels of biopterin, neopterin and related pterins and plasma levels of folate in infantile autism.' *Journal of Autism and Developmental Disorders*, **22**, 295–308.

Fattal-Valevski, A., Kramer, U., Leitner, Y., Nevo, Y., Greenstein, Y., Harel, S. (1999) 'Characterization and comparison of autistic subgroups: 10 years' experience with autistic children.' *Developmental Medicine and Child Neurology*, **41**, 21–25.

Felicetti, T. (1981) 'Parents of autistic children: some notes on the chemical connection.' *Milieu Therapy*, **1**, 13–16.

Freeman, W.J. (1997) 'Neurohumoral brain dynamics of social group formation. Implications for autism.' *Annals of the New York Academy of Science*, **807**, 501–503.

Gillberg, C. (1984) 'Infantile autism and other childhood psychoses in a Swedish region: epidemiological aspects.' *Journal of Child Psychology and Psychiatry*, **25**, 35–43.

Gillberg, C., Terenius, L., Lonnerholm, G. (1985) 'Endorphin activity in childhood psychosis.' *Archives of General Psychiatry*, **42**, 780–783.

Gillberg, C., Hagberg, B., Witt-Engerström, I., Eriksson, I. (1990) 'CSF beta-endorphin in childhood neuropsychiatric disorders.' *Brain and Development*, **12**, 88–92.

Goldberg, M., Hattab, J., Meir, D., Ebstein, L., Belmaker, R. (1984) 'Plasma cyclic AMP and cyclic GMP in childhood-onset psychoses.' *Journal of Autism and Developmental Disorders*, **14**, 159–164.

Gupta, S., Aggarwal, S., Rashanravan, B., Lee, T. (1998) 'Th1- and Th2-like cytokines in CD4+ and CD8+ T cells in autism.' *Journal of Neuroimmunology*, **85**, 106–109.

Harrison, K.L., Pheasant, A.E. (1995) 'Analysis of urinary pterins in autism.' *Biochemical Society Transactions*, **23**, 603S.

Hayek, J. (1991) 'Intracellular magnesium in autistic subjects.' *Brain Dysfunction*.

Hérault, J., Petit, E., Martineau, J., Cherpi, C., Perrot, A., Barthélémy, C., Lelord, G., Muh, J.P. (1996) 'Serotonin and autism: biochemical and molecular features.' *Psychiatry Research*, **65**, 33–43.

Himwich, H.E., Jenkins, R.L., Fujimori, M., Narasimhachi, N., Ebersole, M. (1972) 'A biochemical study of early infantile autism.' *Journal of Autism and Childhood Schizophrenia*, **2**, 114–126.

Hollander, E., DelGiudice-Ash, G., Simon, L., Schmeidler, J., Cartwright, C., DeCaria, C.M., Kwon, J., Cunningham-Rundles, C., Chapman, F., Zabriskie, J.B. (1999) 'B lymphocyte antigen D8/17 and repetitive behaviors in autism.' *American Journal of Psychiatry*, **156**, 317–320.

Hollander, E., Novotny, S., Allen, A., Aronowitz, B., Cartwright, C., DeCaria, C. (2000) 'The relationship between repetitive behaviors and growth hormone response to sumatriptan challenge in adult autistic disorder.' *Neuropsychopharmacology*, **22**, 163–167.

Hoshino, Y., Kumashiro, H., Kaneko, M., Numata, Y., Honda, K., Yashima, Y., Tachibana, R., Watanabe, M. (1979) 'Serum serotonin, free tryptophan and plasma cyclic AMP in autistic children – with special reference to their hyperkinesia.' *Fukushima Journal of Medical Science*, **26**, 79–91.

Hoshino, Y., Ohno, Y., Murate, S., Yokoyama, F., Kaneko, M., Kumashiro, H. (1980) 'Plasma cyclic AMP level in psychiatric diseases of childhood.' *Folia Psychiatrica et Neurologica Japonica*, **34**, 9–16.

Hoshino, Y., Watanabe, M., Tachibana, R., Kaneko, M., Kumashiro, H. (1984) 'The hypothalamo-pituitary function in autistic children.' *Neurosciences*, **110**, 285–291.

212

Insel, T.R., O'Brien, D.J., Leckman, J.F. (1999) 'Oxytocin, vasopressin and autism: is there a connection?' *Biological Psychiatry*, **45**, 145–157.

Jensen, J.B., Realmuto, G.M., Garfinkel, B.D. (1985) 'The dexamethasone suppression test in infantile autism.' *Journal of the American Academy of Child Psychiatry*, **24**, 263–265.

László, A., Horváth, E., Eck, E., Fekete, M. (1994) 'Serum serotonin, lactate and pyruvate levels in infantile autistic children.' *Clinica Chimica Acta*, **229**, 205–207.

Leboyer, M., Bouvard, M.P., Recasens, C., Philippe, A., Guilloud-Bataille, M., Bondoux, D., Tabuteau, F., Dugas, M., Panksepp, J., Launay, J.M., *et al.* (1994) 'Difference between plasma N- and C-terminally directed beta-endorphin immunoreactivity in infantile autism.' *American Journal of Psychiatry*, **151**, 1797–1801.

Leboyer, M., Philippe, A., Bouvard, M., Guilloud-Bataille, M., Bondoux, D., Tabuteau, F., Feingold, J., Mouren-Simeoni, M.C., Launay, J.M. (1999) 'Whole blood serotonin and plasma beta-endorphin in autistic probands and their first degree relatives.' *Biological Psychiatry*, **45**, 158–163.

Lekman, A., Skjeldal, O., Sponheim, E., Svennerholm, L. (1995) 'Gangliosides in children with autism.' *Acta Paediatrica*, **84**, 787–790.

Lesch, K.P., Walozin, B.L., Murphy, D.L., Reiderer, P. (1993) 'Primary structure of the human platelet serotonin uptake site: identity with the brain serotonin transporter.' *Journal of Neurochemistry*, **60**, 2319–2322.

Levy, P.Q., Bicho, M.P. (1997) 'Platelet serotonin as a biological marker of autism.' (In Portuguese) *Acta Medica Portuguesa*, **10**, 927–931.

Lishman, W.A. (1987) *Organic Psychiatry. 2nd Edn.* Oxford: Blackwell Scientific.

Lombes, A., Romero, N.B., Touati, G., Frachon, P., Cheval, M.A., Giraud, M., Simon, D., Ogier de Baulny, H. (1996) 'Clinical and molecular heterogeneity of cytochrome c oxidase deficiency in the newborn.' *Journal of Inherited Metabolic Disease*, **19**, 286–295.

Lord, C. (1998) 'What is melatonin? Is it a useful treatment for sleep problems in autism?' *Journal of Autism and Developmental Disorders*, **28**, 345–346.

Lucarelli, S., Frediani, T., Zingoni, A.M., Ferruzzi, F., Giardini, O., Quintieri, F., Barbato, M., D'Eufemia, P., Cardi, E. (1995) 'Food allergies and infantile autism.' *Panminerva Medica*, **37**, 137–141.

McCarthy, D.M., Coleman, M. (1979) 'Response of intestinal mucosa to gluten challenge in autistic subjects.' *Lancet*, **2**, 877–878.

McDougle, C.J., Naylor, S.T., Cohen, D.J., Aghajanian, G.K., Heninger, G.R., Price, L.H. (1996a) 'Effects of tryptophan depletion in drug-free adults with autistic disorder.' *Archives of General Psychiatry*, **53**, 993–1000.

McDougle, C.J., Naylor, S.T., Cohen, D.J., Volkmar, F.R., Heninger, G.R., Price, L.H. (1996b) 'A double-blind, placebo-controlled study of fluvoxamine in adults with autistic disorder.' *Archives of General Psychiatry*, **53**, 1001–1008.

McDougle, C.J., Epperson, C.N., Price, L.H., Gelernter, J. (1998) 'Evidence for linkage disequilibrium between serotonin transporter protein gene (SLC6A4) and obsessive compulsive disorder.' *Molecular Psychiatry*, **3**, 270–273.

McFadden, S.A. (1996) 'Phenotypic variation in xenobiotic metabolism and adverse environmental response: focus on sulfur-dependent detoxification pathways.' *Toxicology*, **111**, 43–65.

McKean, C.M. (1971) 'Effects of a totally synthetic, low phenylalanine diet on adolescent phenylketonuria patients.' *Archives of the Diseases of Childhood*, **46**, 608.

Mahanand, D., Wypych, M.K., Calcagno, P.L. (1976) 'Serum zinc and copper levels in autistic patients and controls.' *In:* Coleman, M. (Ed.) *The Autistic Syndromes.* New York: Elsevier, pp. 73–76.

Maher, K.R., Harper, J.F., Macleay, A., King, M.G. (1975) 'Peculiarities in the endocrine response to insulin stress in early infantile autism.' *Journal of Nervous and Mental Disorders*, **161**, 180–184.

Martin, G., Eglen, R., Hamblin, M., Hoyer, D., Yocca, F. (1998) 'The structure and signalling properties of 5HT receptors: an endless diversity?' *Trends in Pharmacological Science*, **19**, 2–4.

Martineau, J., Hérault, J., Petit, E., Guerin, P., Hameury, L., Perrot, A., Mallet, J., Sauvage, D., Lelord, G., Muh, J.P. (1994) 'Catecholaminergic metabolism and autism.' *Developmental Medicine and Child Neurology*, **36**, 688–697.

Menage, P., Thibault, G., Martineau, J., Hérault, J., Muh, J.P., Barthélémy, C., Lelord, G., Bardos, P. (1992) 'An IgE mechanism in autistic hypersensitivity.' *Biological Psychiatry*, **31**, 210–212.

Messahel, S., Pheasant, A.E., Pall, H., Ahmed-Choudhury, J., Sungum-Paliwal, R.S., Vostanis, P. (1998) 'Urinary levels of neopterin and biopterin in autism.' *Neuroscience Letters*, **241**, 17–20.

213

Minderaa, R.B., Anderson, G.M., Volkmar, F.R., Akkerhuis, G.W., Cohen, D.J. (1994) 'Noradrenergic and adrenergic functioning in autism.' *Biological Psychiatry*, **36**, 237–241.

Miwa, S., Watanabe, Y., Koshimura, K., Masaki, T. (1992) 'A novel function of tetrahydrobiopterin.' (In Japanese) *Nippon Yakurigaku Zasshi*, **100**, 367–381.

Miyazaki, M., Hashimoto, T., Yoneda, Y., Saijio, T., Mori, K., Ito, M., Kuroda, Y. (1998) 'Adrenocorticotropic hormone therapy for infantile spasms alters pyruvate metabolism in the central nervous system.' *Brain Development*, **20**, 312–318.

Modahl, C., Fein, D., Waterhouse, L., Newton, N. (1992) 'Does oxytocin deficiency mediate social deficits in autism?' *Journal of Autism and Developmental Disorders*, **22**, 449–451.

Modahl, C., Green, L., Fein, D., Morris, M., Waterhouse, L., Feinstein, C., Levin, H. (1998) 'Plasma oxytocin levels in autistic children.' *Biological Psychiatry*, **43**, 270–277.

Money, J., Bobrow, N.A., Clarke, F.C. (1971) 'Autism and autoimmune disease: a family study.' *Journal of Autism and Childhood Schizophrenia*, **1**, 146–160.

Moos, M., Goldberg, N.D. (1988) 'Cyclic AMP opposes IP3-induced calcium release from permeabilized platelets.' *Second Messengers and Phosphoproteins*, **12**, 163–170.

Moreno-Fuenmayor, H., Borjas, L., Arrieta, A., Valera, V., Socorro-Candanoza, L. (1996) 'Plasma excitatory amino acids in autism.' *Investigacion Clinica*, **37**, 113–128.

Mouridsen, S.E. (1989) 'Pervasive developmental disorder and idiopathic precocious puberty in a 5-year-old girl.' *Journal of Autism and Developmental Disorders*, **19**, 351–353.

Nagamitsu, S., Matsuishi, T., Kisa, T., Komori, H., Miyazaki, M., Hashimoto, T., Yamashita, Y., Ohtaki, E., Kato, H. (1997) 'CSF beta-endorphin levels in patients with infantile autism.' *Journal of Autism and Developmental Disorders*, **27**, 155.

Narayan, M., Srinath, S., Anderson, G.M., Meundi, D.B. (1993) 'Cerebrospinal fluid levels of homovanillic acid and 5-hydroxyindoleacetic acid in autism.' *Biological Psychiatry*, **33**, 630–635.

Nir, I., Meir, D., Zilber, N., Knobler, H., Hadjez, J., Lerner, Y. (1995) 'Brief report: Circadian melatonin, thyroid-stimulating hormone, prolactin and cortisol levels in serum of young adults with autism.' *Journal of Autism and Developmental Disorders*, **25**, 631–654.

Nordin, V., Lekman, A., Johansson, M., Fredman, P., Gillberg, C. (1998) 'Gangliosides in cerebrospinal fluid in children with autism spectrum disorders.' *Developmental Medicine and Child Neurology*, **40**, 587–594.

O'Neill, M., Jones, R.S. (1997) 'Sensory-perceptual abnormalities in autism; a case for more research?' *Journal of Autism and Developmental Disorders*, **27**, 283–293.

Panksepp, J. (1979) 'A neurochemical theory of autism.' *Trends in Neuroscience*, **2**, 174–177.

—— (1993) 'Commentary on the possible role of oxytocin in autism.' *Journal of Autism and Developmental Disorders*, **23**, 567–569.

Panksepp, J., Siviy, S., Normansell, L. (1985) 'Brain opioids and social emotions.' *In:* Reite, M., Fields, T. (Eds) *The Psychobiology of Attachment and Separation*. Orlando, Florida: Academic Press.

Perry, T., Hansen, S., Christie, R.G. (1978) 'Amino compounds and organic acids in the CSF, plasma and urine in autistic children.' *Biological Psychiatry*, **13**, 575–586.

Ragusa, L., Elia, M., Scifo, R. (1993) 'Growth hormone deficit in autism.' *Journal of Autism and Developmental Disorder*, **23**, 421–422.

Raiten, D.J., Massaro, T. (1986) 'Perspectives on the nutritional ecology of autistic children.' *Journal of Autism and Developmental Disorders*, **16**, 133–144.

Realmuto, G.M., Jensen, J.B., Reeve, E., Garfinkel, B.D. (1990) 'Growth hormone response to L-Dopa and clonidine in autistic children.' *Journal of Autism and Developmental Disorders*, **20**, 455–465.

Rocchigiani, M., Sestini, S., Micheli, V., Pescaglini, M., Jacomelli, G., Hayek, G., Pompucci, G. (1995) 'Purine and pyridine nucleotide metabolism in the erythrocytes of patients with Rett syndrome.' *Neuropediatrics*, **26**, 288–292.

Rolf, L.H., Haarmann, F.Y., Grotemeyer, K.H., Kehrer, H. (1993) 'Serotonin and amino acid content in platelets of autistic children.' *Acta Psychiatrica Scandinavica*, **87**, 312–316.

Rosengren, L.E., Ahlsen, G., Belfrage, M., Gillberg, C., Haglid, K.G., Hamberger, A. (1992) 'A sensitive ELISA for glial fibrillary acidic protein: application in CSF of children.' *Journal of Neuroscience Methods*, **44**, 113–119.

Ross, D., Pickar, D., DeJong, J., Karoum, F., Linnoila, M. (1987) 'Reduction of elevated CSF beta-endorphin by fenfluramine in infantile autism.' *Pediatric Neurology*, **3**, 83–86.

Saladino, C.F., Sankar, D.V. (1973) 'Studies in erythrocyte magnesium and potassium levels in children, schizophrenia and growth.' *Physicians Drug Manual*, **4–5**, 107–110.

214

Sandman, C.A., Barron, J.L., Chicz-DeMet, A., DeMet, E.M. (1991) 'Brief report: Plasma beta-endorphin and cortisol levels in autistic patients.' *Journal of Autism and Developmental Disorders*, **21**, 83–87.

Shaw, W., Kassen, E., Chaves, E. (1995) 'Increased urinary excretion of analogs of the Krebs cycle metabolites and arabinose in two brothers with autistic features.' *Clinical Chemistry*, **41**, 1094–1104.

Singh, V.K. (1996) 'Plasma increase of interleukin-12 and interferon-gamma. Pathological significance in autism.' *Journal of Neuroimmunology*, **66**, 143–145.

Singh, V.K., Warren, R.P., Odell, J.D., Cole, P., Warren. I. (1993) 'Antibodies to myelin basic protein in children with autism.' *Brain Behavior and Immunity*, **7**, 97–103.

Singh, V.K., Singh, E.A., Warren, R.P. (1997a) 'Hyperserotoninemia and serotonin receptor antibodies in children with autism but not mental retardation.' *Biological Psychiatry*, **41**, 753–755.

Singh V.K., Warren, R.P., Averett, R., Ghaziuddin, M. (1997b) 'Circulating autoantibodies to neuronal and glial filament proteins in autism.' *Pediatric Neurology*, **17**, 88–90.

Steinemann, T.L., Christiansen, S.P. (1998) 'Vitamin A deficiency and xeropthalmia in an autistic child.' *Archives of Opthalmology*, **116**, 392–393.

Stubbs, G. (1995) 'Interferonemia and autism.' (Letter) *Journal of Autism and Developmental Disorders*, **25**, 71–73.

Stubbs, E.G., Crawford, M.L., Burger, D.R., Vandenbark, A.A. (1977) 'Depressed lymphocyte responsiveness in autistic children.' *Journal of Autism and Childhood Schizophrenia*, **7**, 49–55.

Stubbs, E.G., Litt, M., Lis, E., Jackson, R., Voth, W., Lindberg, A., Litt, R. (1982) 'Adenosine deaminase activity decreased in autism.' *Journal of the American Academy of Pediatrics*, **21**, 71–74.

Takesada, M., Nakane, A., Yamazaki, K., Noguchi, T., Watanabe, Y., Hayaishi, O. (1987) Therapeutic effect of tetrahydrobiopterin in infantile autism. *Proceedings of Japanese Academy Series B*, **63**, 231–239.

Tani, Y., Fernell, E., Watanabe, Y., Kanai, T., Langstrom, B. (1994) 'Decrease in 6R-5,6,7,8-tetrahydrobiopterin content in cerebrospinal fluid of autistic children.' *Neuroscience Letters*, **7**, 169–172.

Todd, R.D. (1992) 'Neural development is regulated by classical neurotransmitters: dopamine D2 receptor stimulation enhances neurite outgrowth.' *Biological Psychiatry*, **31**, 794–807.

Tordjman, S., Anderson, G.M., McBride, P.A., Hertzig, M.E., Snow, M.E., Hall, L.M., Ferrari, P., Cohen, D.J. (1995) 'Plasma androgens in autism.' *Journal of Autism and Developmental Disorders*, **25**, 295–304.

Tordjman, S., Ferrari, P., Sulmont, V., Duyme, M., Roubertoux, P. (1997a) 'Androgenic activity in autism.' *American Journal of Psychiatry*, **154**, 1626–1627.

Tordjman, S., Anderson, G.M., McBride, P.A., Hertzig, M.E., Snow, M.E., Hall, L.M., Thompson, S.M., Ferrari, P., Cohen, D.J. (1997b) 'Plasma beta-endorphin, adrenocorticotropin hormone and cortisol in autism.' *Journal of Child Psychology and Psychiatry*, **38**, 705–715.

Van Gent, T., Heijnen, C.J., Treffers, P.D. (1997) 'Autism and the immune system.' *Journal of Child Psychology and Psychiatry*, **38**, 337–349.

Wakefield, A.J., Murch, S.H., Anthony, A., Linnell, J., Casson, D.M., Malik, M., Berelowitz, M., Dhillon, A.P., Thomson, M.A., Harvey, P., Valentine, A., Davies, S.E., Walker-Smith, J.A. (1998) 'Ileal-lymphoid-nodular hyperplasia, non-specific colitis and pervasive-developmental disorder in children.' *Lancet*, **351**, 637–641.

Waring, R H , Ngong, J.M., Klovrza, L., Green, S., Sharp, H. (1996) 'Biochemical parameters in autistic children.' *Developmental Brain Dysfunction*, **10**, 40–43.

Warren, R.P., Margaretten, N.C., Pace, N.C., Foster, A. (1986) 'Immune abnormalities in patients with autism.' *Journal of Autism and Developmental Disorders*, **16**, 189–197.

Warren, R.P., Foster, A., Margaretten, N.C. (1987) 'Reduced natural killer cell activity in autism.' *Journal of the American Academy of Child and Adolescent Psychiatry*, **26**, 333–335.

Warren, R.P., Yonk, L.J., Burger, R.A., Cole, P., Odell, J.D., Warren, W.L., White, E., Singh, V.K. (1990) 'Depression of suppressor-inducer (CD4+CD45R+) T cells in autism.' *Immunological Investigations*, **19**, 245–251.

Warren, R.P., Burger, R.A., Odell, D., Torres, A.R., Warren, W.L. (1994) 'Decreased plasma concentrations of the C4B complement protein in autism.' *Archives of Pediatric and Adolescent Medicine*, **148**, 180–183.

Warren, R.P., Yonk, J., Burger, R.W., Odell, D., Warren, W.L. (1995) 'DR-positive T cells in autism: association with decreased plasma level of the complement C4B protein.' *Neuropsychobiology*, **31**, 53–57.

Warren, R.P., Singh, V.K., Averett, R.E., Odell, J.D., Maciulis, A., Burger, R.A., Daniels, W.W., Warren, W.L. (1996) 'Immunogenetic studies in autism and related disorders.' *Molecular and Chemical Neuropathology*, **28**, 77–81.

215

Warren, R.P., Odell, J.D., Warren, W.L., Burger, R.A., Maciulis, A., Daniels, W.W., Torres, A.R. (1997) 'Brief report: Immunoglobulin A deficiency in a subset of autistic subjects.' *Journal of Autism and Developmental Disorders*, **27**, 187–192.

Weizman, A., Weizman, R., Szekely, G.A., Wijsenbeck, H., Livni, E. (1982) 'Abnormal immune response to brain tissue antigen in the syndrome of autism.' *American Journal of Psychiatry*, **139**, 1462–1465.

Weizman, R., Gil-Ad, I., Dick, J., Tyano, S., Szekely, G., Laron, Z. (1988) 'Low plasma immunoreactive beta-endorphin.' *Journal of the American Academy of Child and Adolescent Psychiatry*, **27**, 430–433.

Wiedel, L., Coleman, M. (1976) 'The autistic and control population of this study.' *In:* Coleman, M. (Ed.) *The Autistic Syndromes*. New York: Elsevier, pp. 11–20.

Willemsen-Swinkels, S.H., Buitelaar, J.K, Weijnen, F.G, Thijssen, J.H., van Engeland, H. (1996) 'Plasma beta-endorphin concentrations in people with learning disability and self-injurious and/or autistic behaviour.' *British Journal of Psychiatry*, **168**, 105–109.

Winsberg, B.G., Sverd, J., Castells, S., Hurwic, M., Perel, J.M. (1980) 'Estimation of monoamine and cyclic-AMP turnover and amino acid concentrations in spinal fluid of autistic children.' *Neuropediatrics*, **11**, 250–255.

Yamazaki, K., Saito, Y., Okada, F., Fujieda, T., Yamashita, I. (1975) 'An application of neuro-endocrinological studies in autistic children and Heller's syndrome.' *Journal of Autism and Childhood Schizophrenia*, **5**, 323–332.

Yonk, L.J., Warren, R.P., Burger, R.A., Cole, P., Odell, J.D., Warren, W.L., White, E., Singh, V.K. (1990) 'CD4+ helper T cell depression in autism.' *Immunology Letters*, **25**, 341–346.

Yuwiler, A., Shih, J.C., Chen, C.H., Ritvo, E.R., Hanna, G., Ellison, G.W., King, B.H. (1992) 'Hyperserotoninemia and antiserotonin antibodies in autism and other disorders.' *Journal of Autism and Developmental Disorders*, **22**, 33–45.

14
STRUCTURAL INFORMATION – FROM BRAIN IMAGING AND NEUROPATHOLOGY

With the development of modern imaging techniques, combined with newer studies in neuropathology, a great deal has been learned about the structural changes in the brains of patients with autism. However, as is the problem with so much data collected about a putative single disease called autism, there are often inconsistent results from good or excellent laboratories, probably not because of technical problems, but because they are dealing with different populations of diseases under the umbrella of the autistic syndrome.

Clinical reports of structural abnormalities
SPACE-OCCUPYING LESIONS SUCH AS TUMORS AND CYSTS

Space-occupying lesions are reported infrequently in children with autism. Knobloch and Pasamanick (1975) described a case of hydrocephalus secondary to a papilloma of the choroid plexus in a child with autism. A cystic ganglioglioma in the right posterior temporal lobe and an interpeduncular cistern epidermoid cyst have been reported (Gaffney and Tsai 1987). A pineal cyst has been seen by MRI (Nowell *et al.* 1990). In a Spanish survey of a population of children with autism, two of the patients had brain tumors (Carod *et al.* 1995). A tumor in the left temporal lobe, an oligodendroglioma, has been reported in a young boy who met DSM-III-R criteria for PDD (Hoon and Reiss 1992). A temporal lobe tumor on the right side was found in a patient with a severe autistic regression, and there was evidence of subclinical seizure activity in both temporal lobes (Neville *et al.* 1997); it is not unusual for unilateral temporal lobe lesions to cause bilateral dysfunction.

Arachnoid cysts located in the middle fossa pressing on the temporal lobe have been described in some children with autism (Segawa *et al.* 1986). Bilateral arachnoid cysts in both temporal fossae, with marked hypoplasia of both temporal lobes, have been reported in a 3½-year-old girl with autistic behavior, intractable seizures and very severe psychomotor retardation (Pascual-Castroviejo and Pascual-Pascual 1994). The pathophysiology of an arachnoid cyst is a congenital malformation of the leptomeninges. Whether these cysts, at least when unilateral, are directly relevant to the patient's symptoms of autism is yet to be established, since the middle fossa is the most common location of such cysts and they are described in a number of other disease entities. In addition to headaches and seizures, arachnoid cysts are the most common presenting symptoms of the attention deficit disorder associated with the temporal lobe arachnoid cyst. It is called the temporal arachnoid cyst/attention deficit disorder (TAC/ADD) syndrome (Millichap 1997).

One of the first cases of autism evaluated from a biological point of view revealed a child with widening of the ventricular system, or what appeared to be arrested (occult) hydrocephalus (Schain and Yannet 1960). The ventricular system can be enlarged either due to atrophy of the surrounding structures or due to pressure inside the ventricles as a result of abnormal pressure (hydrocephalus). A number of patients with autistic features and a wider ventricular system have been added to the early literature (Knobloch and Pasamanick 1975, Damasio *et al.* 1980, Campbell *et al.* 1982, Gillberg and Svendsen 1983, Garreau *et al.* 1984, Coleman and Gillberg 1985). In the Knobloch and Pasamanick (1975) cases, the etiology of the hydrocephalus was known – the Dandy-Walker syndrome, secondary to meningitis or to a papilloma of the choroid plexus. But in most of the cases the mechanism leading to the widening of the ventricular system has not been established. The only consistent feature is that the widening of the ventricular system/ hydrocephalus is occult or mild rather than severe.

Exactly where the ventricular system had been widened was also evaluated, but the results were not consistent from study to study. Patients with different disease entities and of different ages probably help to account for this wide variation. Studies have indicated that there is widening in the area of the temporal lobes (Steffenburg 1991), the third ventricle which encompasses the thalamus and hypothalamus area (Hoshino *et al.* 1984, Jacobson *et al.* 1988), the caudate nuclei bilaterally (Jacobson *et al.* 1988), the pontine/ midbrain area (Steffenburg 1991) and the fourth ventricle (Gaffney and Tsai 1987, Courchesne *et al.* 1988).

Neuroimaging studies
The development of imaging techniques enables us to peer inside the living brain. The techniques used today are CT (computer tomography), MRI (magnetic resonance imaging) and functional MRI (FMRI), MRS (magnetic resonance spectroscopy), PET (positron emission tomography), SPECT (single photon emission computed tomographic imaging) and SPET (single photon emission tomography). With the newest techniques (PET, FMRI, SPECT and SPET), the brain can actually be seen in action while performing specific mental tasks, by measuring cerebral blood flow (CBF) or regional cerebral blood flow (rCBF). These techniques even allow the study of pathways of specific neurotransmitters such as dopamine (Ernst *et al.* 1997) and serotonin (Chugani *et al.* 1997) in the brains of persons with autism.

As seen over and over again in studies of autism, results from excellent centers often fail to confirm each other's results. The basic principle in medicine of clarifying problem areas by authors replicating each other's work does not seem to be working well. A reasonable explanation for this problem is not that the differing studies are technically inaccurate but rather that each center has its own mix of patients with different diseases and of different ages; autism is not one disease.

The imaging studies will be reviewed in two sections in an attempt to make more coherent the abundance of available data which can only be described as unclear. First, studies limited to two categories within the autistic syndrome will be discussed: individuals with high-functioning autism and those with Asperger syndrome. The remaining studies, which do not distinguish with regard to level of functioning in individuals within the autistic syndrome, will then be reviewed. This does not mean that the general studies of autism are any less valid than those limited to high-functioning patients. However, studies limited to high-functioning individuals might possibly be more revelatory for the purposes of attempting to tease out what features might be specific only to the behavioral component of autism. Of course, it is important to put in the caveat, known to everyone who works with children with autism, that apparently lower-functioning individuals with autism may, in fact, have quite high levels of functioning hidden beneath their defensive sensory postures. So this distinction is an artificial one limited to this chapter.

IMAGING STUDIES LIMITED TO PERSONS WITH HIGH-FUNCTIONING AUTISM
Regarding the cerebral cortex in high-functioning adults with autism, some studies are available. MRI studies of high-functioning individuals with autism have recorded evidence of developmental cortical abnormalities. In a study of 14 patients with high-level autism, Gaffney and Tsai (1987) found 6 persons with detectable lesions by MRI. They included left occipital heterotopic grey matter, a right temporal ganglioglioma, an interpeduncular cistern epidermoid cyst, an unidentified lesion in the right parietal area, as well as dilatation of lateral ventricles. In a study of high-functioning males with autism, Piven et al. (1990) reported that more than half (7 out of 13) had evidence of cerebral cortical malformations. The lesions were polymicrogyria, macrogyria and schizencephaly. Berthier et al. (1990) have also described left frontal macrogyria and bilateral opercular polymicrogyria in two cases with Asperger syndrome – evidence of malformations of cortical development.

MRI scans read as negative may not be definitive. A study of SPET with correlative MRI found focal areas of decreased perfusion in the thalami (19/23), posterior parietal lobe (10/23), temporal lobe (7/23), cerebellar hemisphere (20/23) and basal ganglia (5/23) in 23 young children (mean age: 54 months) who met DSM-IV criteria of autism (Ryu et al. 1999). By contrast, all the children had normal MRI findings in these areas. The limitations of interpretation of an MRI scan were also pointed out by Schifter et al. (1994), who demonstrated that an FDG-PET may provide evidence of metabolic dysfunction after an MRI scan has initially been read as unremarkable. They report that malformations of cortical development such as focal pachygyria were found in three children with autism only after the FDG-PET provided evidence of a regional metabolic abnormality. In that same study, there were three other children with evidence of metabolic abnormalities and seven children with normal imaging studies. Of course, it should be noted that descriptions of abnormalities that can be interpreted as malformations of cortical development are not limited to high-functioning patients, but are also described in general studies of patients with autism (Nowell et al. 1990).

One of the first studies to use metabolic rates for glucose (resting CMR ratios) determined by PET was a study based on men with autism, almost all of whom were high-functioning (Horowitz et al. 1988). This study discovered an imbalance in mutually inhibitory frontal–parietal interactions as well as evidence of disruption of thalamic–neocortical interactions. The authors raise the question of whether, in autism, the inward-directed frontal lobe might dominate the outward-directed parietal lobe.

In a seminal study, 11 high-functioning individuals with autism, aged 12-36 years, were matched with a control group selected for age, gender, IQ, race and socioeconomic status by Minshew *et al.* (1993). The study used *in vivo* 31P nuclear MRS to determine alterations in high energy phosphate and membrane phospholipid metabolism in the dorsal prefrontal brain. In the persons with autism, the studies showed a hypermetabolic energy state with undersynthesis and enhanced degradation of brain membranes. When this energy status was compared to neuropsychological and language test scores, correlations were observed in the autistic group which paralleled their clinical severity. Such correlations were not seen in the controls. The tests found to correlate in individuals with autism were the Wisconsin Card Sorting Test, Test of Language Competence, semantic language comprehension tests and delayed recall memory tests. There are a number of possible interpretations of this interesting data, including the observation by Johns (1998) that altered phosphorus MRS is a possible finding in mitochondrial encephalopathies. While the Minshew group found abnormalities in the dorsal prefrontal cortex, another study of 14 adults by Siegel *et al.* (1995) found abnormalities in the medial frontal cortex. Using PET, they found negative correlations of the glucose metabolic rate in the medial frontal cortex with a test of sustained attention.

The dentato-thalamo-cortical pathway has been evaluated in four high-functioning autistic men (Müller *et al.* 1998a) using [^{15}O]-water PET. The dorsolateral prefrontal area 46 and the thalamus in the left hemisphere and the right dentate nucleus showed overall less activation for receptive and expressive language conditions. This study is further confirmation by this group of an earlier study of the same pathway using a serotonin precursor (Chugani *et al.* 1997).

Regarding the cerebral cortex in Asperger syndrome, left occipital hypoperfusion by PET has been reported in a case with Asperger syndrome (Ozbayrak *et al.* 1991). McKelvey *et al.* (1995) studied three persons with Asperger syndrome and demonstrated right hemisphere abnormalities by SPECT – a developmental anomaly, abnormalities of profusion in the temporal and polar frontal areas, and diffusely decreased right hemisphere uptake. An attempt to duplicate a "theory of mind" experiment by PET, which activated the left medial prefrontal cortex in healthy volunteers, failed when it was attempted in five people with Asperger syndrome (Happé *et al.* 1996). However, normal PET activity was observed in areas immediately adjacent to the left medial prefrontal cortex in the individuals with Asperger syndrome during the duplicate experiment.

Regarding specific gyri, the anterior rectal gyrus was shown to have an abnormal left>right asymmetry in 16 high-functioning adults compared to healthy controls, by Siegel *et al.* (1992) using PET. (The normal asymmetry in that region is left<right.) A high glucose metabolic rate by 18-fluoro-2-deoxyglucose PET was found in the right posterior calcarine cortex in 16 high-functioning adults compared to healthy controls (Siegel *et al.* 1992). The anterior cingulate gyrus has been studied using a combination of MRI and PET in seven high-functioning patients with autism and age, sex-matched

healthy controls (Haznedar *et al.* 1997). These authors found that the right anterior cingulate area 24' was significantly smaller in volume, and both area 24 and area 24' were less metabolically active in the patients with autism. The study used glucose, whose uptake is primarily in dendrites; planning future work, it should be noted that anterior cingulate regions are extremely rich in serotonin receptor density.

Regarding the basal ganglia, an unidentified bilateral lesion in the globus pallidus has been seen on MRI (Gaffney and Tsai 1987). The left posterior putamen was reported to have a depressed glucose metabolic rate in the PET study by Siegel *et al.* (1992). In a retrospective review in young children aged 28–92 months who met DSM-IV criteria, SPET with correlative MRI found focal areas of decreased perfusion in the basal ganglia in 5 out of the 23 children, even though the children had normal MRI findings (Ryu *et al.* 1999).

Regarding the brainstem, Gaffney *et al.* (1988) described 13 high-functioning patients with a smaller size of the pons on MRI. Hashimoto *et al.* (1992a) found that the size of the pons did not differ from controls in their MRI studies on retarded children with autism. With higher-functioning children, Hashimoto *et al.* (1993) reported evidence of a significantly smaller size of the midbrain and medulla oblongata by MRI; their studies indicated that anatomical changes in the posterior fossa structures probably took place in the prenatal period, since the later rate of development of these structures was more rapid than in controls (Hashimoto *et al.* 1994). They found, however, that the smaller size of the midbrain and medulla oblongata existed irrespective of the IQ or DQ of the children, although it was more marked in the lower DQ group (Hashimoto *et al.* 1992b).

Regarding research on the cerebellum, in 1992 two outstanding centers tested 15 (Piven *et al.* 1992) and 18 (Holttum *et al.* 1992) high-functioning individuals with autism compared to carefully selected controls. Neither group was able to confirm gross structural abnormalities of the cerebellum. Another study of high-functioning individuals with autism compared them with two sets of controls – healthy controls and brain-damaged survivors of acute lymphoblastic leukemia (ALL) who had brain sequelae from radiation and chemotherapy (Ciesielski *et al.* 1997). The study used MRI and neuropsychological tests. MRI tests revealed modest but consistent hypoplasia of vermal lobules I-V and more marked reduction of VI-VII in both autistic and ALL groups compared to controls. The authors point out that the cerebellum is more vulnerable than earlier maturing areas of the brain to continuing deleterious insults in early childhood. Regarding the subject of specificity of VI and VII hypoplasia, a quantitative MRI study by Schaefer *et al.* (1996) looked at 102 patients with a variety of neurogenetic abnormalities and found that hypoplasia of cerebellar vermal lobules VI and VII is a non-specific finding that occurs in several conditions without autistic behavior.

OTHER IMAGING STUDIES

An important point of contention in autism of all developmental levels is whether there are identifiable abnormalities in the cerebral cortex, particularly in the frontal and prefrontal cortex and the temporal lobe. In 1991, a SPECT study by Lelord *et al.* found decreased perfusion in the frontal, parietal and left temporal lobes in 31 patients with autism. A SPECT study using xenon-133 failed to demonstrate abnormalities of rCBF in frontal, temporal and sensory association cortices (Zilbovicius *et al.* 1992). However, in a SPECT study with a newer technique using technetium-99m-HMPAO in four adults, George *et al.* (1992) found total brain perfusion significantly decreased, most marked in the right lateral temporal and right, left and midfrontal lobes. Gillberg *et al.* (1993) also used a SPECT method with technetium-99m-HM-PAO and found evidence of hypoperfusion of the temporal lobes which was bilateral in 10 of their 16 patients. Also using the same SPECT technique to examine rCBF, Mountz *et al.* (1995) studied 12 annular cortical regions in severely autistic children compared to age-matched controls. They reported that temporal and parietal lobes had abnormal rCBF in their six patients, with the left cerebral hemisphere showing greater abnormalities than the right. A similar study – a single study on an autistic patient with a 20/22 chromosomal translation and an interstitial deletion of chromosome 22q11, with technetium-99m-HM-PAO – showed hypoperfusion of the left temporoparietal cortex (Carratala *et al.* 1998). The Zilbovicius group (1995) studied age as a factor in interpreting studies of metabolism in the cortex in autism. They published a challenging study where they compared rCBR at two different ages in the same children. The first study was performed when the children were 3–4 years of age, the second study three years later. They found a transient frontal hypoperfusion at the younger age, which had disappeared three years later. By the age of 6–7 years, the autistic children's frontal perfusion had attained normal values.

SPET is another technique that has been used in studies of patients with autism. A study by Ryu *et al.* (1999) did a retrospective review of studies using the technetium-99m ethyl cysteinate dimer. They limited their report to 23 very young children aged between 28 and 82 months who met DSM-IV criteria, and compared the SPET results with MRI in the same children. Because of the very young age group, this study may pertain to either high-functioning or all-level-functioning children. The Ryu group found focal areas of decreased perfusion in the cerebellar hemisphere (20/23), thalami (19/23), posterior parietal (10/23), temporal (7/23) and the basal ganglia (5/23). By contrast, all patients had normal MRI findings.

Another study, using the techniques of PET to measure accumulation of a dopamine precursor fluorine-18-labeled fluorodopa (FDOPA), checked children with autism and carefully matched controls all close to the age of 13 years (Ernst *et al.* 1997). These researchers made a ratio of regions rich in dopamine terminals compared to the occipital cortex, known as a region poor in dopamine terminals. In children with autism, the regional FDOPA ratio was reduced by 39 per cent in the anterior medial prefrontal cortex but not in other areas studied.

Regarding the measurement of the frontal lobes by MRI, one study found the frontal, lateral and orbital regions to be normal in size (Courchesne *et al.* 1993). Another study found the frontal lobes diminished in size compared to other cerebral lobes in a study of macrocephalic children with autism (Piven *et al.* 1996). The parietal lobe was studied by MRI in 21 autistic patients compared to three sets of controls. Nine of the 21 patients were found to have parietal lobes that were abnormal in appearance bilaterally, mostly due to cortical volume loss, although three also had white matter volume loss. Temporal lobe enlargement has been found in autistic children and adults on MRI, and seems predominantly right-sided (Piven *et al.* 1996); another study found it normal in size (Courchesne *et al.* 1993). An MRI study that included limbic structures found them normal in size (Courchesne *et al.* 1993). When measurements were made by detailed (1.5 mm) MRI of the hippocampus, a study of 35 subjects with autism and 36 control subjects showed no differences in the volumes (Piven *et al.* 1998).

The report, in many patients, of enlarged fourth ventricles (Gaffney and Tsai 1987, Gaffney *et al.* 1988) and diminished size of cerebellar lobules VI and VII (Courchesne *et al.* 1988) led to a number of studies which could be summarized by saying that these findings are sometimes present and sometimes not present, undoubtedly depending upon each patient's underlying disease process. In one large study, Nowell *et al.* (1990) found that 9 per cent (5 out of 53) of patients who met the criteria of autism had significant cerebellar vermian atrophy. In a study of the volume of the total cerebellum and the area of cerebellar lobules I through VII by detailed (1.5 mm) MRI in 35 subjects with autism, Piven *et al.* (1997) found no abnormalities in the size of the lobules, but reported that the volume of the total cerebellum was increased. Hsu *et al.* (1991) could not find any difference between the size of the midbrain and pons between normal and autistic children.

Neuropathology

The attempt to find what all patients with autism actually do have in common, which results in their autistic behavior patterns, is quite a challenging problem. Clinical/ neuropathological correlations are the traditional way in medicine of deciphering underlying disease processes. However, this is still a distant goal in the field of autism. We do not have an accurate diagnosis in many – perhaps most – individuals during life, and there is a paucity of careful postmortem studies even in patients identified during life as having an autistic syndrome.

Each disease entity of autism presumably has its own neuropathological picture which includes, in addition to its own specific brain abnormalities, the particular lesions related to the behavior syndrome of autism. What is clearly needed is neuropathological studies comparing the specific disease entities within the autistic syndrome to try to pinpoint what lesions they might share in common. To our knowledge, only one autopsy has been performed on a patient who had a definite medical diagnosis during life. In their neuro pathological study of four retarded persons with autistic behavior, Williams *et al.* (1980) included an individual who had been diagnosed during life as having phenylketonuria (PKU). (Another patient in this series may have had Rett syndrome, although not diagnosed during life and not definite.) The Williams *et al.* (1980) team looked at the cerebral cortex of the four patients – including hippocampus, parahippocampal gyrus, thalamus, striatum, hypothalamus and midbrain tectum – with the rapid Golgi method and electron microscopy. In the brains of two patients, nothing of interest was found. In the brains of the other two, including the PKU patient, there were only subtle findings. These authors reported a diminution in dendritic caliber and spine density of layer V pyramidal neurons of the mid-frontal gyrus, even though these neurons were oriented normally and had richly branched dendritic arbors. This is not much in the way of neuropathological findings in view of the devastating clinical picture of these individuals.

Because of the many diseases that may cause autistic symptoms, documented throughout this book, it will come as no surprise that the neuropathological studies available in patients diagnosed as autistic – often done by outstanding centers – do not report the same findings. Many of the postmortem studies were performed on patients with seizure disorders, which brings into question the effect of seizures themselves as well as anti-epileptic drugs on the cerebellum and other brain structures. The most consistent finding of three major studies to date (Ritvo *et al.* 1986, Bailey *et al.* 1998, Kemper and Bauman 1998) is a reduction in the number of Purkinje cells. However, even here, there is a case which met DSM-IV criteria where the patient had Purkinje cells that were normal in size and number in spite of epilepsy (Guerin *et al.* 1996). It should be noted that the Guerin *et al.* (1996) case was hardly a typical patient with autism; she was a severely retarded epileptic patient with dysmorphic features who had a microcephalic brain; neuropathologically, she had a thin corpus callosum and ventricular dilatation.

Regarding the cerebral cortex and subcortical areas, imaging studies have suggested that some brains may show evidence that suggests abnormalities in cortical neuronal proliferation, migration and organization (see Table 14.1). Neuropathological studies, more modest in number, do confirm this possibility. Unusually small and more closely packed neurons have been reported in anterior cingulate cortex in 8 or 9 brains (Kemper and Bauman 1993, 1998). Polymicrogyria has been reported in two postmortem cases (Ritvo *et al.* 1986, Kemper 1988). Neuronal hetertopias, focally increased numbers of single neurons in the white matter, neuronal disorganization, increases in cortical thickness and high neuronal density are described among their six cases by Bailey *et al.* (1998).

The limbic system is a major focus of interest in autism. Kemper and Bauman (1998) found small, densely distributed neurons in the amygdala, the entorhinal cortex, the septal nuclei, and the hippocampus (especially in fields CA1 and CA4). These are the kind of results expected for an earlier stage of maturation for the individuals involved. The authors pointed out that this maturational delay is different from that recorded in mental retardation inasmuch as it appeared to be confined to the limbic system. Bailey *et al.* (1998) were aware of these reports yet they note that they failed to find consistent hippocampal abnormalities in the six brains they studied. Kemper and Bauman (1998) reported that the neurons of the dentate nucleus were enlarged in the brains of younger autistic individuals.

Evidence of neuronal ectopia and other developmental abnormalities has been identified in the brainstem (Bailey *et al.* 1998). Detailed examination of the brainstem of one patient by Rodier *et al.* (1996) showed a marked reduction in the number of neurons in the facial nucleus and superior olive, as well as shortening of the brainstem between the trapezoid body and inferior olive. Kemper and Bauman (1993) reported that there were abnormalities in the size of the inferior olivary nuclei and that some of the neurons of the inferior olive tended to cluster at the periphery of the inferior convolution. In the study by Bailey *et al.* (1998), the inferior olives were malformed in three brains and olivary dysplasia was associated with enlarged arcuate nuclei in two cases. However, in these cases, the neuronal size of the olive appeared unremarkable and there was no tendency for olivary cells to cluster at the periphery of the convolutions.

Evidence of abnormal migration has been identified in two cases in the cerebellum (Bailey *et al.* 1998). In the Bailey *et al.* study, which included 4 out of 6 patients with a seizure disorder, there was no significant cerebellar atrophy or apparent granule cell loss even though Purkinje cell density was decreased in all the adult cases, similar to findings by Ritvo *et al.* (1986) and Kemper and Bauman (1998). A most interesting report of the Bailey group was the finding of cytoplasmic inclusion bodies in the Purkinje cells of one childhood case.

New methods of investigation of human brain tissue may help to resolve the conflicting results available to date. One such study, using quantitative analysis of confocal laser-scanning microscopy (CLSM) to measure the distribution and density of a synaptic vesicle protein – synaptophysin (p38) – evaluated the frontal, temporal, motor, visual and entorhinal cortices of brains from individuals with autism and Rett syndrome (Belichenko *et al.* 1996). They reported that the p38 immunofluorescence was diminished in the patients' brains compared to controls.

Macrocrania

Are the cranial circumferences of children with autism unusually large? This section will discuss the recent interest in the literature regarding macrocrania. However, this is nothing new – both more large and more small heads have long been noted in children with autism. A 1976 study of 78 children with autism, paired with 78 age- and sex-matched healthy controls, found that "head circumferences were significantly larger or smaller than the mean circumference for each age group examined" (Walker 1976). A recent study has confirmed this increased incidence of both macrocephaly and microcephaly in patients with autism (Fombonne *et al.* 1999).

Macrocrania is defined as an increased cranial circumference above two standard deviations. A study of 91 children who met DSM-III-R criteria for PDD reported that this group of children had head circumferences above the mean when compared to standardized growth curves (Chudley *et al.* 1998). Woodhouse *et al.* (1996) report that when autistic children are limited to the PDD diagnosis, about one-third have macrocrania. In another study, 25 children with childhood autism were compared to non-autistic children, referred for developmental deviancy, who were matched to the autistic children by sex, age and intellectual level; macrocrania was found only among the children with autism (Skjeldal *et al.* 1998). Studies of children with autism have found that 18 per cent (Davidovitch *et al.* 1996) to 37 per cent (Bailey *et al.* 1993, Lainhart *et al.* 1997) of them have macrocrania by early or middle childhood. An even higher figure of 42 per cent (9 out of 19) has been reported in an autistic twin epidemiological study (Bailey *et al.* 1995). In most instances the infant is not born macrocephalic but develops the condition by early childhood. Non-autistic children may, of course, sometimes have macrocrania; these studies simply emphasize the distinct possibility of macrocrania in autism.

What could cause an increased cranial circumference in an individual with autism? Macrocrania does not define a homogeneous grouping of autistic individuals according to

225

clinical features (Lainhart *et al.* 1997). The main reasons that have been documented for macrocrania in autism are Sotos syndrome (see Chapter 11), occult hydrocephalus (discussed earlier in this chapter) and megalencephaly. Megalencephaly is an enlarged and heavier brain.

A 1992 MRI study of the mid-sagittal area of the cerebellum and pons found this area significantly enlarged compared to two different control groups (Piven *et al.* 1992). A detailed (1.5 mm) MRI of the brains of 22 male autistic subjects compared to volunteer controls found that the enlargement was the result of both greater brain tissue and greater lateral ventricle volume (Piven *et al.* 1995). Of the neuropathological studies published, there are several where the majority of brain weights meet the criteria of megalencephaly. In the study by Bailey *et al.* (1998), 4 out of 6 brains met megalencephaly criteria. (It is assumed that the cases described by Bailey *et al.* (1993) are subsumed into the larger 1998 series.) Kemper and Bauman (1998) also reported that 8 out of 11 brains of children aged less than 12 years had a significant increase in weight compared to controls, although

TABLE 14.1
Malformations of cortical development*
(those described to date in patients with autism)

  I Malformations due to abnormal neuronal and glial proliferation
      B Focal or multifocal
          (3) Abnormal proliferation (abnormal cell types)
              (a) Non-neoplastic
                  (i) Tuberous sclerosis, types 1 and 2
                  (ii) Hypomelanosis of Ito
                  (iii) Neurofibromatosis, type 1
              (b) Neoplastic (associated with disordered cortex)
                  (ii) Ganglioglioma

  II Malformations due to abnormal neuronal migration
      A Generalized
          (4) Heterotopia
      B Focal or multifocal malformations in neuronal migration
          (2) Focal or multifocal heterotopia
               (e) Marginal glioneuronal heterotopia
                  (i) Fetal alcohol syndrome
          (3) Focal or multifocal heterotopia with organizational abnormality of the cortex
              (c) Focal mixed subcortical/subependymal
                  (ii) Peroxisomal disorders
          (4) Excessive single ectopic white matter neurons

  III Malformations due to abnormal cortical organization
      C Focal or multifocal
          (1) Polymicrogyria/schizencephaly**
              (b) Asymmetric polymicrogyria
               (c) Schizencephaly and mixed schizencephaly/polymicrogyria

---

  * classification scheme created by Barkovich *et al.* 1996
** in this scheme, schizencephaly is assumed to be an extreme form of polymicrogyria; pachygyria is assumed to be regions of fusion of the molecular layer of polymicrogyria

they did not find the same phenomenon in older patients. A recent study based on brain weights of 21 postmortem cases, however, found three that were megalencephalic and one that was microcephalic; the rest were within normal limits for brain weight for age (Courchesne *et al.* 1999). Other neuropathological reports in autism which include megalencephaly are those of Darby (1976), Williams *et al.* (1980) and Rodier *et al.* (1996).

Exactly why some brains are megalencephalic is unknown. A provocative hypothesis has been proposed by Chugani *et al.* (1999) based on manipulation of serotonin in developing animals which recapitulates some of the pathological findings in autism. These authors wonder whether the increased neuronal cell numbers in the hippocampus as reported by Bauman and Kemper might possibly result from serotonin depletion during critical fetal developmental periods. One of the most challenging aspects of interpreting megalencephaly in autism is the dissociation between cortical and callosal size. The corpus callosum, which connects the two cortical hemispheres, instead of being enlarged, appears, by MRI studies, to have reduced volume in some patients. This has been best documented in the posterior subregions of the corpus callosum. Exactly what this means, particularly in the context of megalencephaly, remains to be determined (for fuller discussion, see Chapter 19).

Are megalencephalic brains more common in younger children? Kemper and Bauman (1998) noted that the weights of 6 out of 8 brains of individuals over 18 years of age were lower than expected, although the difference did not reach statistical significance. In contrast to Bailey *et al.* (1998), who did report megalencephaly in adult brains, Kemper and Bauman (1998) did not find heavy weights in adult brains compared to controls. Based on this finding and other histological details, Kemper and Bauman raise the question of whether the cases they studied began with a disease process in prenatal development and retained an ongoing pathological process that continued into adult life. A theoretical explanation of such a process would be failure of the usual overgrowth followed by pruning, a pattern that is seen when the brains of normal children are compared to the brains of normal adults (Minshew 1996). This might indicate a mistake in the programmed cell death that normally occurs in the central nervous system of children.

Conclusion

Combining the information obtained from both modern neuroimaging studies and the available neuropathological studies, it is overwhelmingly apparent that autism is a syndrome of many disparate disease entities. The elusive one anatomical section of the brain leading to that final common pathway in the central nervous system causing autistic symptoms is not identified. As was already known, autism is a heterogeneous disease entity containing different clinical subgroups, which do not manifest similar imaging pictures (Nowell *et al.* 1990).

Looking at the information available from structural studies, it is striking how much evidence there is in favor of neurodevelopmental lesions. If the Barkovich *et al.* (1996) classification of Malformations of Cortical Development (see Table 14.1) is scanned with autistic patients in mind, information from imaging studies, neuropathological reports, and a number of the double syndromes fit into this table. The table is based on the three fundamental embryological events of cortical formation – proliferation, migration and organization. As scientific techniques improve, neocortical malformations are being identified much more often than was previously suspected; they are already known to be a common cause of epilepsy and developmental delay in children and young adults. In the past, these disorders tended to all be labeled as neuronal migration disorders; however, it is becoming clear that many involve abnormal formation in the germinative zone or abnormal cortical organization. It is quite complicated to understand; there may be more to it than meets the eye (from looking at an imaging study). This is because the mere presence of heterotopia may not be enough to prove an origin of the clinical symptoms, since it has been demonstrated that, in some situations, heterotopic cortex may demonstrate preserved function (Müller *et al.* 1998b).

REFERENCES

Bailey, A., Luthert, P., Bolton, P., Le Couteur, A., Rutter, M., Harding, B. (1993) 'Autism and megalencephaly.' (Letter) *Lancet*, **341**, 1225–1226.

Bailey, A., Le Couteur, A., Gottesman, I., Bolton, P., Simonoff, E., Yudza, E., Rutter, M. (1995) Autism as a strongly genetic disorder: evidence from a British twin study. *Psychological Medicine*, **25**, 63–77.

Bailey, A., Luthert, P., Dean, A., Harding, B., Janota, I., Montgomery, M., Rutter, M., Lantos, P. (1998) 'A clinicopathological study of autism.' *Brain*, **121**, 889–905.

Barkovich, A.J., Kuzniecky, R.I., Dobyns, W.B., Jackson, G.D., Becker, L.E., Evrard, P. (1996) 'A classification scheme for malformations of cortical development.' *Neuropediatrics*, **27**, 59–63.

Bauman, M.L. (1996) 'Neuroanatomic observations of the brain in pervasive developmental disorders.' (Review) *Journal of Autism and Developmental Disorders*, **26**, 199–203.

Bauman, M.L., Kemper, T.L. (1985) 'Histoanatomic observations of the brain in early infantile autism.' *Neurology*, **35**, 866–874.

Belichenko, P.V., Fedorov, A.A., Dahlstrom, A.B. (1996) 'Quantitative analysis of immunofluorescence and lipofuscin distribution in human cortical areas by dual-channel confocal laser scanning microscopy.' *Journal of Neuroscience Methods*, **69**, 155–161.

Berthier, M.L., Starkstein, S.E., Leiguarda, R. (1990) 'Developmental cortical anomalies in Asperger's syndrome.' *Journal of Neuropsychiatry and Clinical Neurosciences*, **2**, 197–201.

Campbell, M., Rosenbloom, S., Perry, R., George, A.E., Kricheff, I.I., Anderson, L., Small, A.M., Jennings, S.J. (1982) 'Computerized axial tomography in young autistic children.' *American Journal of Psychiatry*, **139**, 510–512.

Carod, F.J., Prats, J.M., Garaizar, C., Zuazo, E. (1995) 'Clinical-radiological evaluation of infantile autism and epileptic syndromes associated with autism.' (In Spanish) *Review Neurologique*, **23**, 1203–1207.

Carratala, F., Galan, F., Moya, M., Esstivill, X., Pritchard, M.A., Llevadot, R., Nadal, M., Gratacos, M. (1998) 'A patient with autistic disorder and a 20/22 chromosomal translocation.' *Developmental Medicine and Child Neurology*, **40**, 492–495.

Chudley, A.E., Gutierrez, E., Jocelyn, L.J., Chodirker, B.N. (1998) 'Outcomes of genetic evaluation in children with pervasive developmental disorder.' *Journal of Developmental and Behavioral Pediatrics*, **19**, 321–325.

Chugani, D.C., Muzik, O., Rothermel, R.D., Behen, M.E., Chakraborty, P.K., Mangner, T.J., da Silva, E.A., Chugani, H.T. (1997) 'Altered serotonin synthesis in the dentato-thalamo-cortical pathway in autistic boys.' *Annals of Neurology*, **14**, 666–669.

Chugani, D.C., Muzik, O., Behen, M., Rothermel, R., Janisse, J.J., Lee, J., Chugani, H.T. (1999) 'Developmental changes in brain serotonin synthesis capacity in autistic and nonautistic children.' *Annals of Neurology*, **45**, 287–295.

Ciesielski, K.T., Harris, R.J., Hart, B.L., Pabst, H.F. (1997) 'Cerebellar hypoplasia and frontal lobe cognitive deficits in disorders of early childhood.' *Neuropsychologia*, **35**, 643–655.

Coleman, M., Gillberg, C. (1985) *The Autistic Syndromes. 1st Edn.* New York: Praeger, p. 165.

Courchesne, E., Yeung-Courchesne, R., Press, G.A., Hesselink, J.R., Jernigan, T.L. (1988) 'Hypoplasia of cerebellar vermal VI and VII in autism.' *New England Journal of Medicine*, **318**, 1349–1354.

Courchesne, E., Press, G.A., Yeung-Courchesne, R. (1993) 'Parietal lobe abnormalities detected with MR in patients with infantile autism.' *AJR American Journal of Roentgenology*, **160**, 387–393.

Courchesne, E., Muller, R.A., Saitoh, O. (1999) 'Brain weight in autism: normal in the majority of cases, megalencephalic in rare cases.' *Neurology*, **52**, 1057–1059.

Damasio, H., Maurer, R.G., Damasio, A.R., Chui, H.C. (1980) 'Computerized tomographic scan findings in patients with autistic behavior.' *Archives of Neurology*, **37**, 504–510.

Darby, J.K. (1976) 'Neuropathologic aspects of psychosis in children.' *Journal of Autism and Childhood Schizophrenia*, **6**, 339–352.

Davidovitch, M., Patterson, B., Gortside, P. (1996) 'Head circumference measurements in children with autism.' *Journal of Child Neurology*, **11**, 389–393.

Ernst, M., Zametkin, A.J., Matochik, J.A., Pascualvaca, D., Cohen, R.M. (1997) 'Low medial prefrontal dopaminergic activity in autistic children.' (Letter) *Lancet*, **351**, 454.

Fombonne, E., Roge, B., Claverie, J., Courty, S., Fremolle, J. (1999) 'Microcephaly and macrocephaly in autism.' *Journal of Autism and Developmental Disorders*, **29**, 113–119.

Gaffney, G., Tsai, L. (1987) 'Brief report: Magnetic resonance imaging of high level autism.' *Journal of Autism and Developmental Disorders*, **17**, 433–438.

Gaffney, G., Kuperman, S., Tsai, L., Minchin, S. (1988) 'Morphologic evidence for brainstem involvement in infantile autism.' *Biological Psychiatry*, **24**, 578–586.

Garreau, B., Barthélémy, C., Sauvage, D., Leddet, I., Lelord, G. (1984) 'A comparison of autistic syndromes with and without associated neurological problems.' *Journal of Autism and Developmental Disorders*, **14**, 105–111.

George, M.S., Costa, D.C., Kouris, K., Ring, H.A., Ell, P.J. (1992) 'Cerebral blood flow abnormalities in adults with infantile autism.' *Journal of Nervous and Mental Diseases*, **180**, 413–417.

Gillberg, C., Svendsen, P. (1983) 'Childhood psychosis and computed tomographic brain scan findings.' *Journal of Autism and Developmental Disorders*, **13**, 19–32.

Gillberg, I.C., Bjure, J., Uvebrant, P., Vestergren, E., Gillberg, C. (1993) 'SPECT (Single photon emission computed tomography) in 31 children and adolescents with autism and autistic-like conditions.' *European Child and Adolescent Psychiatry*, **2**, 50–59.

Guerin, P., Lyon, G., Barthélémy, C., Sostak, E., Chevrollier, V., Garreau, B., Lelord, G. (1996) 'Neuropathological study of a case of autistic syndrome with severe mental retardation.' *Developmental Medicine and Child Neurology*, **38**, 203–211.

Happé, F., Ehlers, S., Fletcher, P., Frith, U., Johansson, M., Gillberg, C., Dolan, R., Frackowiak, R., Frith, C. (1996) '"Theory of mind" in the brain. Evidence from a PET scan study of Asperger syndrome.' *Neuroreport*, **8**, 197–201.

Hashimoto, T., Murakawa, K., Miyazaki, M., Tayama, M., Kuroda, Y. (1992a) Magnetic resonance imaging of the brain structures in the posterior fossa in retarded autistic children. *Acta Paediatrica*, **81**, 1030–1034.

Hashimoto, T., Tayama, M., Miyazaki, M., Sakurama, N., Yoshimoto, T., Murakawa, K., Kuroda, Y. (1992b) 'Reduced brainstem size in children with autism.' *Brain Development*, **14**, 94–97.

Hashimoto, T., Tayama, M., Miyazaki, M., Murakawa, K., Shimakawa, S., Yoneda, Y., Kuroda, Y. (1993) 'Brainstem involvement in high-functioning autistic children.' *Acta Neurologica Scandinavica*, **88**, 123–128.

Hashimoto, T., Tayama, M., Murakawa, K., Miyazaki, M., Yoshimoto, T., Harada, M., Kuroda, Y. (1994) 'Development of the brainstem and cerebellum in autistic children.' (In Japanese) *No To Hattatsu*, **26**, 480–485.

Haznedar, M.M., Buchsbaum, M.S., Metzger, M., Solimando, A., Spiegel-Cohen, J., Hollander, E. (1997) 'Anterior cingulate gyrus volume and glucose metabolism in autistic disorder.' *American Journal of Psychiatry*, **154**, 1047–1050.

Holttum, J.R., Minshew, N.J., Sanders, R.S., Phillips, N.E. (1992) 'Magnetic resonance imaging of the posterior fossa in autism.' *Biological Psychiatry*, **32**, 1091–1101.

Hoon, A.H., Reiss, A.L. (1992) 'The mesial-temporal lobe and autism.' *Developmental Medicine and Child Neurology*, **34**, 252–259.

Horowitz, B., Rumsey, J.M., Grady, C.L., Rapoport, S.I. (1988) 'The cerebral metabolic landscape in autism.' *Archives of Neurology*, **45**, 749–755.

Hoshino, Y., Manome, T., Kaneko, M., Yashima, Y., Kumashiro, H. (1984) 'Computed tomography of the brain in children with early infantile autism.' *Folia Psychiatrica et Neurologica Japonica*, **38**, 33–43.

Hsu, M., Yeung-Courchesne, R., Courchesne, E., Press, G.A. (1991) 'Absence of magnetic resonance imaging evidence of pontine abnormality in infantile autism.' *Archives of Neurology*, **48**, 1160–1163.

Jacobson, R., Le Couteur, A., Howlin, P., Rutter, M. (1988) 'Selective subcortical abnormalities in autism.' *Psychological Medicine*, **18**, 39–48.

Johns, D.R. (1998) 'The genetic basis of mitochondrial disease.' *In:* Jameson, J.L. (Ed.) *Principles of Molecular Medicine*. Totowa, NJ: Humana Press.

Kemper, T.L. (1988) 'Neuroanatomic studies of dyslexia and autism.' *In:* Swann, J.W., Messer, A. (Eds) *Disorders of the Developing Nervous System: Changing Views on their Origins, Diagnoses and Treatments*. New York: Alan R. Liss, pp. 125–154.

Kemper, T.L., Bauman, M.L. (1993) 'The contribution of neuropathologic studies to the understanding of autism.' *Neurology Clinics*, **11**, 175–187.

Kemper, T.L., Bauman, M. (1998) 'Neuropathology of infantile autism.' *Journal of Neuropathology and Experimental Neurology*, **57**, 645–652.

Knobloch, H., Pasamanick, B. (1975) 'Some etiologic and prognostic factors in early infantile autism and psychosis.' *Journal of Pediatrics*, **55**, 182–191.

Lainhart, J.E., Piven, J., Wzorek, M., Landa, R., Santangelo, S.L., Coon, H., Folstein, S.E. (1997) 'Macrocephaly in children and adults with autism.' *Journal of the American Academy of Child and Adolescent Psychiatry*, **36**, 282–290.

Lelord, G., Garreau, B., Syrota, A., Bruneau, N., Pourcelot, L., Zilbovicius, M. (1991) 'SPECT-rCHF, Doppler transcranial ultrasonography and evoked potential studies in pervasive developmental disorders.' *Biological Psychiatry (Supplement)*, **29**, 292.

McKelvey, J.R., Lambert, R., Mottron, L., Shevell, M.I. (1995) 'Right-hemisphere dysfunction in Asperger's syndrome.' *Journal of Child Neurology*, **10**, 310–314.

Millichap, J.C. (1997) 'Temporal lobe arachnoid cyst – attention deficit disorder syndrome: role of the electroencephalogram in diagnosis.' *Neurology*, **48**, 1435–1439.

Minshew, N.J. (1996) 'Brief report: Brain mechanisms in autism: functional and structural abnormalities.' *Journal of Autism and Developmental Disorders*, **26**, 205–209.

Minshew, N.J., Goldstein, G., Dombrowski, S.M., Panchalingam, K., Pettegrew, J.W. (1993) 'A preliminary 31P MRS study of autism: evidence for undersynthesis and increased degradation of brain membranes.' *Biological Psychiatry*, **33**, 762–773.

Mountz, J.M., Tolbert, L.C., Lill, D.W., Katholi, C.R., Liu, H.G. (1995) 'Functional deficits in autistic disorder: characterization by technetium-99m-HM-PAO and SPECT.' *Journal of Nuclear Medicine*, **36**, 1152–1162.

Müller, R.A., Chugani, D.C., Behen, M.E., Rothermel, R.D., Muzik, O., Chakraborty, P.K., Chugani, H.T. (1998a) 'Impairment of dentato-thalamo-cortical pathway in autistic men: language activation data from positron emission tomography.' *Neuroscience Letters*, **245**, 1–4.

Müller, R.A., Rothermel, R.D., Behen, M.E. *et al.* (1998b) 'Participation of neuronal heterotopia in cognitive processing.' (Abstract) *Neuroimage*, **7**, s495.

Neville, B.G., Harkness, W.F., Cross, J.H., Cass, H.C., Burch, V.C., Lees, J.A., Taylor, D.C. (1997) 'Surgical treatment of severe autistic regression in childhood epilepsy.' *Pediatric Neurology*, **16**, 137–140.

Nowell, M.A., Hackney, D.B., Muraki, A.S., Coleman, M. (1990) 'Varied MR appearance of autism: fifty-three pediatric patients with the full autistic syndrome.' *Magnetic Resonance Imaging*, **8**, 811–816.

Ozbayrak, K.R., Kapucu, O., Erdem, E., Aras, T. (1991) 'Left occipital hypoperfusion in a case with the Asperger syndrome.' *Brain and Development*, **13**, 454–456.

Pascual-Castroviejo, I., Pascual-Pascual, S.I. (1994) 'Bilateral arachnoid cysts, seizures and severe encephalopathy: Case report.' *Neuropediatrics*, **25**, 42–43.

Piven, J., Berthier, M.L., Starkstein, S.E., Nehme, E., Pearlson, G., Folstein, S. (1990) 'Magnetic resonance imaging evidence for a defect of cerebral cortical development in autism.' *American Journal of Psychiatry*, **147**, 734–739.

Piven, J., Nehme, E., Simon, J., Barta, P., Pearlson, G., Folstein, S.E. (1992) 'Magnetic resonance imaging in autism: measurement of the cerebellum, pons, and fourth ventricle.' *Biological Psychiatry*, **31**, 491–504.

Piven, J., Arndt, S., Bailey, J., Havercamp, S., Andreasen, N.C., Palmer, P. (1995) 'An MRI study of brain size in autism.' *American Journal of Psychiatry*, **152**, 1145–1149.

230

Piven, J., Arndt, S., Bailey, J., Andreasen, N. (1996) 'Regional brain enlargement in autism: a magnetic resonance imaging study.' *Journal of the American Academy of Child and Adolescent Psychiatry*, **35**, 530–538.

Piven, J., Saliba, K., Bailey, J., Arndt, S. (1997) 'An MRI study of autism: the cerebellum revisited.' *Neurology*, **49**, 546–551.

Piven, J., Bailey, J., Ranson, B.J., Arndt, S. (1998) 'No difference in hippocampus volume detected on magnetic resonance imaging in autistic individuals.' *Journal of Autism and Developmental Disorders*, **28**, 105–110.

Ritvo, E.R., Freeman, B.J., Scheibel, A.B., Duong, T., Robinson, H., Guthrie, D. (1986) 'Lower Purkinje cell counts in the cerebella of four autistic subjects: initial findings of the UCLA-NSAC autopsy research report.' *American Journal of Psychiatry*, **146**, 862–866.

Rodier, P.M., Ingram, J.L., Tisdale, B., Nelson, S., Romano, J. (1996) 'Embryological origin for autism: developmental anomalies of the cranial nerve motor nuclei.' *Journal of Comparative Neurology*, **370**, 247–261.

Ryu, Y.H., Lee, J.D., Yoon, P.H., Kim, D.I., Lee, H.B., Shin, Y.J. (1999) 'Perfusion impairments in infantile autism on technetium-99m ethyl cysteinate dimer brain single-photon emission tomography: comparison with findings on magnetic resonance imaging.' *European Journal of Nuclear Medicine*, **26**, 253–259.

Schaefer, G.B., Thompson, J.N., Bodensteiner, J.B., McConnell, J.M., Kimberling, W.J., Gay, C.T., Dutton, W.D., Hutchings, D.C., Gray, S.B. (1996) 'Hypoplasia of the cerebellar vermis in neurogenetic syndromes.' *Annals of Neurology*, **39**, 382–385.

Schain, R., Yannet, H. (1960) 'Infantile autism: an analysis of 50 cases and a consideration of certain relevant neuropsychological concepts.' *Journal of Pediatrics*, **57**, 560–567.

Schifter, T., Hoffman, J.M., Hatten, H.P. Jr., Hanson, M.W., Coleman, R.E., DeLong, G.R. (1994) 'Neuroimaging in infantile autism.' *Journal of Child Neurology*, **9**, 155–161.

Segawa, M., Nomura, Y., Nagata, E., Hata, K., Saitoch, S. (1986) 'Autism with middle fossa arachnoid cyst.' *Journal of Child Neurology*, **1**, 276.

Siegel, B.V., Jr., Asarnow, R., Tanguay, P., Call, J.D., Abel, L., Ho, A., Lott, I., Buchsbaum, M.S. (1992) 'Regional cerebral glucose metabolism and attention in adults with a history of childhood autism.' *Journal of Neuropsychiatry and Clinical Neuroscience*, **4**, 406–414.

Siegel, B.V., Jr., Nuechterlein, K.H., Abel, L., Wu, J.C., Buchsbaum, M.S. (1995) 'Glucose metabolic correlates of continuous performance test performance in adults with a history of infantile autism, schizophrenia, and controls.' *Schizophrenia Research*, **17**, 85–94.

Skjeldal, O.H., Sponheim, E., Ganes, T., Jellum, E., Bakke, S. (1998) 'Childhood autism: the need for physical investigations.' *Brain Development*, **20**, 227–233.

Steffenburg, S. (1991) 'Neuropsychiatric assessment of children with autism: a population-based study.' *Developmental Medicine and Child Neurology*, **33**, 495–511.

Walker, H.A. (1976) 'Incidence of minor physical anomalies in autistic patients.' *In:* Coleman, M. (Ed.) *The Autistic Syndromes.* Amsterdam: North-Holland.

Williams, R.S., Hauser, S.L., Purpura, D.P., DeLong, G.R., Swisher, C.N. (1980) 'Autism and mental retardation. Neuropathological studies performed in four retarded persons with autistic behavior.' *Archives of Neurology*, **37**, 749–753.

Woodhouse, W., Bailey, A., Rutter, M., Bolton, P., Baird, G., Le Couteur, A. (1996) 'Head circumference in autism and other pervasive developmental disorders.' *Journal of Child Psychology and Psychiatry*, 37: 665–671.

Zilbovicius, M., Garreau, B., Tzourio, N., Mazoyer, B., Bruck, B., Martinot, J.L., Raynaud, C., Samson, Y., Syrota, A., Lelord, G. (1992) 'Regional blood flow in autism: a SPECT study.' *American Journal of Psychiatry*, **149**, 924–930.

Zilbovicius, M., Garreau, B., Samson, Y., Remy, P., Barthelemy, C., Syrota, A., Lelord, G. (1995) 'Delayed maturation of the frontal cortex in childhood autism.' *American Journal of Psychiatry*, **152**, 248–252.

231

15
THE GENETICS OF AUTISM

There is a consensus developing that the autistic spectrum of disease groupings – which includes autism (Bailey *et al*. 1995), PPD (Szatmari *et al*. 1998) and Asperger syndrome (Volkmar *et al*. 1998) – is composed mainly of underlying diseases that have a strong genetic component. There is a good review of the subject by Szatmari *et al*. (1998). Of course, this generalization cannot be definitely proven until, at some future time, most patients with an autistic syndrome have a specific diagnosis. The ability to give specific diagnoses to patients with autism involves a great deal of medical knowledge of rare diseases and access to modern laboratory facilities. As Swillen *et al*. (1996) wrote, "Although family and twin studies have shown that hereditary factors play a role in autism, clinicians should not only rely on these epidemiological findings" but actually work the patients up.

As medical science moves forward, it is highly likely that the disease entities discussed in Chapters 10 and 11 will be – or have already been – shown to have a genetic component, with the exception of the infectious and toxic etiologies. In many of these disorders, Mendelian genetics (autosomal dominant, autosomal recessive, sex-linked recessive) have been established. In some of the disease entities, a "double hit" hypothesis has been postulated, where the inherited allele is only expressed if a second somatic mutation occurs. Also, the new genetics as revealed by molecular biology (disorders of trinucleotide repeats, imprinting or mitochondrial DNA) have been demonstrated in some of the patients with autism. Regarding the remainder of the patients, who have no specific diagnosis as yet, a polygenic inheritance model has been put forward by some investigators. This theoretically might involve up to six genes acting in concert and has been proposed as one explanation for some of the findings of the twin, sib-pair and family, broader phenotype studies discussed below.

Family studies have shown that the frequency of autism among siblings of probands with autism is between 2 and 5 per cent, *i.e.* 20–60 times more frequent than in the general population. The high concordance of monozygotic twins with autism was initially identified by Rimland (1964). He reported 11 pairs of monozygotic twins who were concordant, and discussed the implications. Comparing the identical twins with autism to identical-twin studies in schizophrenia, he concluded "the genetic element in autism would appear to be unusually strong." However, he noted that in several cases of identical twins stricken with autism, the degree of affliction, while invariably severe, was not quite identical, raising the question of modifying factors. He also reported two sets of fraternal twins, one discordant, the other set concordant.

Later twin studies have also shown that monozygotic concordance rates exceed the dizygotic concordance rate (Folstein and Rutter 1977, Ritvo *et al*. 1985, Steffenburg *et al*.

1989). When the first British twin sample was combined with a newer British sample, the results of the combined sample showed 60 per cent concordance for 25 pairs of monozygotic twins and no concordance for 20 pairs of dizygotic twins (Bailey *et al.* 1995). The authors report that this finding gives rise to an estimate of heritability of 91 to 93 per cent. When a broader spectrum of related cognitive and social abnormalities was applied to the same combined sample, 92 per cent of the monozygotic twins were concordant versus 10 per cent of the dizygotic twins. According to Szatmari *et al.* (1996), siblings with autism and PDD from the same family also tend to have a high correlation of IQ and social behaviors

The findings of the study by Bailey *et al.* (1995) are that there is no correlation at all for autism among dizygotic twins, and that there is very little correlation in the dizygotic twin of an autistic proband with the broader spectrum related to social abnormalities. On the other hand, some studies of multiple-incidence (multiplex) families suggest that the genetic liability for autism may be expressed in some of the non-autistic relatives in a phenotype that is milder but qualitatively similar to the symptoms of autism (Le Couteur *et al.* 1996, Bailey *et al.* 1998). The broader phenotype, which includes milder social and language based cognitive deficits, appears to be inherited. A British family study found that 20 per cent of first-degree relatives were affected with autism or with milder social and/or cognitive disorders (Bolton *et al.* 1994). A study of siblings of children with autism in multiplex families found significant evidence of social impairment in the expression and understanding of facial expressions of emotion, and increased behaviors related to rituals and repetitive play (Spiker *et al.* 1994). In the study of the relatives of disabled probands by Piven *et al.* (1997), 25 multiple-incidence autism families were compared with 30 Down syndrome families. These authors evaluated social and communication deficits as well as stereotyped behavior and found higher rates in the relatives of probands with autism. Lower performance of verbal skills was reported for brothers of autistic females by Plumet *et al.* (1995) when they were compared to the siblings of Down syndrome females.

No longer is autism thought of as a single disease; it is now clear that it has a multifactorial etiology. Those studying the genetic form of autism concede that more than one gene appears to be involved (De Braekeleer *et al.* 1996). These reports agree that several genes may be involved (Maestrini *et al.* 1998), or that 3–4 loci may be involved, with up to 10 loci (Pickles *et al.* 1995), or 15 loci (Risch *et al.* 1999) possible. Many different forms of genetic transmission have now been documented in patients with autism. Some of the family trees presented in the literature as having autosomal dominant inheritance actually demonstrate strict matrilineal transmission, raising the question of a disorder of mitochondrial DNA. For the record, Hallmayer *et al.* (1996b) have documented six families that have male-to-male transmission.

More and more disease entities are being found that do not strictly fit Mendelian models of inheritance. The discovery that expanding trinucleotide repeats are a form of mutation is a radical departure from the traditional genetic principles of inheritance based on stable transmission of DNA sequences. The concept that a gene may be altered from tissue to tissue in a single individual, or from one generation to the next, and that it may confer increasing mutability on itself has provided insight into the clinical phenomenon of anticipation as manifested by increasing severity, declining age of onset and increasing penetrance in certain inherited disorders. Autism, as a disorder of infancy, can be an expression of anticipation in a family if that family has older members with neuro-psychiatric disease. So far, research appears to have shown that disorders of trinucleotide repeat expansion have two consistent features – neuropsychiatric symptoms and the phenomenon of genetic anticipation. One of the double syndromes (see Chapter 11), the fragile X syndrome, has been shown to be a trinucleotide repeat disease entity.

Other fragile sites are reported in some patients with autism. With the exception of fragile X, the meaning of fragile sites on chromosomes is not established at the time of writing, and the significance, if any, to autistic symptoms remains unknown. (See the discussion of the fragile X syndrome in this chapter for the meaning of a fragile site in that syndrome.) In a study of Basque children with autism, a statistically significant increase of autosomal folate-sensitive fragile sites was found, compared to a control sample (Arrieta *et al.* 1996). They found three fragile sites (2q13, 6p23, 12q13), expressed only in individuals with autism, in their series. However many fragile sites are commonly seen in the laboratory and can be induced in normal individuals. When fragile sites on the chromosomes of patients with the autistic syndrome are listed in this chapter, their meaning is considered unknown and they are mentioned for the sake of completeness. A study of fragile sites in 104 people with autism in Taiwan compared to normal individuals found no difference in frequency (Li *et al.* 1993).

Chromosomal translocations are rare among children with the autistic syndrome; only a few have been described. Because translocations pinpoint exact areas of a chromosome where genes may be located, they are an important tool in genetic analysis. Balanced translocations are not usually symptomatic but studies have shown that there is some risk (Fryns *et al.* 1986). Possible putative mechanisms that might make a balanced trans-location symptomatic are a minimal loss of genetic material or a subdivision of a genetic site disrupting the function of that gene product.

In this chapter, under each chromosome, there are two sections. One lists the actual chromosome aberrations found in patients with autism. They were usually identified in the peripheral blood lymphocytes. The second section describes molecular biological studies. These include areas screened in looking for candidate genes as well as the actual genes located. There have been many studies looking at regions of potential susceptibility in genome-wide scans for autism. The International Molecular Genetic Study of Autism Consortium studied 99 families with evidence of a genetic load and regions identified under each of the chromosomes; they reported regions on chromosomes 4, 10, 22 as well as 2q, 7q, 16p, and 19p (IMGSAC 1998). The PARIS group studied 51 multiplex families and found overlapping results on 2q, 7q, 16p and 19p, plus regions on chromosomes 4q, 5p, 6q, 10q, 18q and Xp (Philippe *et al.* 1999). The South Carolina Autism Project of 100 cases identified a ring 7, a deletion of 20p, a pericentric inversion 12 as well as four cases with abnormalities on 15q (Schroer *et al.* 1998). The Johns Hopkins study identified a region on 7q31–33 as well as chromosome 13 (Barrett *et al.* 1999).

The background mutation rate for genes – the rate at which a gene spontaneously mutates – is typically about one in 50,000 to one in 100,000. There are cases in which the gene is more error prone, resulting in a higher frequency of mishaps. This is particularly true in the mitochondrial genes and is also true in a nuclear gene which is uncommonly long in size. The effects of any given mutation on behavior may involve changes at the cellular or molecular level that are several steps removed from their initial point of action. Almost all of the single genes identified to date as responsible for a disease – monogenetic diseases – cause *rare* diseases.

CHROMOSOMES AND GENES: THE AUTOSOMES

Chromosome 1
CHROMOSOMAL ABERRATIONS
Most fetuses with major aberrations of the longer chromosomes do not survive. Chromosome 1 is the longest of all. Terminal deletions of the long arm – del (1q) – cause a characteristic combination of minor physical anomalies, seizures, severe mental retardation and autistic-like behaviors (Halal *et al.* 1990, Murayama *et al.* 1991). These behaviors include no interest in people, gaze avoidance, muteness, lack of emotionality, "cri-du-chat" shrill cry, Rett-like hand-wringing, autistic-type hand-flapping, and head-shaking. This syndrome has been described in boys and in girls, but possibly with a preponderance in females.

Deletions of the short arm – del (1p) – are very rare. A terminal deletion of 1p35 has been described in a boy who appeared to have a normal infancy (Wenger *et al.* 1988). However, by 30 months of age, language delay, social difficulties and hyperactivity became apparent. After several psychiatric hospital admissions, he was placed in a special classroom for children with autism. At the age of 9 years, his weight increased from the 50th to the 90th percentile in a year.

A boy with DSM-III-R criteria of autism, at the age of 4 years had moderate mental retardation without major dysmorphic features, focal neurological abnormalities or seizures. He was found to have a complex chromosome rearrangement involving trans-location of portions of chromosome 1p22 and 7q on to chromosome 21q (Lopreiato and Wulfsberg 1992). Both parents had normal karyotypes.

Chromosome 2
CHROMOSOMAL ABERRATIONS
A boy with DSM-III-R autism and seizures had a deletion of the long arm of chromosome 2 – del (2q37) – in combination with partial trisomy 6p (with duplications ranging from 6p21 to 6p25). The authors (Burd *et al.* 1988) point out that the trisomy 6p syndrome has not been reported to be associated with autism or seizures, raising a question about the deleted area of the second chromosome. Two additional cases of del (2q37) have recently been reported (Ghaziuddin and Burmeister 1999).

A region on the long arm of chromosome 2 was identified by the IMGSAC and PARIS studies.

A folate-sensitive fragile site at 2q13 has been reported in individuals with autism (Jayakar *et al.* 1986, Arrieta *et al.* 1996) and Asperger syndrome (Saliba and Griffiths 1990). In most cases, the fragile sites were also identified in a parent of the child.

Chromosome 3

CHROMOSOMAL ABERRATIONS

A 17-year-old male with an IQ in the 20–30 range met the DSM-III criteria for autism (Mariner *et al*. 1986). His CARS score was 35.5, indicating moderately severe autism. He was aloof with no eye contact, echolalic speech, severe hyperactivity, a catastrophic reaction to change and a fascination for watches. He also had hypertelorism and skin lesions, including hand scarring from self-biting and scattered lesions that were both hypo- and hyperpigmented, as well as prominent low-set ears, dental malocclusion and pectus excavatum. He had a complicated chromosomal aberration of chromosome 3 – deletion of the p13-14 region, duplication of the p21-24 region, and an inversion of the G positive band material proximal to the centromere; there was also an interstitial deletion on the short arm of chromosome 17. Parental chromosomes were normal. He had some of the symptoms of the Smith–Magenis syndrome, which is associated with the aberration on chromosome 17.

A boy with autistic behavior, severe mental retardation and seizures was found to have a translocation involving the short arm of chromosome 3 and the long arm of chromosome 12 (Fahsold *et al*. 1991). At 9 years of age, adenoma sebaceum began to develop and CT findings of the skull were characteristic for tuberous sclerosis, a known double syndrome. The translocation was: t(3;12)(p26.3;q23.3).

THE GENES (MOLECULAR BIOLOGY)

The translocation case described above apparently did not have either of the known genes for tuberous sclerosis on chromosomes 9 and 16, raising the question of whether there may be a third locus for tuberous sclerosis in 3p26 or 12q23 areas.

Chromosome 4

CHROMOSOMAL ABERRATIONS

A 17-year-old girl who met DSM-III-R criteria, with an IQ measured at 52, was found to have a balanced translocation (4q11;10p5.3) (Pearl and Coleman 1996). She had an overriding fourth toe and the right-wrist area was scarred from self-biting. She had an unusual rote memory for music. She had become severely aggressive at puberty and had compulsive eating and drinking. A region on the long arm of chromosome 4 was identified by the genome-wide scan of autism performed by the PARIS group.

Chromosome 5

CHROMOSOMAL ABERRATIONS

Translocations involving chromosome 5 have been reported in several patients with autism. An unbalanced translocation was reported in a 19-year-old man without dysmorphic features who met criteria for DSM-III-R autistic disorder and ICD-10 for childhood autism (Vostanis *et al*. 1994). The translocation was between the short arm of chromosome 5 and the long arm of the Y chromosome (Yq12). This translocation resulted in monosomy for part of the short arm of chromosome 5 (5pter→5p15.3).

A balanced reciprocal translocation from the long arm of chromosome 5 to the long

236

arm of chromosome 11 was identified in a female with an IQ of 33 who was tested as part of an epidemiological study of autism in the state of Utah (Ritvo *et al.* 1990). Her father also had this translocation.

A boy with DSM-III-R autistic disorder was described (Herder 1993) who had a karyotype involving extra material on the long arm of chromosome 5 (46,XY,5q+). Mariner *et al.* (1986) described a patient with extra chromosomal material on the short arm of chromosome 5 (46,XY,5p+); the facial features were not dysmorphic and the boy had a CARS score of 33 (mild to moderate autism).

A profoundly mentally retarded woman of 43 years, who was reported to meet ICD-10 criteria for childhood autism, was referred for laboratory testing because of her autism. She was found to have an interstitial deletion on the long arm of chromosome 5 – del(5)(q15q22.3) (Barber *et al.* 1994).

A cytogenetic survey of 67 mentally retarded individuals with autistic behaviors in a state institution identified two unrelated men whose chromosomes identified them as having the cri-du-chat syndrome (the 5p- syndrome) (Cantú *et al.* 1990). They had del 5 (p14) and del 5 (p15); this is one of the most common deletion syndromes found in humans. These individuals had not been previously diagnosed or identified as having physical stigmata of enough significance to warrant chromosomal testing; they were included in the survey because of their autistic traits. Autistic symptoms have been described as an early developmental feature of many persons with the cri-du-chat syndrome (Wilkins *et al.* 1983). A region on the short arm of chromosome 5 has been identified by the genome-wide scan of autism performed by the PARIS group.

THE GENES (MOLECULAR BIOLOGY)
In the Barber *et al.* case (1994), where a mentally retarded woman had been referred for testing because of autism, molecular analysis revealed deletions of the MCC (carcinoma coli) and APC (adenomatous polyposis coli) genes, probably located in the 5q22.1 subband. Adenomatous polyposis coli and carcinoma of the rectum, known to be associated with deletions in this subband, were subsequently diagnosed in the patient. The abnormality was inherited from her mother who had an intrachromosomal insertion within the long arm of chromosome 5 and at the age of 75 years had had an adeno-carcinoma of the rectum excised.

Chromosome 6
CHROMOSOMAL ABERRATIONS
More than a dozen patients have been described with partial trisomy 6p; their breakpoint in the duplicated segment ranged from 6p21 to 6p25. A boy who met DSM-III-R criteria for infantile autism with seizures had a partial trisomy 6p with a breakpoint at 6p23; he also had a deletion of 2q37 (Burd *et al.* 1988). His mother had a balanced translocation. None of the other patients with partial trisomy 6p described to date have autism or an associated deletion on another chromosome.

Three children with DSM-III infantile autism (one boy and two girls) and severe mental retardation – two of whom also had a seizure disorder – had a fragile site at 6q26 in a small percentage of examined lymphocytes, together with fragile sites on other chromosomes (Gillberg and Wahlström 1985). One of the girls had been detected in an epidemiological study of autism in Sweden. One case of 6q deletion (del(6)(q25.1q25.3)) has been diagnosed as autistic (Sulumar *et al.* 1999). A region on the long arm of chromosome 6 has been identified in the genome-wide scan of autism performed by the PARIS group (Philippe *et al.* 1999).

THE GENES (MOLECULAR BIOLOGY)
Decreased plasma C4B complement protein levels – resulting from a null allele of the C4B gene located in the middle of the major histocompatibility complex (MHC) – have been reported in a major subset of patients with autism (Warren *et al.* 1994). The C4B null allele has been associated with increased viral and bacterial infections. Since the C4B null allele is known to be part of the ancestral haplotype (B44-SC30-DR4), the extended haplotype was investigated in 45 patients with autism and found to be represented in 40 per cent of the patients and/or their mothers, while in only 2 per cent of controls (Daniels *et al.* 1995). Taking this a step further, Warren and Singh (1996) compared serum serotonin levels in patients with and without MHC and found a positive relationship of the complex to elevated levels of serotonin.

Chromosome 7
CHROMOSOMAL ABERRATIONS
Twins with autism and mental retardation associated with a balanced (7;20) translocation have been described by a Spanish group (de la Barra *et al.* 1986).

A boy with DSM-III-R autistic disorder was demonstrated to have a deletion and an inversion on the short arm of chromosome 7 (del(7)(p21), inv(7)(p13p21)) (Herder 1993). A family with two boys with autism inheriting a paracentric inversion in chromosome 7 (inv(7)(q22–q31.2) has been reported (Ashley-Koch *et al.* 1999).

The Danish Cytogenetic Central Register study identified 7q21 as a possible candidate region for autism (Lauritsen *et al.* 1999). A portion of chromosome 7q was included in the complicated karyotype of the Lopreiato and Wulfsberg (1992) case described under chromosome 1. A region on chromosome 7q has been identified by the IMGSAC and PARIS studies, and the South Carolina Autism Project found a ring 7. The same susceptibility locus 7q31–33 was also identified by the Johns Hopkins team (Barrett *et al.* 1999).

Chromosome 8
CHROMOSOMAL ABERRATIONS
Most individuals reported in the literature with a chromosomal 8 error are mosaics; they have a 46/47 + 8 (normal/trisomy 8) mosaicism. A partial trisomy of the distal tip of chromosome 8 and a probable partial deletion of the middle of the short arm of chromosome 8 have been described in a male with autism and an IQ of 36 (Ritvo *et al.* 1990). No evidence of mosaicism is mentioned.

A patient with the diagnosis of PDDNOS was found to have a deletion on the long arm of chromosome 8 (Weidmer-Mikhail *et al.* 1998).

A boy with the Hypomelanosis of Ito and atypical autism/Asperger syndrome had low normal intelligence (Åkefeldt and Gillberg 1991). His karyotype showed several variant cells – one with an 8q-marker chromosome, one with monosomy of chromosome 8, one with the loss of the Y chromosome, others with monosomy 18 and monosomy 19.

A translocation – t(X;8)(p22.13;q22.1) – has been described in a young adult female with autism diagnosed by DSM-IV and ICD-10 (Bolton *et al.* 1995). Her mother and brother had normal karyotypes. She had multiple exostoses and an IQ of 35. There is no comment one way or the other regarding the possibility of steatorrhea in this patient. Clinically she did not resemble Cohen syndrome – one of the double syndromes mapped to 8q22–q23 – nor any known X chromosome syndrome. The molecular biology in this case is discussed below.

THE GENES (MOLECULAR BIOLOGY)
In the patient with the X;8 translocation described above, the translocation breakpoint was isolated and confirmed to be reciprocal within a 5'-GGCA-3' sequence found on both X and 8 chromosomes without gain or loss of a single nucleotide (Ishikawa-Brush *et al.* 1997). The breakpoint on chromosome 8 occurred approximately 30 kb distal to the 3' end of the syndecan-2 (SDC2) gene. The translocation breakpoint on the X chromosome occurred in the first intron of the gastrin-releasing peptide receptor (GRPR) gene. The gene was shown to have escaped X-inactivation. The gene GRPR exhibits a wide range of activities, including regulation of gastrointestinal hormone release and growth regulation in various tissues. Because the patient is autistic, it is of interest that the gene is expressed in the limbic system of the brain and is involved in neural activity. The orientation of these two genes with respect to the translocation was incompatible with the formation of a fusion gene, making these genes potential candidate genes. To date, the GRPR locus has been checked in 37 individuals with Rett syndrome with negative results (Heidary *et al.* 1998). To our knowledge, it has not been checked in a patient with the autism/steatorrhea syndrome.

Chromosome 9
CHROMOSOMAL ABERRATIONS
A deletion in the short arm of chromosome 9 (9p-) has been described in a male with autism with an IQ of 60 (Ritvo *et al.* 1990).

A balanced translocation of material from the long arm of chromosome 9 and the long arm of chromosome 17 has been described in a boy with autism who inherited the translocation from his phenotypically normal father (Ho and Kalousek 1989). The actual translocation is: t(9;17)(q12;q21).

Autism is a common behavioral feature of tuberous sclerosis (see Chapter 11) which has one of its genetic loci on chromosome 9.

THE GENES (MOLECULAR BIOLOGY)
Chromosome 9 has been implicated in the etiology of some cases of tuberous sclerosis with autism (Ritvo *et al.* 1990). Among families with tuberous sclerosis, about half have

been found to carry a gene located at chromosome 9q34 called TSC1 (Fryer *et al.* 1987) (while a gene on chromosome 16p13 called TSC2 is found in most of the other families). About two-thirds of all cases arise as *de novo* mutations, presumably in one of these two genes (Halley 1996). The gene product from TSC1 is called hamartin but its function has not yet been established. It may participate in an evolutionarily conserved pathway of eukaryotic cell-growth regulation (van Slegtenhorst *et al.* 1997). There is evidence that it may behave as a tumor suppressor gene (Smalley 1998).

Chromosome 10
Chromosomal Aberrations
A girl with a balanced translocation (4q11;10p5.3) has been reported (Pearl and Coleman 1996) and is described under chromosome 4. The Danish Cytogenetic Central Register study identified 10q21.2 as a possible candidate region for autism (Lauritsen *et al.* 1999). A region on chromosome 10q has been identified by the PARIS study.

Chromosome 11
Chromosomal Aberrations
A balanced reciprocal translocation from the long arm of chromosome 5 to the long arm of chromosome 11 has been described in a female with autism (Ritvo *et al.* 1990). See above, under chromosome 5, for a fuller description.

The Genes (Molecular Biology)
The short arm of chromosome 11 in the p15.5 area has become an area of interest in autism. In 55 unrelated French children with autism, positive associations were identified at two markers – one localized to the 3' terminus coding sequence of the *c-Harvey-ras* (HRAS) gene, and an additional marker on exon 1 (Hérault *et al.* 1995). The products of *ras* genes are involved in the proliferation and differentiation of neural cells. Comings *et al.* (1996) sought to verify this finding by studying the HRAS Msp 1 polymorphism. They confirmed a just significant increase in the prevalence of the >2.1 kb alleles in autism, and also found a significant trend toward higher scores for preselected symptom clusters with obsessive-compulsive and phobic symptoms in >2.1 kb homozygotes. There were negative results with Tourette syndrome.

Chromosome 12
Chromosomal Aberrations
A boy with tuberous sclerosis and autistic behavior has been described with the translocation: t(3;12)(p26.3)(q23.3). The case is discussed above under chromosome 3. A case with autism and a pericentric inversion 12 was reported by the South Carolina Autism Project.

The Genes (Molecular Biology)
In addition to the translocation breakpoint in the child with tuberous sclerosis (see above), the long arm of chromosome 12 also contains the human phenylalanine hydroxylase

(PAH) gene responsible for the metabolic disease phenylketonuria, a double syndrome (see Chapter 11). The PAH gene spans about 90,000 base pairs of DNA and has 13 exons. More than 50 RFLP haplotypes have been reported at the human PAH locus (Woo 1988). There have been 31 different PKU mutations documented and five instances of PKU mutation occurring more than once (Scriver 1991).

Chromosome 13

CHROMOSOMAL ABERRATIONS

Trisomy 13 (Patau syndrome) is a well-described syndrome usually characterized by major malformations in the brain such as arhinencephaly or holoprosencephaly. A boy with an autistic disorder, severe mental retardation, minor physical anomalies, and a cardiac malformation was found to have trisomy 13 (Steffenburg 1991), as was a child in Canada (Konstantareas and Homatidis 1999).

The 13 deletion syndrome (13q-;13r) is also a well-known syndrome, usually with facial dysmorphisms and microcephaly, as well as holoprosencephaly in half the cases. Retinoblastoma is common. A patient with autism and retinoblastoma was found to have a deletion at 13q13; he also had reduced esterase D activity (Ritvo et al. 1988). However, this patient had a second cousin with autism who had normal chromosomes. In a Swedish epidemiological study of autistic disorder, a boy meeting both DSM-III and DSM-III-R criteria for autism was shown to have a deletion of chromosome 13; however, this time it was the short arm (13p-). His father, who had normal chromosomes, was mildly retarded, as was the boy himself (Steffenburg 1991).

Possible susceptibility loci have been identified on chromosome 13 by the Johns Hopkins team (Barrett et al. 1999).

Chromosome 15

THE ROLE OF 15q11–q13

How the genes on the long arm of chromosome 15 in the q11–13 portion relate to autism is a fascinating question. First, there are the cases with deletions or other evidence of silencing in this chromosomal area. A woman with DSM-III-R autistic disorder, "profound" mental retardation and an atypical bipolar disorder (with a positive response to lithium) was found to have a deletion of chromosome 15q12 (Kerbeshian et al. 1990). There is a patient placed in a residential home in Belgium because of an autistic syndrome who had a translocation 46,XY,t(1;15)(p35;q12.33) with one of the breaks on chromosome 15 at q12.33 (Swillen et al. 1996). Sabry and Farag (1998) have reported a micro-deletion in the 15q11–12 region in a patient who met DSM-IV criteria. It is relevant to note that the rearrangements described in these three patients could well encompass regions outside the specific Angelman region. Also, it is known that patients affected in one of the double syndromes, Angelman syndrome (see Chapter 11), have an error in chromosome 15q11–q13. These patients often have autistic characteristics (Steffenburg et al. 1996); it has been found that the gene causing their syndrome (see below) is silenced.

Then there are the cases of too much chromosomal material in the q11–13 section of chromosome 15. There is a patient who met the criteria for autistic disorder who had a complete tetrasomy of chromosome 15 (Weidmer-Mikhail *et al.* 1998). There have been at least 15 other cases of children and adults, reported from five different autism centers, with partial tetrasomy 15q11–q13, meeting stringent criteria for autistic disorder/ childhood autism (Gillberg 1998). Partial trisomies of the same region (15q11–q13) are also reported in patients with autism. The patients with autism and excessive chromosomal material in the q11–13 region have been described by Schinzel (1990), Cantú *et al.* (1990), Gillberg *et al.* (1991), Ghaziuddin *et al.* (1993b), Bakker *et al.* (1994), Bundey *et al.* (1994), Leana-Cox *et al.* (1994), Crolla *et al.* (1995), Hotopf and Bolton (1995), Flejter *et al.* (1996), Cook *et al.* (1997a) and Wang *et al.* (1998). Since all of these studies raised questions about the relationship of excessive chromosomal material of this region to autism, Rineer *et al.* (1998) performed a study of patients identified because they had excess material on the 15th chromosome. They started with 29 children and young adults with a supernumerary isodicentric chromosome 15, and performed standard assessments for autism on this patient group. Molecular studies were not reported. The assessments resulted in 20 of the 29 individuals with "a high probability" of being autistic. Of the remaining 9 children, 8 were under 5 years of age. The chromosomal region duplicated in these cases involves megabase regions, raising the possibility of unknown candidate genes.

The syndrome suffered by individuals with a definite diagnosis of autism and excessive chromosomal material in the 15q11–13 section does not, at this time, appear to be specific enough to be determined by clinical criteria alone. Mental retardation is described as ranging from mild to profound. There are several cases with a seizure disorder. The facial anomalies, if present, appear to be subtle. In the Gillberg *et al.* (1991) series, minor motor epilepsy and spinal deformities were present in several cases.

The region on 15q11–q13 has been identified by the candidate gene studies in autism in the Pericak-Vance *et al.* (1997), Schroer *et al.* 1998 and PARIS studies. (It is probably coincidence, but there is a great deal of interest in schizophrenia research regarding a locus close by at chromosome 15q14 (Leonard *et al.* 1998).)

In summary, the duplication data suggest a locus for autism in proximal 15q but no candidate gene(s) has/have yet been definitely identified.

THE GENES (MOLECULAR BIOLOGY)

Chromosome 15q11–q13 is known to have three subregions: a proximal region containing genes that are expressed from the paternally inherited chromosome only; a central region containing genes expressed from the maternally inherited chromosome only; and a distal region containing genes that are expressed from both alleles (Nicholls 1998). The gene causing the Angelman syndrome may be from the central region and has been identified as UBE3A; it encodes for E6-AP ubiquitin-protein ligase. The malfunction or silencing of this gene can be caused in several different ways. It can be due to a deletion, a point mutation (seen in familial cases), an imprinting mutation or uniparental disomy. Although there are multiple molecular genetic mechanisms that can lead to silencing of the gene, each leads to a common gene deficit which involves the silencing of the maternal allele. Therefore the absence of expression of an active maternal gene leads to the Angelman syndrome. This gene has been found to be preferentially maternally expressed in the human brain and expressed solely from the murine maternal chromosome in the hippocampus and cerebellar Purkinje cells (Albrecht *et al.* 1997), regions implicated in the neuropathology of autism (see Chapter 14).

In the case of the duplicated 15q11–q13 material in individuals meeting strict criteria for autism, molecular biological studies have been performed on the chromosomes of patients described in several of the published studies. In the patients described by Gillberg *et al.* (1991), the research showed that the marker chromosome consisted of an inverted duplication of chromosome 15p13q12 and that it originated in the maternal meiotic process rather than in an early mitosis in the developmental process of the embryo (Martinsson *et al.* 1996). In patients described by Ghaziuddin *et al.* (1993b), the marker chromosome involved duplication of chromosome 15, which extended at least into the band 15q13. Flejter *et al.* (1996) investigated two patients with inv dup(15) chromosomes. Cook *et al.* (1997b) reported an intrachromosomal duplication of proximal 15q present in a phenotypically normal mother and inherited by the two of her children who had autism or atypical autism. The duplication is thought to have arisen *de novo* from the mother's paternal chromosome 15. The patients described by Wang *et al.* (1998) had either isodicentric duplications of chromosome 15q13–pter or extra chromosomal 15q13–pter arising from a maternal 4/15 balance translocation. All of these molecular studies demonstrated that the extra chromosomal material was maternally derived. Haplotype analysis is reported to have identified a meiotic recombination hot spot in the q11–13 region on the maternal chromosome (Wang *et al.* 1998). A Schroer *et al.* (1998) case also had a maternally derived aberration of chromosome 15q. Based on these preliminary results, it appears that the presence of extra dosages of maternal genes located in the 15q11–13 region has the distinct possibility of being involved in the expression of autistic behavior.

In 138 families, a linkage-disequilibrium mapping of autistic disorder with 15q11–13 markers turned up GABRB3 or genes adjacent to it as candidate genes for further investigation; in this study no evidence was found for parent-of-origin effects on allelic transmission (Cook *et al.* 1998). However, two studies focused on the GABRB3 gene in 139 (Salmon *et al.* 1999) and 94 (Maestrini *et al.* 1999) autism muliplex families were negative. A patient with non-specific retardation and partial agenesis of the corpus callosum has been found to have two copies of the paternal allele and one copy of the maternal allele in an interstitial duplication of proximal 15q involving the Angelman syndrome region (Mohandas *et al.* 1999).

Chromosome 16
CHROMOSOMAL ABERRATIONS

Partial trisomy of chromosome 16p (with a breakpoint at 16p13.1) has been found in a 14-year-old boy who was mildly dysmorphic and had an IQ of about 80 (Hebebrand *et al.* 1994). This patient met the criteria for both DSM-III-R and Tourette disorder. His parents had normal chromosomes.

A 4-year-old boy with autistic-like behavior was found to have a deletion on the long

243

arm of chromosome 16 (16q23.1) (Monaghan *et al.* 1997). His autism, bilateral cataracts and iris coloboma had not been previously reported in patients with 16q deletions. His hypotonia, psychomotor retardation, high forehead, hypertelorism, upward slanting palpebral fissures, low-set abnormally modeled ears, and talipes equinovarus are known aspects of the 16q- syndrome.

A woman who was diagnosed as autistic by a psychiatrist at the age of 10 years, and received a diagnosis of DSM-III criteria for infantile autism, residual state, at 26 years, was found to have an aberration of chromosome 16 (Mariner *et al.* 1986). She had mild dysmorphic features including relative macrocephaly and an IQ of 50. Her chromosomes showed an inversion/duplication of chromosome 16q13-22; her parents' chromosomes were normal.

In a Swedish epidemiological study of chromosomes in DSM-III infantile autism, 12 per cent of the children had fragile sites at 16q23 in a few per cent of their lymphocytes (Gillberg and Wahlström 1985). Since this is one of the most common fragile sites seen in any population, the meaning of this finding is unclear. However, as the authors point out, the fact that two of the affected boys were first cousins implies that the finding cannot be summarily dismissed as unimportant.

Autism is a common behavioral feature of tuberous sclerosis (see Chapter 11) and has one of its genetic loci on chromosome 16.

THE GENES (MOLECULAR BIOLOGY)
In about half of the families with tuberous sclerosis, the gene (TSC2) associated with the disease is located on the short arm of the 16th chromosome at 16p13. The TSC2 gene was identified in 1993 and shown to code for a protein product, tuberin, which is thought to function as a GTPase activating protein (GAP) (European Chromosome 16 Tuberous Sclerosis Consortium 1993). GAP proteins are a class of proteins that determine the on–off state of the GTPases (GAPs) – a function which serves to negatively regulate GTPase activity – which is important in cell growth and differentiation. TSC2 encodes a 5.5kb transcript that has a region of sequence homology with GTPase-activating proteins, known to regulate rap1GAP. Rap1GAP is a protein that can induce DNA synthesis – thus tuberin is suspected to play an important role in neuronal migration, differentiation and/or development (Smalley 1998). Although exactly how disruption in tuberin function leads to hamartomas, hamartias and neoplasms is unknown, investigations suggest that tuberin (and hamartin, the product of TSC1) may behave as tumor suppressor genes.

An area on the short arm of chromosome 16 near the telomere was identified in the IMGSAC and PARIS studies. This area was the second most significant in the IMGSAC study.

Chromosome 17
CHROMOSOMAL ABERRATIONS
In a chromosomal study of children with autism, searching for the fragile X syndrome, a boy was located who had a balanced translocation (9;17)(q12;q21) which he had inherited from a phenotypically normal father (Ho and Kalousek 1989). A 10-year-old boy with

Asperger syndrome and presumed normal intelligence had a balanced *de novo* trans-location: t(17;19)(p13.3;p11) (Anneren *et al.* 1995).

Two double syndromes, neurofibromatosis type 1 and the Smith–Magenis syndrome, both have loci on chromosome 17 (see Chapter 11 for a description of the syndromes and the cases with autism). In the case of neurofibromatosis type 1, the gene is located on the long arm at q11.2. The Smith–Magenis syndrome has been found to have an interstitial deletion on the short arm of the chromosome at p11.2.

Trisomy 17 has never been reported in a live birth to date. There has been a case of a boy with trisomy 17 mosaicism – with blood lymphocytes normal but up to 80 per cent of the cells in skin fibroblast culture with trisomy 17. The child was said to be autistic-like but the clinical description in the published paper is too brief to be sure that criteria for autism were met. The patient had mental and growth retardation, seizures, microcephaly, minor anomalies, hearing loss and increased pain tolerance (Shaffer *et al.* 1996).

THE GENES (MOLECULAR BIOLOGY)

The gene for neurofibromatosis type 1, is called the NF1 gene; it is located at 17q11.2. Deletions, insertions, base substitutions and splice site mutations in the NF1 gene have been described in a number of cases. No one hot spot for mutations on the gene has yet been identified. The majority of mutations result in a truncated and presumably non-functional protein. The NF1 gene encodes for a protein of 2818 amino acids called neurofibromin, whose sequence homology suggests that it is a member of the GTPase-activating protein (GAP) family. Thus it appears that neurofibromin may suppress tumor formation in normal cells by a complex mechanism. There is evidence that inappropriately high levels of NF1 mRNA editing play a role in NF1 tumorigenesis (Cappione *et al.* 1997).

The Smith–Magenis syndrome is caused by an interstitial deletion of chromosome 17p11.2. Molecular evaluation strongly suggests that it is a contiguous gene syndrome. To date there have been 12 genes localized to that region of the interstitial deletion (Smith *et al.* 1998).

In the case of trisomy 17 mosaicism discussed by Shaffer *et al.* (1996), molecular analysis using 13 highly polymorphic markers spanning the length of chromosome 17 demonstrated the extra chromosome 17 in the skin to be of a parental origin. Three alleles were never seen in the trisomic cell line, suggesting that the extra chromosome arose through a mitotic duplication error after conception (a somatic error). Uniparental disomy was excluded in the euploid blood sample.

The human serotonin transporter gene on chromosome 17 has polymorphic sites in the gene which have been associated with mood disorders, anxiety-related personality traits and late-onset Alzheimer's disease, although some non-replications have been reported. A recent candidate gene study revealed evidence of an association between autistic disorder and a variant of the promoter region of the human serotonin transporter gene (HTT) in 86 trios consisting of the patient and both parents (Cook *et al.* 1997b). The polymorphism in the promoter region of the gene (SLC6A4) encoding this protein was reported to affect protein expression.

This work may have implications for the development of treatments in autism. The serotonin transporter is a prime target for drugs called selective serotonin reuptake inhibitors (SSRIs) which are under investigation for therapeutic use in autism (see Chapter 17). There is already a study reporting that the efficacy of fluvoxamine, one of the SSRIs under investigation in autism, appears to be related to allelic variation within the promoter region in adult patients with delusional depression (Smeraldi *et al.* 1998).

Chromosome 18

CHROMOSOMAL ABERRATIONS

The long arm of chromosome 18 – particularly in the 18q21.1–18q21.2 area – has had deletions reported in a number of children with autism. In 1989, a boy with an interstitial deletion of 18(q12.1–q21.1) in his lymphocytes was reported (Wilson and Al Saadi 1989). The boy had autistic tendencies and developed obesity at 3 years of age. Deletions on the long arm of chromosome 18 at an almost identical site were found in two unrelated moderately retarded children with some autistic tendencies (Poissonnier *et al.* 1992). A boy of 2 years 8 months who was completely non-verbal met DSM-III-R criteria for PDD of the autistic disorder subtype. He was not dysmorphic but had a deletion of chromosome 18 – 18(pter→21.2) (Seshadri *et al.* 1992). László *et al.* (1994) have reported a 16-year-old patient who met DSM-III criteria and had 18q deletion; this retarded patient also had hyperuricemia. In a review of 27 patients with 18q deletion syndromes (with breakpoints ranging from 18q21.2 through 18q22.3), Mahr *et al.* (1996) found one additional individual who met the criteria for childhood autism. If it turns out that there is a specific locus for autistic symptoms on the long arm, finer tuning is needed to identify the exact site. The 18q deletion syndrome is an established syndrome with many dysmorphic features but what is striking about these 18q deletion patients who also have autistic features is the relative lack of stigmata. A region of chromosome 18q was identified in the IMGSAC and PARIS studies.

Mosaic patterns involving chromosome 18 and autism have been described. A deletion of the short arm of chromosome 18 – 18p11.3 – was found in about 50 per cent of the examined cells from peripheral blood in a mildly obese girl with DSM-III-R autistic disorder and moderate mental retardation. In another cell-line in the girl, comprising about 50 per cent of the cells, a duplication of the long arm of chromosome 18 was reported (Ghaziuddin *et al.* 1993a). Ring chromosome 18 mosaicism associated with severe autistic behavior and mental retardation has been reported in a 2-year-old boy (50 per cent/50 per cent) and a 37-year-old woman (75 per cent/25 per cent) (Fryns and Kleczkowska 1992). Both patients had an almost normal physical phenotype.

Chromosome 19

THE GENES (MOLECULAR BIOLOGY)

Dynamic expansion of the CTG trinucleotide repeat sequence in the gene-dense region on chromosome 19q3.3 causes myotonic dsytrophy; one case had autism and two such cases have been found to have Asperger syndrome (see Chapter 11). A region on 19q was identified in both the IMGSAC and PARIS studies.

Chromosome 20

A boy with autism and Hirschsprung disease was found to have an interstitial deletion of chromosome 20 (p11.22–p11.23) (Michaelis *et al.* 1997). His parents had normal chromosomes; the deleted chromosome of the child was maternally derived. See below for a discussion of plausible genes in this case.

A mute 3-year-old boy who met 10 criteria of an autistic condition (DSM-IV) has been found to have a 20/22 translocation and an interstitial deletion within the 22q11 region (Carratala *et al.* 1998). His chromosomes were 45,XY,-22,+der(20),t(20;22)(q13.3;q11.2). This boy had none of the symptoms of the DiGeorge syndrome usually seen with 22q11 deletions. He had mildly dysmorphic facies, pectum excavatum and a short thumb.

A deletion of 20p has been found by the South Carolina Autism Project in a single case.

THE GENES (MOLECULAR BIOLOGY)

In the patient described by Michaelis *et al.* (1997), with an interstitial deletion of 20p11.22–p11.23, microsatellite analysis showed a deletion involving a 5-6 cM region from the maternally derived chromosome 20. The deleted region is proximal to, and does not overlap, the recently characterized Alagille syndrome region. The deleted region is known to contain three genes that could plausibly contribute to abnormal neural development in a fetus. They are: SSTR4, most likely involved in signal transduction in neurons that receive somatostatinergic input; ZNF133, a zinc-finger gene which encodes a transcription regulator that could influence neural development; and the gene that encodes the brain-specific form of glycogen phosphorylase.

Chromosome 21

Trisomy of part of the 21st chromosome is the etiology of Down syndrome. In most patients with the syndrome, there is full trisomy of the entire 21st chromosome. A small group of patients have a mixture of two types of cells in their bodies – trisomy 21 with 47 chromosomes and the usual cell number of 46 chromosomes; they are called mosaics. Translocations and ring chromosomes have also been found in patients with Down syndrome; they always involve the 21st chromosome. In several large series of patients with autism, 2 per cent also had Down syndrome (Ritvo *et al.*1990, Collacott *et al.*1992). However, as discussed in Chapter 11, there is little hard evidence that children with Down syndrome are more prone to autism than other forms of mental handicap. Because of the high frequency of both Down syndrome and the autistic syndrome, there is inevitable overlap in some persons, which it is likely is a major factor in the many double syndrome cases reported. There are so many cases reported that Down syndrome/autism is now classified as a double syndrome with its own specialized preventive medicine work-ups and educational programming for these children (see Chapter 11).

A child with autistic behaviors but without Down syndrome was found to be mosiac 46XX/47XX + mar21 (Sun *et al.* 1995). The marker chromosome was a ring-like structure deriving from chromosome 21. She had mental retardation and short stature.

The long arm of chromosome 21 is responsible for the many recognizable features of Down syndrome, and genes have been identified, particularly in the 21q22 band, that contribute to the syndrome. However, the relevance of any of this molecular biological work to patients with the double syndrome of Down syndrome/autism remains far from clear.

In the case reported by Sun *et al.* (1995), molecular biological techniques were used to identify the marker chromosome as material from the 21st chromosome.

Chromosome 22

Chromosomal Aberrations

There appear to have been cases of trisomy 22 associated with autism in the medical literature in the 1960s, although at the early technological stage that they were described it is not entirely clear that the chromosomes were actually chromosome 22 (Turner and Jennings 1961, Biesele *et al.* 1962). There has been a case of a female patient with autism and a translocation between chromosome 22 and a chromosome characterized at that state of technology as belonging to the "D group" (13,14,15) (Hansen *et al.* 1977).

Since modern techniques have become available, a retarded boy of 13 years who met DSM-IV criteria for the autistic syndrome was found to have a ring chromosome 22 – 46,XY,r22 (Assumpcão 1998), as was an 11-year-old boy (MacLean *et al.* 2000). There is also a family described with a chromosomal variation – elongation of the short arm of chromosome 22 (Wilcox 1998). The proband and a cousin had a full autistic syndrome; other family members had asocial behavior, isolation and toe-walking. Only the affected family members had the chromosomal elongation. The deletion at 22q11.21, the identified site for the velocardiofacial syndrome, has been reported in two children with PDDNOS (Eliez *et al.*, in press).

One form of purine autism involves an inborn error of adenylosuccinate lyase (see Chapter 10). The gene for adenylosuccinate lyase has been mapped to chromosome 22q13.1→q13.2 (Fon *et al.* 1993). A region on chromosome 22p was identified by the IMGSAC study.

THE GONOSOMES (THE SEX CHROMOSOMES)

X chromosome

Chromosomal Aberrations

The fragile X syndrome – a double syndrome with a chromosomal abnormality on the long arm of the X chromosome – is discussed in Chapter 11. In 1969, Lubs described a chromosomal abnormality in the form of a constriction close to the distal end of the long arm of the X chromosome in afflicted males and in obligate female carriers. It was found that the fragile site was at q27.3. In 1977, Sutherland formulated the laboratory culture conditions, involving the depletion of folate, in which the fragile X karyotype could be cultivated in the leukocytes of carriers. For a description of the molecular biology of the fragile X syndrome, see below.

Regarding the short arm of the X chromosome, there is a report of a 3-year-old boy who was diagnosed with a severe autistic disorder and severe mental retardation, who had a terminal Xp duplication (Rao *et al.* 1994). The final karyotype was 46,dir dup(X)(pter→p22.3::p22.3→p22.2::p22.3→qter),Y. The chromosomal aberration was inherited from his mother; the clinical description is not detailed enough to decide how many specific criteria for autism were met. There is a young adult woman with autism who has a translocation involving Xp22. Her karyotype is t(X;8)(p22.13;q22.1); her case is discussed under chromosome 8. Small deletions of the short arm of the X chromosome have been reported in three females with the features of autism; they were part of a larger group of eight females with Xp deletions (Thomas *et al.* 1999). This study suggested that a critical region for autism in females with Xp deletion may lie between the pseudo-autosomal boundary and DXS7103. A fragile site at Xp22 has been reported to be common in Rett syndrome and in autism (Gillberg *et al.* 1984a). A region on chromosome Xp was identified in the PARIS study (Philippe *et al.* 1999).

On the long arm of the X chromosome, in the Xq28 region, the gene for Rett syndrome – MECP2 – has been identified (see Chapter 11).

Regarding extra X chromosomes, most of the well-established aneuploidy syndromes have been reported to be sometimes associated with the full syndrome of autism. The Klinefelter syndrome (47,XXY) is one of the most common syndromes; therefore, it is not known if the cases of autism described with this syndrome (Hagerman 1989, Konstantareas and Homatidis 1999) occurred by chance. One case of autism and the XXX syndrome has been reported from a study in which 25 individuals with autism were screened for chromosomal aberrations (Wolraich *et al.* 1970).

A missing X chromosome, seen in Turner syndrome, is not usually associated with major psychiatric disorder in childhood. However, there was one case of 45,X described in 1995 by Lewis *et al.*, a woman with DSM-III autism and mental retardation was identified in a cytogenetic survey of a large psychiatric in-patient clientele. Five individuals with a ring X chromosome have been described as having "autistic-like features" (El Abd *et al.* 1999). A mosaic case (45,X/46,XX) has also been reported in an autistic individual with the Hypomelanosis of Ito (Åkefeldt and Gillberg 1991). Two cases of autism were reported in a series of 27 cases of 45X/46,XY mosaicism (Telvi *et al.* 1999). In Noonan syndrome, a partial clinical mimic of Turner syndrome, patients have been described with autism (see Chapter 11).

THE GENES (MOLECULAR BIOLOGY)

Fragile sites on the X chromosome

The fragile X syndrome is one of the developmental disorders where the pathogenesis from gene to behavioral manifestations is best understood. It does not follow classical Mendelian genetics but is part of the new and growing understanding of diseases related to trinucleotide repeats. In 1991, FMR1, the mutated gene responsible for the fragile X karyotype and its clinical manifestations, was located and identified by Verkerk *et al.* (1991). Its site is called FRAXA. The most common mutation resulting in the fragile X syndrome consists of an expansion of the number of cytosine-guanine-guanine (CGG) trinucleotide repeats within the promoter region of the FMR1 gene. In the normal FMR1 gene, the number of CGG repeats at the critical site varies between 5 and 52. In certain susceptible individuals, the number of CGG repeats increases to a range of approximately 52–200. This increased number is often referred to as a "premutation." Both the normal and premutation forms of the FMR1 gene are functionally effective in transcribing messenger RNA and producing FMRP, the protein product of the gene.

However the premutation is meiotically and mitotically unstable, particularly in female carriers, and is prone to yet further expansion to even larger numbers of CGG repeats in their children, both boys and girls. When the number of repeats goes over about 200, and the gene becomes partially or completely inactive in producing FMRP, then the FMR1 gene is designated as a "full mutation." There may be between 230 and 4000 CGG repeats. The mechanism of inactivation is not fully understood but there appear to be additional factors besides just the absolute number of repeats (Hagerman *et al.* 1994). Also, sometimes, the degree of CGG repeat expansion may vary from one cell to another in the offspring. This mosaic pattern can result in cases where some of the child's cells carry the fully mutated FMR1 allele while other cells in the same child carry the premutation.

In general, over succeeding generations there is an increase in the expansion of the CGG repeat sequences through female carriers toward the full mutation, resulting in pedigrees with increasing frequency and severity of the fragile X syndrome (Feinstein and Reiss 1998). This is the phenomenon of *genetic anticipation*.

The expanded CGG repeats have different effects in boys and girls. In boys who have the full mutation, since they have only one X chromosome, they suffer an inevitable full or partial (if they are mosaic) failure to produce FMRP. Thus they have the clinical fragile X syndrome. Girls with the fragile X syndrome have a back-up system of two X chromosomes; one of their X chromosomes may have the FMR1 mutation while there may be a normal FMR1 allele in the other chromosome. Thus their symptoms tend to be more variable and generally less severe. An interesting study by Mazzocco *et al.* (1997) found that variations in the degree of FMRP reduction in females with the fragile X syndrome correlated with decreases in the size of lobules VI and VII of the posterior cerebellar vermis, and increased scores of deviance in stereotypic and restricted repertoires of behavior.

The emerging evidence that FMR1 plays a role in cytoplasmic mRNA metabolism, possibly in control of translation, is somewhat at odds with the pathophysiology of fragile X syndrome. The disorder has profound consequences on the brain, yet few structural abnormalities are found. It might be expected that loss of a protein involved in a fundamental process such as translational control would lead to much more widespread anomalies. It may be that for most tissues redundancy of function is provided by other similar proteins. A knockout model of fragile X is similarly mildly affected with subtle learning defects and enlarged testes. It is likely that the brain and the testes are particularly important sites of action of FMRP. The hippocampus and the cerebellum – two brain areas of interest for the fragile X syndrome and the autistic syndrome – appear to have particularly high expression of FMR1.

Other fragile X sites have been found distal to FRAXA, the site of the FMR1 gene responsible for the fragile syndrome. FRAXE and FRAXF, both folate-sensitive, were distinguished from FRAXA only after the development of DNA probes at FRAXA. FRAXF appears to cause no abnormalities in individuals carrying expanded trinucleotide repeats. In the case of FRAXE, a large gene, FMR2, whose expression is reduced by FRAXE expansion has been recently identified; its function has not yet been determined. Although these additional fragile sites have been studied in boys with autism and their mothers, and the triplet repeat numbers were found to be within the normal range in one study (Holden *et al.* 1996), it is still possible that FRAXE may be associated with high-functioning autism (Abrams *et al.* 1997). On the long arm of the X chromosome, between the sites of FRAXE and FRAXF, lies the site of the gene defective in Hunter syndrome.

Two additional autosomal folate-sensitive fragile sites have been characterized at the molecular level. These are FRA16A and FRA11B. Each results from an expansion of a polymorphic CGG repeat sequence with strong similarity to the expansion seen at FRAXA, FRAXE, and FRAXF. FRA16A, like FRAXF, is not known to be associated with pathology in the expanded form. On the other hand, FRA11B appears to predispose to the loss of the terminal portion of 11q in the gametes of carriers of the fragile site. The resulting offspring develop 11q- (the Jacobsen syndrome), a disorder resulting from haploidy for this region of chromosome 11 (11q23→qter).

Markers on the X chromosome
Petit *et al.* (1996) tested several markers on the X chromosome in autistic and control populations by association study. For the DXS287 marker, chi 2 analysis showed a different allele distribution between control and patient groups. Hallmayer *et al.* (1996a) also studied the X chromosome and concluded that in their population "We were able to exclude any moderate or strong gene effect causing autism on the X chromosome." Smaller gene effects could not be excluded – in particular, a gene of small effect located between DXS453 and DSX1001.

It should be noted that one or more loci have been found on the human X chromosome (probably on Xq or close to the centromere on Xp) that influence social cognition (Skuse *et al.* 1997). The imprinted locus is only expressed from a paternally inherited X chromosome, which means that boys do not express it since their only X chromosome comes from their mother. This study has started a discussion about whether imprinting might help explain why boys are more vulnerable to the developmental disorders that affect social behavior, such as autism (Scourfield *et al.* 1997).

Y chromosome
Structural variants of the Y chromosome have been reported. An unbalanced translocation between Yq12 and chromosome 5p15.3 (Vostanis *et al.* 1994) was discussed under chromosome 5. The Y chromosome has been reported to be exceptionally long in several cases of autism (Judd and Mandell 1968; Hoshino *et al.* 1979, Gillberg and Wahlström 1985); the meaning of this finding is unknown in view of the fact that 2 to 3 per cent of all men show considerable variation in the length of the Y chromosome. A 3-year-old with

autism and severe retardation was demonstrated to have a normal X chromosome and an abnormal Y chromosome containing two centromeres (Blackman *et al.* 1991). The abnormality was interpreted as an isochromosome composed of two copies of material from Ypter to Yq11.21; the parents had normal chromosomes.

Regarding supernumerary Y chromosome, the XYY syndrome is a well-studied syndrome. A number of cases of autism/autistic disorder have been found to have the extra Y chromosome (Abrams and Pergament 1971, Mallin and Walker 1972, Nielsen *et al.* 1973, Gillberg *et al.* 1984b, Weidmer-Mikhail *et al.* 1998). In the study by Nielsen *et al.*, poor social-relatedness was reported in 13 of the 21 cases not given the autism diagnosis. Also, there have been some reports of XYY mosaicism in autism (Gillberg and Wahlström 1985) and in Asperger syndrome (Gillberg *et al.* 1987).

MITOCHONDRIAL DISEASES AFFECTING THE RESPIRATORY CHAIN

The mitochondrial encephalomyopathies are a diverse group of disorders that result from structural, biochemical or genetic derangement of mitochondria (DiMauro and Moraes 1993). Mitochondrial DNA represents a well-recognized non-Mendelian genetic system (Johns 1998). Mitochondria are the organelles in the cytoplasm of the cell that generate the energy needed for cellular processes. Over 95 per cent of total brain ATP, the chemical energy of cells, is produced in the mitochondria by the process of oxidative phosphorylation (OXPHOS). The regions of the brain that are the most functionally active, such as the temporal lobe, are sites of increased mitochondrial activity.

Mitochondria are the only animal cellular organelles that contain their own extrachromosomal DNA (distinct from the DNA found in the chromosomes in the nucleus of the cell). Mitochondrial DNA (mtDNA) differs from nuclear DNA in a number of ways: it has a slightly different genetic code and contains very few introns (non-coding sequences). Several unique features of mtDNA compared to nuclear DNA help explain its role in the pathogenesis of disease. Because mtDNA has virtually no introns, any random mutation will usually strike a coding DNA sequence. Also, mtDNA mutates more than 10 times more rapidly than nuclear DNA, it has greater exposure to oxidative stress (it is exposed to oxygen-free radicals generated by OXPHOS), and there is an absence of a protective histone coat. A particularly unfortunate aspect is that mtDNA has no effective repair system for DNA damage. MtDNA is strictly maternally inherited and does not recombine; thus, mitochondrial mutations sequentially accumulate along maternal lineages. Mitochondrial DNA mutations are usually deletions, duplications or maternally inherited point mutations.

Having explained all this, it is necessary to point out that mitochondrial diseases affecting the respiratory chain can also be due to mutations in the nuclear genome, resulting in Mendelian patterns of inheritance. Those due to nuclear mutations can affect genes encoding enzymatic or structural mitochondrial proteins, translocases, mitochondrial protein importation and intergenomic signaling (DiMauro *et al.* 1998). Lombard (1998) has published a medical hypothesis giving the arguments why autism might be a disorder of mitochondrial origin. The presenting signs of known mitochondrial respiratory chain diseases (Jackson *et al.* 1995) include a number that are seen in some individuals with autism. Perhaps the most striking evidence of a disturbance of brain energy metabolism in autism is provided by imaging studies (see Chapter 14). Other suggestive symptoms are patients with a family history of psychiatric dysfunction through maternal transmission, seizures, apparent deafness, ataxia and the laboratory abnormality of lactic acidosis. In a series of children with mitochondrial disorders, a case of autism is reported (Nissenkorn *et al.* 2000).

László *et al.* (1994) have described a child of 5 years of age who met DSM-III criteria for autism as suffering from a mitochondrial encephalopathy and infantile spasms caused by cytochrome c oxidase deficiency, an autosomal recessive Mendelian disorder. The heterogeneity of cytochrome c oxidase deficiency is established (Lombes *et al.* 1996). It can underlie infantile spasms with hypsarrhythmia (Bakker *et al.* 1996, Tsao *et al.* 1997), as in the child with autism described above.

Also, a patient has been described who had autistic regression and a point mutation of the mitochondrial tRNA lys gene (G8363a) in blood (Graf *et al.* 1998). The boy developed normally until 18 months of age and then gradually lost language abilities. He lost his ability to concentrate and developed toe walking, stereotypies and self-injurious behavior. The mutation was originally found in the boy's sister who presented with lactic acidosis, Leigh syndrome, progressive ataxia, chorea and myoclonic seizures. This family illustrates the principle that it can be difficult to link a mitochondrial mutation to a clinical disease because there is often dissociation of the phenotype and genotype; the same mutation can be associated with different phenotypes, as seen in this family. Besides the boy with autism, the 8363 mitochondrial mutation has, to date, been associated with three other phenotypes – Leigh syndrome, cardiomyopathy with hearing loss, and myoclonic epilepsy with ragged red fibers.

OXPHOS disease, most frequently found in Complex I, has been identified in an additional 20 individuals with autism (Shoffner, personal communication). Because these findings are corroborated by secondary abnormalities in fatty acid oxidation – palmitate and myristate – these results are likely to be correct. Whether the actual genetic defect in each case is in mitochondrial DNA or nuclear DNA is unknown.

CONCLUSION

It is highly likely that there is no such thing as an exclusive chromosome carrying the genes for autism. All the chromosomes except 14 have at least one patient with autism associated with them, either through chromosomal aberration or genetic mutation, although direct correspondence between behavioral symptoms and an error on a chromosome can never be automatically inferred. Regarding chromosomal aberrations themselves, the autistic syndromes are more likely to be associated with chromosomal deletions, in contrast to mental retardation syndromes which are often associated with full trisomies; although, of course, there are numerous exceptions to this general statement. In possibly the largest epidemiological study of autism ever undertaken (in which 233 individuals with autism were located in the state of Utah), 5 per cent of the group were found to have chromosomal aberrations (Ritvo *et al.* 1990). This is similar to the rate found in another large epidemiological sample taken in Sweden (Gillberg and Wahlström 1985). Patients with chromosomal aberrations are often karyotyped because of physical stigmata. In children with autism and chromosomal errors, these stigmata range from very marked to the other extreme of being so mild that they are not even noted. Patients with autism and the distinctive cri-du-chat syndrome are an example of those with stigmata sufficiently subtle that they are missed (Cantú *et al.* 1990).

Molecular genetics has begun to contribute to the understanding of autism. Besides the apparently monogenetic disorders with a variety of mutations, molecular techniques have uncovered genetic patterns other than classical Mendelian genetics. Uniparental disomy or genetic imprinting appears possible as a factor in some of the cases of autism found with errors of chromosome 15q11–q13. Trinucleotide repeat disorders – the type seen in the fragile X syndrome – present as diseases of the brain presenting in infancy from families containing older disturbed individuals; such a familial pattern is called the phenomenon of anticipation. There is a medical hypothesis that autism may be caused by lengthier expansions of trinucleotide repeats while schizophrenia results from smaller repeat expansions (Fischer 1998). The origin of the fragile site has already been demonstrated as a trinucleotide repeat in the fragile X syndrome; trinucleotide repeats may well apply to other types of autism with that particular familial pattern of anticipation. Also, there are autistic children who come from families with patterns of maternal inheritance of psychiatric disabilities; this opens up the possibility of errors of mitochondrial DNA, a research area for patients with lactic acidosis and autism. The future holds great promise for further understanding.

REFERENCES

Abrams, M.T., Doheny, K.F., Mazzocco, M.M., Knight, S.J., Baumgardner, T.L., Freund, L.S., Davies, K.E., Reiss, A.L. (1997) 'Cognitive, behavioral and neuroanatomical assessment of two unrelated male children expressing FRAXE.' *American Journal of Medical Genetics*, **74**, 73–81.

Abrams, N., Pergament, E. (1971) 'Childhood psychoses combined with XYY abnormalities.' *Journal of Genetic Psychology*, **118**, 13–16.

Åkefeldt, A., Gillberg, C. (1991) 'Hypomelanosis of Ito in three cases with autism and autistic-like conditions.' *Developmental Medicine and Child Neurology*, **33**, 737–743.

Albrecht, U., Sutcliffe, J.S., Cattanach, B.M., Beechey, C.V., Armstrong, D., Eichele G., Beaudet, A.L. (1997) 'Imprinted expression of the murine Angelman syndrome gene, UBE3A, in hippocampal and Purkinje neurons.' *Nature Genetics*, **17**, 75–78.

Annerén, G., Dahl, N., Uddenfelt, U. (1995) 'Asperger syndrome in a boy with a balanced de novo translocation t(17;19)(p13.3;p11).' (Letter to the editor) *American Journal of Medical Genetics*, **56**, 1–8.

Arrieta, I., Nunez, T., Gil, A., Flores, P., Usobiaga, E., Martinez, B. (1996) 'Autosomal folate sensitive fragile sites in an autistic Basque sample.' *Annales de Genetique*, **39**, 69–74.

Ashley-Koch, A., Wolpert, C.M., Menold, M.M., Zaeem, L., Basu, S., Donnelly, S.L., Ravan, S.A., Powell, C.M., Qumsiyeh, M.B., Aylsworth, A.S., Vance, J.M., Gilbert, J.R., Wright, H.H., Abramson, R.K., DeLong, G.R. Cuccaro, M.L., Pericak-Vance, M.A. (1999) 'Genetic studies of autistic disorder and chromosome 7.' *Genomics*, **61**, 227–236.

Assumpcão, F.B., Jr. (1998) 'Brief report: A case of chromosome alteration associated with autistic syndrome.' *Journal of Autism and Developmental Disorders*, **28**, 253–256.

Bailey, A., Le Couteur, A., Gottesman, I., Bolton, P., Simonoff, E., Yuda, E., Rutter, M. (1995) 'Autism as a strongly genetic disorder: evidence from a British twin study.' *Psychological Medicine*, **25**, 63–77.

Bailey, A., Palferman, S., Heavey, L., Le Couteur, A. (1998) 'Autism: the phenotype in relatives.' *Journal of Autism and Developmental Disorders*, **28**, 369.

Baker, P., Piven, J., Schwartz, S., Patil, S. (1994) 'Brief report: Duplication of chromosome 15q11–13 in two individuals with autistic disorder.' *Journal of Autism and Developmental Disorders*, **24**, 529–535.

Bakker, H.D., Van den Bogert, C., Drewes, J.G., Barth, P.G., Scholte, H.R., Wanders, R.J., Ruitenbeek, W. (1996) 'Progressive generalized brain atrophy and infantile spasms associated with cytochrome c oxidase deficiency.' *Journal of Inherited Metabolic Disease*, **19**, 153–156.

Barber, J.C., Ellis, K.H., Bowles, L.V., Delhanty, J.D., Ede, R.F., Male, B.M., Eccles, D.M. (1994) 'Adenomatous polyposis coli and a cytogenetic deletion of chromosome 5 resulting from a maternal intrachromosomal insertion.' *Journal of Medical Genetics*, **31**, 312–316.

Barrett, S., Beck, J.C., Bernier, R., Bisson, E., Braun, T.A., Casavant, T.L., Childress, D., Folstein, S.E., Garcia, M., Gardiner, M.B., Gilman, S., Haines, J.L., Hopkins, K., Landa, R., Meyer, N.H., Mullane, J.A., Nishimura, D.Y., Palmer, P., Piven, J., Purdy, J., Santangelo, S.L., Searby, C., Sheffield, V., Singleton, J., Slager, S., Struchen, T. (1999) 'An autosomal genomic screen for autism.' *American Journal of Medical Genetics*, **88**, 609–615.

Biesele, J.J., Schmid, W., Lawlis, M.G. (1962) 'Mentally retarded schizoid twin girls with 47 chromosomes.' *Lancet*, **2**, 403–405.

Blackman, J.A., Selzer, S.C., Patel, S., van Dyke, D.C. (1991) 'Autistic disorder associated with an iso-dicentric Y chromosome.' *Developmental Medicine and Child Neurology*, **33**, 153–166.

Bolton, P., Macdonald, H., Pickles, A., Rios, P., Goode, S., Crowson, M., Bailey, A., Rutter, M. (1994) 'A case–control family history study of autism. *Journal of Child Psychology and Psychiatry*, **35**, 877–900.

Bolton, P., Powell, J., Rutter, M., Buckle, V., Yates, J.R., Ishikawa-Brush, Y., Monaco, A.P. (1995) 'Autism, mental retardation, multiple exostoses and short stature in a female with 46,X,t(X,8)(p22.13;q22.1).' *Psychiatric Genetics*, **5**, 51–55.

Bundey, S., Hardy, V., Vickers, S., Kilpatrick, M.W., Corbett, J.A. (1994) 'Duplication of the 15q11–13 region in a patient with autism, epilepsy and ataxia.' *Developmental Medicine and Child Neurology*, **36**, 736–742.

Burd, L., Martsolf, J.T., Kerbeshian, J., Jalal, S.M. (1988) 'Partial 6p trisomy associated with infantile autism.' *Clinical Genetics*, **33**, 356–359.

Cantú, E.S., Stone, J.W., Wing, A.A., Langee, H.R., Williams, C.A. (1990) 'Cytogenetic survey for autistic fragile X carriers in a mental retardation center.' *American Journal on Mental Retardation*, **94**, 442–447.

Cappione, A.J., French, B.L., Skuse, G.R. (1997) 'A potential role for NF1 mRNA editing in the pathogenesis of NF1 tumors.' *American Journal of Human Genetics*, **60**, 305–312.

Carratala, F., Galan, F., Moya, M., Estivill, X., Pritchard, M.A., Llevadot, R., Nadal, M., Gratacos, M. (1998) 'A patient with autistic disorder and a 20/22 chromosomal translation.' *Developmental Medicine and Child Neurology*, **40**, 492–495.

Collacott, R.A., Cooper, S.-A., McGrother, C. (1992) 'Differential rates of psychiatric disorders in adults with Down's syndrome compared to other mentally handicapped adults.' *British Journal of Psychiatry*, **161**, 671–674.

Comings, D.E., Wu, S., Chiu, C., Muhleman, D., Sverd, J. (1996) 'Studies of the c-Harvey-Ras gene in psychiatric disorders.' *Psychiatry Research*, **63**, 25–32.

Cook, E.H., Jr., Lindgren, V., Leventhal, B.L., Courchesne, R., Lincoln, A., Shulman, C., Lord, C., Courchesne, E. (1997a) 'Autism or atypical autism in maternally but not paternally derived proximal 15q duplication.' *American Journal of Human Genetics*, **60**, 928–934.

Cook, E.H., Jr., Courchesne, R., Lord, C., Cox, N.J., Yan, S., Lincoln, A., Haas, R., Courchesne, E., Leventhal, B.L. (1997b) 'Evidence of linkage between the serotonin transporter and autistic disorder.' *Molecular Psychiatry*, **2**, 247–250.

Cook, E.H., Jr., Courchesne, R.Y., Cox, N.J., Lord, C., Gonen, D., Guter, S.J., Lincoln, A., Nix, K., Haas, R., Leventhal, B.L., Courchesne, E. (1998) 'Linkage-disequilibrium mapping of autistic disorder, with 15q11–13 markers.' *American Journal of Human Genetics*, **62**, 1077–1083.

Crolla, J., Harvey, J., Stitch, F., Dennis, N. (1995) 'Supernumerary marker 15 chromosome: a clinical, molecular and FISG approach to diagnosis and prognosis.' *Human Genetics*, **95**, 161–170.

Daniels, W.W., Warren, R.P., Odell, J.D., Maciulis, A., Burger, R.A., Warren, W.L., Torres, A.R. (1995) 'Increased frequency of the extended or ancestral haplotype B44-SC30-DR4 in autism.' *Neuropsychobiology*, **32**, 120–123.

De Braekeleer, M., Tremblay, M., Thivièrge, J. (1996) 'Genetic analysis of genealogies in mentally retarded autistic probands from Saguenay Lac-Saint-Jean (Quebec, Canada).' *Annals of Genetics*, **39**, 47–50.

255

De la Barra, F., Skoknic, V., Alliende, A., Raimann, E., Cortes, F., Lacassie, Y. (1986) 'Gemelas con autismo y retardo mental asociado a translocacion cromosomica balanceada (7;20).' (In Spanish) *Revista de Chilena Pediatria*, **57**, 549–554.

DiMauro, S., Moraes, C.T. (1993) 'Mitochondrial encephalomyopathies.' *Archives of Neurology*, **50**, 1197–1208.

DiMauro, S., Bonilla, E., Davidson, M., Hirano, M., Schon, E.A. (1998) 'Mitochondria in neuromuscular disorders.' *Biochimica et Biophysica Acta*, **1366**, 199–210.

El Abd, S., Patton, M.A., Turk, J., Hoey, H., Howlin, P. (1999) 'Social, communicational, and behavioral deficits associated with a ring X Turner syndrome.' *American Journal of Medical Genetics*, **88**, 510–516.

Eliez, S., Palacio-Espasa, F., Spira, A., Lacroix, M., Pont, C., Luthi, F., Robert-Tissot, C., Feinstein, C. Antonorakis, S.E., Cramer, B. (in press) 'Young children with Velo-Cardio-Facial syndrome.' *European Child and Adolescent Psychiatry*.

European Chromosome 16 Tuberous Sclerosis Consortium. (1993) 'Identification and characterization of the tuberous sclerosis gene on chromosome 16.' *Cell*, **75**, 1305–1315.

Fahsold, R., Rott, H.D., Claussen, U., Schmalenberger, B. (1991) 'Tuberous sclerosis in a child with de novo translocation t(3;13)(p26.3;q23.3).' *Clinical Genetics*, **40**, 326–328.

Feinstein, C., Reiss, A.L. (1998) 'Autism: the point of view from fragile X studies.' *Journal of Autism and Developmental Disorders*, **28**, 393–405.

Fischer, K.M. (1998) 'Expanded (CAG)n, (CGG)n and (GAA)n trinucleotide repeat microsatellites and mutant purine synthesis and pigmentation genes cause schizophrenia and autism.' *Medical Hypothesis*, **51**, 223–233.

Flejter, W.L., Bennett-Baker, P.E., Ghaziuddin, M., McDonald, M., Sheldon, S., Gorski, J.L. (1996) 'Cytogenetic and molecular analysis of inv dup(15) chromosomes observed in two patients with autistic disorder and mental retardation.' *American Journal of Medical Genetics*, **11**, 182–187.

Folstein, S., Rutter, M. (1977) 'Infantile autism: a genetic study of 21 twin pairs.' *Journal of Child Psychology and Psychiatry*, **18**, 297–321.

Fon, E.A., Demczuk, S., Delattre, O., Thomas, G., Rouleau, G.A. (1993) 'Mapping of the human adenylsuccinase lyase gene to chromosome 22q13.1→q13.2.' *Cytogenetics and Cell Genetics*, **64**, 201–203.

Fryer, A.E., Chalmers, A., Connor, J.M., Fraser, I., Povey, S., Yates, A.D., Yates, J.R., Osborne, J.P. (1987) 'Evidence that a gene for tuberous sclerosis is on chromosome 9.' *Lancet*, **8534**, 659–661.

Fryns, J.P., Kleczkowska, A. (1992) 'Autism and ring chromosome 18.' *Clinical Genetics*, **42**, 55.

Fryns, J.P., Kleczkowska, A., Kubien, E., van den Berghe, H. (1986) 'Excess of mental retardation and/or congenital malformation in reciprocal translocations in man.' *Human Genetics*, **72**, 1–8.

Ghaziuddin, M., Burmeister, M. (1999) 'Deletion of chromosome 2q37 and autism: a distinct subtype?' *Journal of Autism and Developmental Disorders*, **29**, 259–263.

Ghaziuddin, M., Sheldon, S., Tsai, L.Y., Alessi, N. (1993a) 'Abnormalities of chromosome 18 in a girl with mental retardation and autistic disorder.' *Journal of Intellectual Disability Research*, **37**, 313–317.

Ghaziuddin, M., Sheldon, S., Venkataraman, S., Tsai, L., Ghaziuddin, N. (1993b) 'Autism associated with tetrasomy 15: a further report.' *European Child and Adolescent Psychiatry*, **2**, 226–230.

Gillberg, C. (1998) 'Chromosomal disorders and autism.' *Journal of Autism and Developmental Disorders*, **28**, 415–425.

Gillberg, C., Wahlström, J. (1985) 'Chromosomal abnormalities in infantile autism and other childhood psychoses: a population study of 66 cases.' *Developmental Medicine and Child Neurology*, **27**, 293–304.

Gillberg, C, Wahlström, J., Hagberg, B. (1984a) 'Infantile autism and Rett's syndrome: common chromosomal denominator' (Letter) *Lancet*, **2**, 1094–1095.

Gillberg, C., Steffenburg, S., Wahlström, J. (1984b) 'The sex chromosomes – one key to autism? An XYY case of infantile autism.' *Applied Research in Mental Retardation*, **5**, 353–360.

Gillberg, C., Steffenburg, S., Jakobsson, G. (1987) 'Neurobiological findings in 20 relatively gifted children with Kanner-style autism or Asperger syndrome.' *Developmental Medicine and Child Neurology*, **29**, 641–649.

Gillberg, C., Steffenburg, S., Wahlström, J., Gillberg, I.C., Sjöstedt, A., Martinsson, T., Liedgren, S., Eeg-Olofsson, O. (1991) 'Autism associated with marker chromosome.' *Journal of the American Academy of Child and Adolescent Psychiatry*, **30**, 489–494.

256

Graf, W.D., Makari, G.S.H., Park, R.D., Marin-Garcia, J. (1998) 'Autistic regression associated with a mutation in mitochondrial tRNA (lys) gene (G8363A).' (Abstract) *Annals of Neurology*, **44**, 533.

Hagerman, R.J. (1989) 'Chromosomes, genes and autism.' *In:* Gillberg, C. (Ed.) *Diagnosis and Treatment of Autism*. New York: Plenum Press, pp. 105–132.

Hagerman, R.J., Hull, C.E., Safanda, J.F., Carpenter, I., Staley, L.W., O'Conner, R.A., Seydel, C., Mazzocco, M.M., Snow, K., Thibodeau, S.N. *et al.* (1994) 'High functioning fragile X males: demonstration of an unmethylated full expanded FRM-1 mutation associated with protein expression.' *American Journal of Medical Genetics*, **51**, 298–308.

Halal, F., Vekemans, M., Kaplan, P., Zeesman, S. (1990) 'Distal deletion of chromosome 1q in an adult.' *American Journal of Medical Genetics*, **35**, 379–382.

Halley, D.J. (1996) 'Tuberous sclerosis; between genetic and physical analysis.' *Acta Geneticae Medicae et Gemellologiae (Rome)*, **45**, 63–75.

Hallmayer, J., Hebert, J.M., Spiker, D., Lotspeich, L., McMahon, W.M., Petersen, P.B., Nicholas, P., Pingree, C., Lin, A.A., Cavalli-Sforza, L.L., Risch, N., Ciaranello, R.D. (1996a) 'Autism and the X chromosome. Multipoint sib-pair analysis.' *Archives of General Psychiatry*, **53**, 985–989.

Hallmayer, J., Spiker, D., Lotspeich, L., McMahon, W.M., Petersen, P.B., Nicholas, P., Pingree, C., Ciaranello, R.D. (1996b) 'Male-to-male transmission in extended pedigrees with multiple cases of autism.' *American Journal of Medical Genetics*, **67**, 13–18.

Hansen, A., Brask, B.H., Nielsen, J., Rasmussen, K., Sillesin, I. (1977) 'A case report of an autistic girl with an extra bisatellited marker chromosome.' *Journal of Autism and Childhood Schizophrenia*, **7**, 263–267.

Hebebrand, J., Martin, M., Korner, J., Roitzheim, B., de Braganca, K., Werner, W., Remschmidt, H. (1994) 'Partial trisomy 16p in an adolescent with autistic disorder and Tourette's syndrome.' *American Journal of Medical Genetics*, **54**, 268–270.

Heidary, G., Hampton, L.L., Schanen, N.C., Rivkin, M.J., Darras, B.T., Battey, J., Francke, U. (1998) 'Exclusion of the gastrin-releasing peptide receptor (GRPR) locus as a candidate gene for Rett syndrome.' *American Journal of Medical Genetics*, **78**, 173–175.

Hérault, J., Petit, E., Martineau, J., Perrot, A., Lenoir, P., Cherpi, C., Barthélémy, C., Sauvage, D., Mallet, J., Muh, J.P., Lelord, G. (1995) 'Autism and genetics: clinical approach and association study with two markers of HRAS gene.' *American Journal of Medical Genetics (Neuropsychiatric Genetics)*, **60**, 276–281.

Herder, G.A. (1993) 'Infantil autisme blant barn i Nordland fylke. Forekomst og arsaksforhold.' (In Norwegian) *Tidsskrift for Norsk Largeforening*, **113**, 2247–2249.

Ho, H.H., Kalousek, D.K. (1989) 'Fragile X syndrome in autistic boys.' *Journal of Autism and Developmental Disorders*, **19**, 343–347.

Holden, J.J., Wing, M., Chalifoux, M., Julien-Inalsingh, C., Schutz, C., Robinson, P., Szatmari, P., White, B.N. (1996) 'Lack of expansion of triplet repeats in the FMR1, FRAXE and FRAXF loci in male multiplex families with autism and pervasive developmental disorders.' *American Journal of Medical Genetics*, **64**, 399–403.

Hoshino, Y., Yashima, Y., Tachibana, R., Kaneko, M., Watanabe, M., Kumashiro, H. (1979) 'Sex chromosome abnormalities in autistic children – long Y chromosome.' *Fukushima Journal of Medical Sciences*, **26**, 31–42.

Hotopf, M., Bolton, P. (1995) 'A case of autism associated with partial tetrasomy 15.' *Journal of Autism and Developmental Disorders*, **25**, 41–49.

IMGSAC (International Molecular Genetic Study of Autism Consortium) (1998) 'A full genome screen for autism with evidence for linkage to a region on chromosome 7q.' *Human Molecular Genetics*, **7**, 571–578.

Ishikawa-Brush, Y., Powell, J.F., Bolton, P., Miller, A.P., Francis, F., Willard, H.F., Lehrach, H., Monaco, A.P. (1997) 'Autism and multiple exostoses associated with an X;8 translocation occurring within the GRPR gene and 3' to the SDC2 gene.' *Human Molecular Genetics*, **6**, 1241–1250.

Jackson, M.J., Bendoff, L.H. *et al.* (1995) 'Presentation and clinical investigation of mitochondrial respiratory chain disease. A study of 51 patients.' *Brain*, **118**, 339–351.

Jayakar, P., Chudley, A.E., Ray, M., Evans, J.A., Perlov, J., Wand, R. (1986) 'Fra(2)(q13) and inv(9)(p11p12) in autism: causal relationship.' *American Journal of Medical Genetics*, **23**, 381–392.

Johns, D.R. (1998) 'Genetic basis of mitochondrial disease.' *In:* Jameson, J.L. (Ed.) *Principles of Molecular Medicine*. Totowa, NJ: Humana Press.

257

Judd, L.L., Mandell, A.J. (1968) 'Chromosome studies in early infantile autism.' *Archives of General Psychiatry*, **18**, 450–457.

Kerbeshian, J., Burd, L., Randall, T., Martsolf, J., Jalal, S. (1990) 'Autism, profound mental retardation and atypical bipolar disorder in a 33-year-old female with a deletion of 15q12.' *Journal of Mental Deficiency Research*, **34**, 205–210.

Konstantareas, M.M., Homatidis, S. (1999) 'Chromosomal abnormalities in a series of children with autistic behavior.' *Journal of Autism and Developmental Delay*, **29**, 275–286.

László, A., Horváth, E., Eck, E., Fekete, M. (1994) 'Serum serotonin, lactate and pyruvate levels in infantile autistic patients.' *Clinica Chimica Acta*, **229**, 205–207.

Lauritsen, M., Mors, O., Mortensen, P.B., Ewald, H. (1999) 'Infantile autism and associated autosomal chromosome abnormalities: a register-based study and a literature survey.' *Journal of Child Psychology and Psychiatry*, **40**, 335–345.

Leana-Cox, J., Jenkins, L., Palmer, C.G., Plattner, R., Sheppard, L., Flejte, W.L., Jackowski, J., Tsien, F., Schwartz, S. (1994) 'Molecular cytogentic analysis of inv dup(15) chromosomes, using probes specific for the Prader Willi/Angelman syndrome critical region: clinical implications.' *American Journal of Human Genetics*, **54**, 748–756.

Le Couteur, A., Bailey, A., Goode, S., Pickles, A., Robertson, S., Gottesman, I., Rutter, M. (1996) 'A broader phenotype of autism: the clinical spectrum in twins.' *Journal of Child Psychology and Psychiatry*, **37**, 785–801.

Leonard, S., Gault, J., Moore, T., Hopkins, J., Robinson, M., Olincy, A., Adler, L.E., Cloninger, C.R., Kaufman, C.A., Tsuang, M.T., Faraone, S.V., Malaspina, D., Svrakic, D.M., Freedman, R. (1998) 'Further investigation on a chromosome 15 locus in schizophrenia.' *American Journal of Medical Genetics (Neuropsychiatric Genetics)*, **81**, 308–312.

Lewis, K.E., Lubetshy, M.J., Wenger, S.L., Steele, M.W. (1995) 'Chromosomal abnormalities in a psychiatric population.' *American Journal of Medical Genetics (Neuropsychiatric Genetics)*, **60**, 53–54.

Li, S.Y., Chen, Y.C., Lai, T.J., Hsu, C.Y., Wang, Y.C. (1993) 'Molecular and cytogenetic analysis of autism in Taiwan.' *Human Genetics*, **92**, 441–445.

Lombard, L.A. (1998) 'Autism: a mitochondrial disorder?' *Medical Hypothesis*, **50**, 497–500.

Lombes, A., Romero, N.B., Touati, G., Frachon, P., Cheval, M.A., Giraud, M., Simon, D., Ogier de Baulny, H. (1996) 'Clinical and molecular heterogeneity of cytochrome c oxidase deficiency in the newborn.' *Journal of Inherited Metabolic Diseases*, **19**, 286–295.

Lopreiato, J.O., Wulfsberg, E.A. (1992) 'A complex chromosome rearrangement in a boy with autism.' *Journal of Developmental and Behavioral Pediatrics*, **13**, 281–283.

Lubs, H.A. (1969) 'A marker X-chromosome.' *American Journal of Human Genetics*, **21**, 231–244.

MacLean, J.E., Teshima, I.E., Szatmari, P., Nowaczyk, M.J. (2000) 'Ring chromosome 22 and autism: report and review.' *American Journal of Medical Genetics*, **90**, 382–385.

Maestrini, E., Marlow, A.J., Weeks, D.E., Monaco, A.P. (1998) 'Molecular genetic investigations of autism.' *Journal of Autism and Developmental Disorder*, **28**, 427–437.

Maestrini, E., Lai, C., Marlow, A., Mathews, N., Wallace, S., Bailey, A., Cook, E.H., Weeks, D.E., Monaco, A.P. (1999) 'Serotonin transporter (S-HTTT) and gamma-aminobutyric acid receptor subunit 3 (GABRB3) gene polymorphisms are not with autism in IMGSA families.' *American Journal of Medical Genetics*, **88**, 492–496.

Mahr, R.N., Moberg, P.J., Overhauser, J., Strathdee, G., Kamholz, J., Loevner, L.A., Campbell, H., Zackai, E.H., Reber, M.E., Mozley, D.P., Brown, L., Turetsky, B.I., Shapiro, R.M. (1996) 'Neuropsychiatry of 18q- syndrome.' *American Journal of Medical Genetics*, **67**, 172–179.

Mallin, S.R., Walker, F.A. (1972) 'Effects of the XYY karyotype in one of two brothers with congenital adrenal hyperplasia.' *Clinical Genetics*, **3**, 490–494.

Mariner, R., Jackson, A.W., Levitas, A., Hagerman, R.J., Braden, M., McBogg, P.M., Smith, A.C., Berry, R. (1986) 'Autism, mental retardation, and chromosomal abnormalities.' *Journal of Autism and Developmental Disorders*, **16**, 425–440.

Martinsson, T., Johannesson, T., Vujic, M., Sjöstedt, A., Steffenburg, S., Gillberg, C., Wahlström, J. (1996) 'Maternal origin of inv dup(15) chromosomes in infantile autism.' *European Child and Adolescent Psychiatry*, **5**, 185–192.

Mazzocco, M.M., Kates, W.R., Baumgardner, T.L., Freund, L.S., Reiss, A.L. (1997) 'Autistic behaviors among girls with fragile X syndrome.' *Journal of Autism and Developmental Disorders*, **27**, 415–435.

Michaelis, R.C., Skinner, S.A., Deson, R., Skinner, C., Moore, C.L., Phelan, M.C. (1997) 'Interstitial deletion of 20p: a new candidate for Hirschsprung disease and autism?' *American Journal of Medical Genetics*, **71**, 298–304.

Mohandas, T.K., Park, J.P., Spellman, R.A., Filano, J.J., Mamourian, A.C., Hawk, A.B., Belloni, D.R., Noll, W.W., Moeschler, J.B. (1999) 'Paternally derived de novo interstitial duplication of proximal 15q in a patient with developmental delay.' *American Journal of Medical Genetics*, **82**, 294–300.

Monaghan, K.G., Van Dyke, D.L., Wiktor, A., Feldman, G.L. (1997) 'Cytogenetic and clinical findings in a patient with a deletion of 16q23.1: first report of bilateral cataracts and a 16q deletion.' *American Journal of Medical Genetics*, **73**, 180–183.

Murayama, K., Greenwood, R.S., Roa, K.W., Aylsworth, A.S. (1991) 'Neurological aspects of del(1q) syndrome.' *American Journal of Medical Genetics*, **40**, 488–492.

Murayama, T., Ito, M., Imoto, S., Matsushita, K., Matozaki, S., Nakagawa, T., Nakao, Y. (1993) 'Idiopathic thrombocytopenic purpura with X chromosome abnormality.' (Letter) *American Journal of Hematology*, **42**, 239–240.

Nicholls, R.D. (1998) 'Prader–Willi and Angelman syndromes.' *In:* Jameson, J.L. (Ed.) *Principles of Molecular Medicine.* Totowa: NJ: Humana Press, pp.1053–1062.

Nielsen, J., Christensen, K.R., Friedrich, U., Zeuthen, E., Ostergaard, O. (1973) 'Childhood of males with XYY syndrome.' *Journal of Autism and Childhood Schizophrenia*, **3**, 5–26.

Nissenkorn, A., Zeharia, A., Lev, D., Watemberg, N., Fattal-Valevski, A., Barash, V., Gutman, A., Harel, S., Lerman-Sagie, T. (2000) 'Neurologic presentations in mitochondrial disorders.' *Journal of Child Neurology*, **15**, 44–48.

Pearl, P., Coleman, M. (1996) 'Autosomal chromosome disorders and autism.' *Developmental Brain Disorders*, **9**, 224–229.

Pericak-Vance, M.A., Wolpert, C.M., Menold, M.M., Blass, M.P., DeLong, G.R., Wright, H.H., Abramson, R.K., Cuccaro, M.L. (1997) 'Linkage evidence supports the involvement of chromosome 15 in autistic disorder.' *American Journal of Human Genetics*, **6**(Suppl.), A4.

Petit, E., Hérault, J., Raynaud, M., Cherpi, C., Perrot, A., Barthélémy, C., Lelord, G., Müh, J.P. (1996) 'X chromosome and infantile autism.' *Biological Psychiatry*, **40**, 457–464.

Philippe, A., Martinez, M., Guilloud-Bataille, M., Gillberg, C., Rastam, M., Sponheim, E., Coleman, M., Zappella, M., Achauer, H., van Malldergeme, L., Penet, C., Feingold, J., Brice, A., Leboyer, M. (1999) 'Genome-wide scan for autism susceptibility genes,' *Human Molecular Genetics*, **8**, 805–812.

Pickles, A., Bolton, P., Macdonald, H., Bailey, A., Le Couteur, A., Sim, C.H., Rutter, M. (1995) 'Latent-class analysis of recurrence risks for complex phenotypes with selection and measurement error: a twin and family history study of autism.' *American Journal of Human Genetics*, **57**, 717–726.

Piven, J., Palmer, P., Jacobi, D., Childress, D., Arndt, S. (1997) 'Broader autism phenotype: evidence from a family history study of multiple incidence families.' *American Journal of Psychiatry*, **154**, 185–190.

Plumet, M.H., Goldblum, M.C., Leboyer, M. (1995) 'Verbal skills in relatives of autistic females.' *Cortex*, **31**, 723–733.

Poissonnier, M., Turleau, C., Olivier-Martin, M., Milleret-Proyart, M.J., Prieur, M., Dubos, M., Cabanis, M.O., Mugneret, F., Blanc, P., Noel, L. (1992) 'Interstitial deletion of the proximal region of the long arm of chromosome 18, del(18q12) a distinct clinical entity? A report of two cases.' *Annals of Genetics*, **35**, 146–151.

Rao, P.N., Klinepeter, K., Stewart, W., Hayworth, R., Grubs, R., Pettenait, M.J. (1994) 'Molecular cytogenetic analysis of a duplication Xp in a male: further delineation of a possible sex influencing region on the X chromosome.' *Human Genetics*, **94**, 149–153.

Rimland, B. (1964) *Infantile Autism: The Syndrome and its Implication for a Neural Theory of Behavior.* Englewood Cliffs, NJ: Prentice-Hall.

Rineer, S., Finucane, B., Simon, E.W. (1998) 'Autistic symptoms among children and young adults with isodicentric chromosome 15.' *American Journal of Medical Genetics*, **81**, 428–433.

Risch, N., Spiker, D., Lotspeich, L., Nouri, N., Hinds, D., Hallmayer, J., Kalaydjieva, L., McCague, P., Dimiceli, S., Pitts, T., Nguyen, L., Yang, J., Harper, C., Thorpe, D., Vermeer, S., Young, H., Hebert, J., Lin, A., Ferguson, J., Chiotti, C., Wiese-Slater, S., Rogers, T., Salmon, B., Nicholas, P., Petersen, P.B., Pingree, C., McMahon, W., Wong, D.L., Cavalli-Sforza, L.L., Kraemer, H.C., Myers, R.M. (1999) 'A genomic screen of autism: evidence for a multifocus etiology.' *American Journal of Human Genetics*, **65**, 493–507.

Ritvo, E., Freeman, B.J., Mason-Brothers, A., Mo, A., Ritvo, A.M. (1985) 'Concordance for the syndrome of autism in 40 pairs of afflicted twins.' *American Journal of Psychiatry*, **142**, 74–77.

Ritvo, E.R., Creel, D., Realmuto, G., Crandall, A.S., Freeman, B.J., Bateman, J.B., Bahr, R., Pingree, C., Coleman, M., Purple, R. (1988) 'Electroretinograms in autism – a pilot study of b-wave amplitudes.' *American Journal of Psychiatry*, **145**, 229–232.

Ritvo, E.R., Mason-Brothers, A., Freeman, B.J., Pingree, C., Jenson, W.R., McMahon, W.M., Petersen, P.B., Jorde, L.B., Mo, A., Ritvo, A. (1990) 'The UCLA-University of Utah epidemiologic survey of autism: the etiologic role of rare diseases.' *American Journal of Psychiatry*, **147**, 1614–1612.

Sabry, M.A., Farag, T.I., (1998) 'Chromosome 15q11–13 region and the autistic disorder.' *Journal of Intellectual Disability Research*, **42**, 259.

Saliba, J.R., Griffiths, M. (1990) 'Brief report: Autism of the Asperger type associated with an autosomal fragile site.' *Journal of Autism and Developmental Disorders*, **20**, 569–575.

Salmon, B., Hallmayer, J., Rogers, T., Kalaydjieva, L., Petersen, P.B., Nicholas, P., Pingree, C., McMahon, W., Spiker, D., Lotspeich, L., Kraemer, H., McCogue, P., Dimiceli, S., Nouri, N., Pitts, T., Yang, J., Hinds, D., Myers, R.M., Risch, N. (1999) 'Absence of linkage and linkage disequilibrium to chromosome 15q11–q13 markers in 139 multiplex families with autism.' *American Journal of Medical Genetics*, **88**, 551–556.

Schinzel, A. (1990) 'Autistic disorder and additional inv dup(15)(pter–q13) chromosome.' *American Journal of Medical Genetics*, **35**, 447–448.

Schroer, R.J., Phelan, M.C., Michaelis, R.C., Crawford, E.C., Skinner, S.A., Cuccaro, M., Simensen, R.J., Bishop, J., Skinner, C., Fender, D., Stevenson, R.E. (1998) 'Autism and maternally derived aberrations of chromosome 15q.' *American Journal of Human Genetics*, **76**, 327–336.

Scourfield, J., McGuffin, P., Thapar, A. (1997) 'Genes and social skills.' *Bioessays*, **19**, 1125–1127.

Scriver, C.R. (1991) 'Phenylketonuria – genotypes and phenotypes.' (Editorial) *New England Journal of Medicine*, **324**, 1280–1281.

Seshadri, K., Wallerstein, R., Burack, G. (1992) '18q- chromosomal abnormality in a phenotypically normal 2½ year old male with autism.' *Developmental Medicine and Child Neurology*, **34**, 1005–1009.

Shaffer, L.G., McCaskill, C., Hersh, J.H., Greenberg, F., Lupski, J.R. (1996) 'A clinical and molecular study of mosaicism for trisomy 17.' *Human Genetics*, **97**, 69–72.

Skuse, D.H., James, R.S., Bishop, D.V., Coppin, B., Dalton, P., Aamodt-Leeper, G., Bacarese-Hamilton, M., Creswell, C., McGurk, R., Jacobs, P.A. (1997) 'Evidence from Turner's syndrome of an imprinted X-linked locus affecting cognitive function.' *Nature*, **387**, 705–708.

Smalley, S.L. (1998) 'Autism and tuberous sclerosis.' *Journal of Autism and Developmental Disorders*, **28**, 407–414.

Smeraldi, E., Zanardi, R., Benedetti, F., Di Bella, D., Perez, J., Catalano, M. (1998) 'Polymorphism within the promoter of the serotonin transporter gene and antidepressant efficacy of fluvoxamine.' *Molecular Psychiatry*, **3**, 508–511.

Smith, A.C., Dykens, E., Greenberg, F. (1998) 'Behavioral phenotype of Smith–Magenis syndrome (del 17p11.2).' *American Journal of Medical Genetics*, **28**, 179–185.

Spiker, D., Lotspeich, L., Kraemer, H.C., Hallmayer, J., McMahon, W., Petersen, P.B., Nicholas, P., Pingree, C., Wiese-Slater, S., Chiotti, C. *et al.* (1994) 'Genetics of autism: characteristics of affected and unaffected children from multiplex families.' *American Journal of Medical Genetics*, **15**, 27–35.

Steffenburg, S. (1991) 'Neuropsychiatric assessment of children with autism: a population-based study.' *Developmental Medicine and Child Neurology*, **33**, 495–511.

Steffenburg, S., Gillberg, C., Hellgren, L., Anderson, L., Gillberg, I.C., Jacobsson, G., Bohman, M. (1989) 'A twin study of autism in Denmark, Finland, Ireland, Norway and Sweden.' *Journal of Child Psychology and Psychiatry*, **3**, 405–416.

Steffenburg, S., Gillberg, C., Steffenburg, U., Kyllerman, M. (1996) 'Autism in Angelman syndrome. A population-based study.' *Developmental Medicine and Child Neurology*, **38**, 131–136.

Sulumar, S., Wang, S., Hoang, K., Vanchiere, C.M., England, K., Fick, R., Pagon, B., Reddy, K.S. (1999) 'Subtle overlapping deletions in the terminal region of chromosome 6q24.2–q26: three cases studied using FISH.' *American Journal of Medical Genetics*, **87**, 17–22.

Sun, Y., Rubinstein, J., Soukup, S., Palmer, C.G. (1995) 'Marker chromosome 21 identified by microdissection and FISH.' *American Journal of Medical Genetics*, **56**, 151–154.

Sutherland, G.R. (1977) 'Fragile sites on human chromosomes: demonstration of their dependence on the type of tissue culture medium.' *Science*, **197**, 265–266.

Swillen, A., Hellemans, H., Steyaert, J., Fryns, J.-P. (1996) 'Autism and genetics: high incidence of specific genetic syndromes in 21 autistic adolescents and adults living in two residential homes in Belgium.' *American Journal of Medical Genetics (Neuropsychiatric Genetics)*, **67**, 315–316.

Szatmari, P., Jones, M.B., Holden, J., Bryson, S., Mahoney, W., Tuff, L., MacLean, J., White, B., Bartolucci, G., Schutz, C., Robinson, P., Hoult, L. (1996) 'High phenotypic correlations among siblings with autism and pervasive developmental disorders.' *American Journal of Medical Genetics*, **67**, 354–360.

Szatmari, P., Jones, M.B., Zwaigenbaum, L., MacLean, J.E. (1998) 'Genetics of autism: overview and new directions.' *Journal of Autism and Developmental Disorders*, **28**, 351–368.

Telvi, L., Lebbar, A., Del Pino, O., Barbet, J.P., Chaussain, J.L. (1999) '45X/45,XY mosaicism: report of 27 cases.' *Pediatrics*, **104**, 304–308.

Thomas, N.S., Sharp, A.J., Browne, C.E., Skuse, D., Hardie, C., Dennis, N.R. (1999) 'Xp deletions associated with autism in three females.' *Human Genetics*, **104**, 43–48.

Tsao, C.Y., Luquette, M., Rusin, J.A., Herr, G.M., Kien, C.L., Morrow, G. 3rd (1997) 'Leigh syndrome, cytochrome C oxidase deficiency and hypsarrhythmia with infantile spasms.' *Clinical Electroencephalography*, **28**, 214–217.

Turner, B., Jennings, A.N. (1961) 'Trisomy for chromosome 22.' *Lancet*, **2**, 49–50.

van Slegtenhorst, M., de Hoogt, R., Hermans, C., Nellist, M., Janssen, B., Verhoef, S., Lindhout, D., van den Ouweland, A., Halley, D., Young, J., Burley, M., Jeremiah, S., Woodward, K., Nahmias, J., Fox, M., Ekong, R., Osborne, J., Wolfe, J., Povey, S., Snell, R.G., Cheadle, J.P., Jones, A.C., Tachataki, M., Ravine, D., Sampson, J., Reeve, M., Richardson, P., Wilmer, F., Munro, C., Hawkins, T., Sepp, T., Ali, J., Ward, S., Green, A., Yates, J., Short, M., Haines, J., Jozwiak, S., Kwiatkowska, J., Henske, E., Kwiatkowski, D. (1997) 'Identification of the tuberous sclerosis gene TSC1 on chromosome 9q34.' *Science*, **277**, 805–808.

Verkerk, A.J., Pieretti, M., Sutcliffe, J.S., Fu, Y.-H., Kuhl, D.P., Pizzuti, A., Reiner, O., Richards, S., Victoria, M.F., Fuping Zhang, M.F.V., Eussen, B.E., van Ommen, G.J.B., Blonden, L.A.J., Riggins, G.J., Chastain, J.L., Kunst, C.B., Galjaard, H., Caskey, C.T., Nelson, D.L., Oostra, B.A., Warren, S.T. (1991) 'Identification of a gene (FMR-1) containing CGG repeat coincident with a breakpoint cluster region exhibiting length variation in fragile X syndrome.' *Cell*, **65**, 905–914.

Volkmar, F., Klin, A., Pauls, D. (1998) 'Nosological and genetics aspects of Asperger syndrome.' *Journal of Autism and Developmental Disorders*, **28**, 457–463.

Vostanis, P., Harrington, R., Prendergast, M., Farndon, P. (1994) 'Case reports of autism with interstitial deletion of chromosome 17 (p11.2p11.2) and monosomy of chromosome 5 (5pter→5p15.3).' *Psychiatric Genetics*, **4**, 109–111.

Wang, C.H., Villaca-Norat, E., Papendick, B.D., Gavrilov, D., Hillman, R., Miles, J. (1998) 'Molecular analysis of the chromosome 15q11-13 region in children with autism.' (Abstract) *Annals of Neurology*, **44**, 546.

Warren, R.P., Singh, V.K. (1996) 'Elevated serotonin levels in autism: association with the major histocompatibility complex.' *Neuropsychobiology*, **34**, 72–75.

Warren, R.P., Burger, R.A., Odell, D., Torres, A.R., Warren, W.L. (1994) 'Decreased plasma concentration of the C4B complement protein in autism.' *Archives of Pediatric and Adolescent Medicine*, **148**, 180–183.

Weidmer-Mikhail, E., Sheldon, S., Ghaziuddin, M. (1998) 'Chromosomes in autism and related pervasive developmental disorders: a cytogenetic study.' *Journal of Intellectual Disability Research*, **42**, 8–12.

Wenger, S.L., Steele, M.W., Becker, D.J., (1988) 'Clinical consequences of deletion 1p35.' (Published erratum appears in *Journal of Medical Genetics* (1992) **2**, 141.) *Journal of Medical Genetics*, **26**, 62–63.

Wilcox, J. (1998) 'Autism associated with chromosome 22.' (Abstract) *American Journal of Medical Genetics*, **81**, 482.

Wilkins, L.E., Brown, J.A., Nance, W.E., Wolfe, B. (1983) 'Clinical heterogeneity in 80 home-reared children with the Cri-du-chat syndrome.' *Journal of Pediatrics*, **103**, 528–533.

Wilson, G.N., Al Saadi, A.A. (1989) 'Obesity and abnormal behavior associated with interstitial deletion of chromosome 18 (q12,2–q21,1).' *Journal of Medical Genetics*, **26**, 62–63.

Wolraich, M., Bzostek, B., Neu, R.L., Gardner, L.I. (1970) 'Lack of chromosome aberrations in autism.' (Letter) *New England Journal of Medicine*, **283**, 1231.

Woo, S.L.C. (1988) 'Collation of RFLP haplotypes at the human phenylalanine hydroxylase (PAH) locus.' *American Journal of Human Genetics*, **43**, 781–783.

16
THE FIRST NEUROPSYCHIATRIC ASSESSMENT

Autism is not a diagnosis; it is a behavioral syndrome of many etiologies. Every child with an autistic syndrome is entitled to a full medical assessment leading to a diagnosis of a specific disease, if possible. The likelihood that a medical diagnosis can be made in a child with autism is no longer remote. This chapter reviews the examination and diagnostic aids to be considered during a medical assessment. The rational approach to selecting treatment is always to begin with an accurate diagnosis.

One important point needs to be emphasized. *It is not enough to talk to the parents and only glance at the child.* Each child with autism is entitled to a one-time comprehensive physical and neurological examination as well as a structured period of behavioral observation. Also, it is important to be alert to general medical conditions, such as abdominal pain, that might be revealed during the examination in these children, whose communication skills are so inadequate.

The examination

History, Including Medical Records and Family History

Family history and gestational history are elementary in evaluating a child with autism. The role of genetics in many cases of autism is becoming increasingly apparent (see Chapter 15). As the malformations of cortical development are now better understood (see Chapter 14), obtaining gestational history is necessary. A most vital bit of information is the age of onset of the initial symptoms. A number of diagnostic instruments are now available to structure the traditional parent interview.

Psychiatric Assessment – see Chapter 2.

Physical Examination

A conscientious physician needs to examine the child in detail in order to reach an accurate diagnosis (Skjeldal *et al.* 1998). This may involve difficult maneuvers, such as placing the cranial circumference tape around the head – often an area of marked haptic defensiveness. Although many children with autism are described as non-stigmatized and exceptionally beautiful, minor physical stigmata have been described in large numbers of children with autism, including hypertelorism, abnormalities of the ears, and partial syndactyly of the second and third toes (Walker 1976, Campbell *et al.* 1978). Some children have more major stigmata. A photograph of the child's face and any other stigmata is indicated. There is now a great deal of information available regarding the meaning of specific stigmata found in a child with autism, as outlined in the Diagnostic Aids below.

When evaluating a child with autism, a Woods lamp should be available for examining skin lesions (and, if positive, the accompanying parents should immediately also be examined, since these disease entities are usually autosomal dominant). Do not forget to look for self-induced abrasions.

NEUROLOGICAL EXAMINATION

Neurological examinations can be very informative in children with autism (Haas *et al.* 1996). Note the level of tactile defensiveness, not only because it is related to certain behaviors and stereotypies (Baranek *et al.* 1997), but also because it can help in planning the order and depth of the examination. In these haptically defensive children, observation is an important skill to cultivate. Difficulties with posture, gait, balance and spontaneous adventitious movements, stereotypies and dyspraxias can be observed and recorded. There should be follow-up formal testing, if possible. Although the great majority of children with autism walk by 18 months (Kokubun *et al.* 1996), hypotonia should be evaluated in those with late walking. Stereotypies – those patterned, repetitive, purpose-less movements performed the same way each time – should ideally be recorded on video. Reflex examination may disclose either immaturity or pathology. The cranial nerve examination, so important in autism, is difficult to complete without a cooperative child. Also, few children with autism will participate in an adequate sensory examination. In speaking children, the content and characteristics of the speech and language should be noted. Ophthalmological and auditory examinations may be part of the examination or may be referred to specialists; they are of value both for diagnosis and for correcting impediments to learning (Rosenhall *et al.* 1999).

NEUROPSYCHOLOGICAL TESTING

This is a standard part of the evaluation of any child with autism (Chapter 9). It can pick up many subtle deficits that are not always obvious. It should be performed by a clinical psychologist with experience in testing (often resistant) children with autism. It is of value both medically and for planning an individual educational program for the child.

LABORATORY TESTING

If a diagnosis has not been reached on completion of the history, medical examinations and neuropsychological stages of the assessment, laboratory testing is indicated. This is the first level of testing:

Blood tests:
- CBC
- chromosomal karyotyping, including fragile X testing
- lead level
- magnesium
- phenylalanine
- pyruvic acid, lactic acid
- serotonin

263

24-hour urine:
- uric acid
- calcium/phosphorus
- creatinine (to monitor accuracy of 24-hour urine)

Sleep electroencephalogram (EEG)
Imaging study
Ophthalmological and auditory testing, if not already done
(Rosenhall *et al.* 1999)

Baseline laboratory testing may guide additional testing. For example, if an imaging study reveals pontocerebellar hypoplasia or progressive cerebellar atrophy, this should initiate an extensive search for hereditary neurometabolic or neurodegenerative conditions (Ramaekers *et al.* 1997). The current emphasis on cost containment indicates that appropriate criteria are needed for the performance of additional specialized tests.

We claim no uniqueness; there are other fine approaches to this assessment (*e.g.* Adrien *et al.* 1989, Part Two of Barthélémy *et al.* 1998/1995, Volkmar *et al.* 1999, Filipek *et al.* 1999).

DIAGNOSTIC AIDS

History
Onset of autistic regression at 18 months or earlier after apparently normal development
- Epilepsy
- Infantile autistic bipolar disorder
- Peroxisomal disorders
- Rett syndrome
- Zappella dysmaturational subgroup with familial complex tics

Signs – general
Short stature
- Chromosomal aberrations
- Noonan syndrome
- Rett syndrome
- Smith–Magenis syndrome
- Williams syndrome

Obesity
- Chromosomal aberrations
- Cohen syndrome

Macrocephaly
- Minor hydrocephalus
- Sotos syndrome

Characteristic facies (often mildly dysmorphic)
- Cohen syndrome
- De Lange syndrome

264

- Fetal alcohol syndrome
- Fragile X syndrome
- Lujan–Fryns syndrome
- Mucopolysaccharidosis
- Noonan syndrome
- Smith–Magenis syndrome
- Sotos syndrome
- Williams syndrome

Skin lesions:
>   *Hypopigmented spots, streaks or whorls*
- Hypomelanosis of Ito
>   *Sebaceous adenoma on the face*
- Tuberous sclerosis
>   *>6 café-au-lait spots*
- Neurofibromatosis 1
>   *Skinfold freckling*
- Neurofibromatosis 1

Unusual or anomalous ears
- Fragile X syndrome
- Goldenhar syndrome

Thick, protruding tongue
- Hypothyroidism
- Joubert syndrome

Visual impairment or blindness
- Leber's hereditary optic neuropathy
- Morning glory syndrome
- Peroxisomal disorders
- Retrolental fibroplasia
- ROP

Hearing impairment or deafness
- Congenital rubella
- Peroxisomal disorders

Voice:
>   *Hoarse cry/voice*
- Hypothyroidism
- Lujan–Fryns syndrome
>   *Shrill, high-pitched in infancy*
- Chromosomal aberrations, especially cri-du-chat

Macroorchidism
- Fragile X syndrome

Symptoms – general
>   *Diarrhea*

- Autism/Steatorrhea syndrome
  Constipation
- Purine autism
  Urinary sediment – pink/orange
- Purine autism

Symptoms – neurological
Infantile spasms
- Cytochrome c oxidase deficiency
- Malformations of cortical development
- Tuberous sclerosis
Other forms of epilepsy
- Angelman syndrome
- Fragile X syndrome
- PKU autism
- Purine autism
- Rett syndrome
- Sanfilippo syndrome
- Tuberous sclerosis
Inappropriate laughter
- Angelman syndrome
- Rett syndrome

Signs – neurological
Hypotonia in infancy
- Cohen syndrome
- Fragile X syndrome
- Joubert syndrome
- Peroxisomal disorders
- Purine autism
- Rett syndrome
Facial diplegia
- Moebius syndrome
- Myotonic dystrophy
Ataxia
- Angelman syndrome
- Joubert syndrome
- Rett syndrome
Tics
- Tourette syndrome
- Zappella dysmaturational subgroup
- Side-effects of neuroleptic drugs
Hand-wringing
- Rett syndrome

- Terminal deletion on chromosome 1q

Respiratory difficulties of central origin
- Joubert syndrome
- Rett syndrome

Self-mutilation
- Chromosomal disorders
- Hypocalcinuria
- Purine autism
- Smith–Magenis syndrome

Follow-up of laboratory abnormalities

Neutropenia
- Cohen syndrome

Lactic acidosis
- Malformations of cortical development
- Mitochondrial disorders

Serotonin:
  Low
- PKU autism
- De Lange syndrome
- Depression/ADD
  High
- Infant hypothyroidism
- Maternal rubella
- Tuberous sclerosis
- Williams syndrome
- Idiopathic

Increased uric acid in urine
- Bratton-Marshal test for adenylosuccinase deficiency (Jaeken *et al.* 1988)

Abnormal retinograms
- Cohen syndrome
- Peroxisomal disorders

Imaging abnormalities:

Malformations of cortical development (includes neuronal migration defects)
- Fetal alcohol syndrome
- Ganglioglioma
- Neurofibromatosis 1
- Peroxisomal disorders
- Tuberous sclerosis
  Cerebellar structural defects
- De Lange syndrome
- Fragile X syndrome
- Gestational cytomegalovirus infection

- Hypomelanosis of Ito
- Joubert syndrome
- Peroxisomal disorders
- Purine autism
- Smith–Magenis syndrome

REFERENCES

Adrien, J.L., Barthélémy, C., Lelord, G., Muh, J.P. (1989) 'Use of bioclinical markers for the assessment and treatment of children with pervasive developmental disorders.' *Neuropsychology*, **22**, 117–124.

Baranek, G.T., Foster, L.G., Berkson, G. (1997) 'Tactile defensiveness and stereotyped behaviors.' *American Journal of Occupational Therapy*, **51**, 91–95.

Barthélémy, C., Hameury, L., Lelord, G. (1998 – English version; 1995 – French version) *Infantile Autism: Exchange and Development Therapy/L'Autisme de l'enfant: La thérapie d'échange et de développement*. Paris: Expansion Scientifique Publications.

Campbell, M., Geller, B., Small, A.M., Petti, T.A., Ferris, S.H. (1978) 'Minor physical anomalies in young psychotic children.' *American Journal of Psychiatry*, **135**, 573–575.

Filipek, P.A., Accardo, P.J., Baranek, G.T., Cook, E.H. Jr., Dawson, G., Gordon, B., Gravel, J.S., Johnson, C.P., Kallen, R.J., Levy, S.E., Minshew, N.J., Prizant, B.M., Rapin, I., Rogers, S.J., Stone, W.L., Teplin, S., Tuchman, R.F., Volkmar, F.R. (1999) 'The screening and diagnosis of autistic spectrum disorders.' *Journal of Autism and Developmental Disorders*, **29**, 439–484.

Haas, R.H., Townsend, J., Courchesne, E., Lincoln, A.J., Schreibman, L., Yeung-Courchesne, R. (1996) 'Neurologic abnormalities in infantile autism.' *Journal of Child Neurology*, **11**, 84–92.

Jaeken, J., Wadman, S.K., Duran, M., van Sprang, F.J., Beemer, F.A., Holl, R.A., Theunissen, P.M., de Cock, P., van den Berghe, G., Vincent, M.F. *et al.* (1988) 'Adenylsuccinase deficiency: an inborn error of purine nucleotide synthesis.' *European Journal of Pediatrics*, **148**, 126–131.

Kokubun, M., Haishi, K., Okuzumi, H., Hosobuchi, T. (1996) 'Factors affecting age of walking by children with mental retardation.' *Perceptual and Motor Skills*, **80**, 547–552.

Ramaekers, V.Th., Heimann, G., Reul, J., Thron, A., Jaeken, J. (1997) 'Genetic disorders and cerebellar structural abnormalities in childhood.' *Brain*, **120**, 1739–1751.

Rosenhall, U., Nordin, V., Sandstrom, M., Ahlsen, G., Gillberg, C. (1999) 'Autism and hearing loss.' *Journal of Autism and Developmental Disorders*, **29**, 349–357.

Skjeldal, O.H., Sponheim, E., Ganes, T., Jellum, E., Bakke, S. (1998) 'Childhood autism: the need for physical investigations.' *Brain Development*, **20**, 227–233.

Volkmar, F., Cook, E.H. Jr., Pomeroy, J., Realmuto, G., Tanguay, P. (1999) 'Practice parameters for the assessment and treatment of children, adolescents and adults with autism and other pervasive developmental disorders. American Academy of Child and Adolescent Psychiatry Working Group on Quality Issues.' *Journal of the American Academy of Child and Adolescent Psychiatry*, **38** (suppl. 12), 32S–54S.

Walker, H. (1976) 'The incidence of minor physical anomalies in autistic children.' *In:* Coleman, M. (Ed.) *The Autistic Syndromes*. Amsterdam: North-Holland, pp. 95–116.

17
MEDICAL THERAPIES

Medical therapies in the autistic syndrome are a subject fraught with difficulty. Accurate evaluation of medical therapies throughout medicine has its limitations because of the difficulty of quantifying the effects of treatments on volatile human beings. The studies are plagued by the placebo effect and a number of other possible misinterpretations due to lack of randomness, inappropriate or imprecise instrumentation, small samples or attrition of participants, statistical regression toward the mean, absence of long-term follow-up, etc. It is not unusual for well-designed studies from excellent medical centers to disagree with each other.

In the case of treatment studies in the behavioral syndrome of autism, there are all the usual culprits compounded by additional ones. A major extra problem is the fact that any behavior measurement is inevitably greatly affected by what actually happens in real life each day to a child with an extraordinarily tuned sensory system. Also, that child is growing up, maturing and changing while the evaluation of the therapy is underway. Another problem is that the medicines are rarely targeted to specific diseases or identified subgroups of patients with autism; they may be tried out on any child who happens to meet a predetermined diagnostic criterion of autism. Under these circumstances, in spite of the careful research designs, with elaborate statistics, in the many studies discussed in this chapter, the results of the evaluations of medical treatments described here would probably be most accurately described as "best guesses."

To our knowledge, there is no established medical treatment that cures any group of patients with autism, with the exception of the PKU diet started at under 6 weeks of age in children who would otherwise develop PKU autism (see Chapter 11). In a study in England, Grafton *et al.* (1998) found that it was the diagnosis of autism, rather than the specific behavior of the child, that often led to trials of antipsychotic medication; this conclusion was reached by comparing autism to conduct disorder – which also has aggression and destructive behavior. Tsai (1999) has written an excellent summary of psychopharmacological research and indications in autism.

There are medical therapies that are reported to be likely to improve the clinical dysfunctions of autism in particular children. These medical therapies of the autistic syndrome fall into three categories. First, wherever possible, is the ideal therapy of actually treating the basic disease process itself which is causing the symptoms of autism – targeting the specific place in the metabolic pathway, etc. This would involve research treatments for the disease entities discussed in Chapter 10. (Any medical therapies available for double syndrome patients are already listed in Chapter 11.) A second approach to medical therapy involves treatment of symptom complexes not specific to, but found within, the autistic syndrome – such as treatment of sleep disorders or hyperactivity.

These are the symptomatic treatments. Finally, there are the non-specific therapies that attempt to treat the core symptoms of the overall syndrome that we call autism, when it is not further defined. In the non-specific therapies, although the drugs are classified by a particular mode of action, it needs to be noted that the full impact of each drug on the brain usually involves other metabolic pathways and is often far from being well understood.

Specific therapies
Infantile Autistic Bipolar Disorders (IABD)
Patients with IABD are candidates for a trial of anti-depressants, with careful attention to dose based on considerations of the weight of the child. There are several classes of pharmacological agents used for depression in adults. Since the tricyclic anti-depressant, imipramine, lowers the seizure threshold (Campbell *et al.* 1971), tricyclics have not been a popular choice in patients with autism. (The relatively new tricyclic drug, clomipramine, is discussed later in this chapter.) There is some preliminary evidence that anti-depressants that inhibit the CNS neuronal uptake of serotonin – another class of pharmacological agents – may be of great value to some of the patients with IABD.

DeLong, who identified and named the IABD group, performed an open trial of a serotonin reuptake inhibitor, fluoxetine, with a group of colleagues (DeLong *et al.* 1998). They studied 37 children whose subgroup of autism had not been identified. The dose of fluoxetine was quite varied, from as low as 0.2 mg/kg/day up to 1.4 mg/kg/day. They reported that 11 children had an excellent response, another 11 had some improvement but remained definitely autistic, and 15 did not improve or worsened, developing hyper-activity, agitation or lethargy. The excellent responders showed behavioral, affective, language and cognitive improvements and were able to attend mainstream classrooms. Nearly all of the children were receiving other therapies, including other drugs and behavior modification. For those children for whom fluoxetine was effective, its effects surpassed those of other treatment modalities. The researchers attempted to withdraw the drug in all but one case and found that discontinuation of successful treatment nearly always resulted in prompt regression. The positive response to fluoxetine correlated with a family history of major affective disorder; of 21 subjects with a family history of major affective disorder (bipolar or unipolar), 18 had a positive response to fluoxetine, and 8 of these were in the group that had excellent results. (Additional studies on serotonin reuptake inhibitors are described later in this chapter.)

Lithium is also a drug to be considered in the IABD group if the family history contains individuals with cycling, bipolar patterns. Studies of lithium carbonate in autism started as early as 1972 and are still continuing intermittently as patients are selected for this therapy (Gram and Rafaelsen 1972, Kerbeshian *et al.* 1987, Steingard and Biederman 1987). Other therapies that can be tried include other mood stabilizers, carbamazepine and valproic acid. Also, buspirone or risperadol sometimes have important benefits.

The ability, after pharmacological intervention, to function in mainstream classes is becoming a reality for some regular or mildly retarded children in this group of patients.

The Dysmaturational Subgroup with Familial Complex Tics

This group of children is responsive to a special therapy. The therapy is based on guiding parents and teachers – in a nursery school for normal children – to interact with the child along the lines of interactional development, with emphasis on the bodily interactions which occur in the first year of life, and on raising the mood of the child and his parents. Also, the child is guided to acquire new abilities with the help of developmental tables of milestones. This therapy, "Motor Activation with Reciprocal Body Interactions," is described by Zappella (1996). Adjunct speech therapy is often indicated. If a young child with autism belongs to this subgroup, he should remain in a normal nursery school, follow the above-mentioned therapeutic approach, and avoid the usual, rigid programs that are usually so helpful to children with other forms of autism.

With the help of the Zappella program, the ability to function in mainstream classes is often a reality for this group of boys.

Purine Autism

Patients with purine autism, no matter whether their metabolic error produces *hypo*uricosuria or *hyperuricosuria*, often appear to have some amelioration of their behavioral and

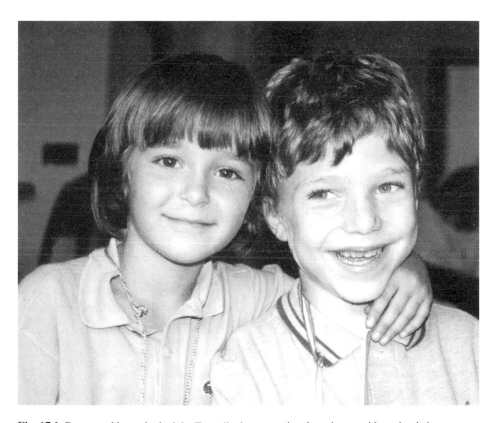

Fig. 17.1 Recovered boy who had the Zappella dysmaturational syndrome with a school chum.

271

seizure symptoms by following a restricted purine diet (Bartels 1943, Landgrebe 1976) (information on the diet is available on the internet at http://www2.dgsys.coml~purinel). Approximately one-fifth of all purines metabolized in the body come directly from the diet. However, even if the diet is helpful, it is not curative. In metabolic disease, a specific way of compensating for the individual enzyme errors must be found. It should be noted that full diets cannot be evaluated by even a pretense of any blindness in a research study. Thus the available open crossover data studying any diet therapy, such as the restricted purine diet in purine autism (Coleman 1989), remains wide open to placebo interpretation.

One hyperuricouric patient with autism who had an unusually good response to the diet was a girl whose first symptom was haptic defensiveness (she could not be touched) as a newborn; she had many classic symptoms of autism (Coleman 1989). She was placed on the restricted purine diet at 5 years of age, with the parents agreeing to an ABAB treatment protocol, a research design with two open crossovers off the diet. However, an attempt at crossover, with the child eating a normal diet after one year on the diet, had to be cut short after three days due to major clinical deterioration; then the parents adamantly refused the second crossover. The young woman is now a college student. Recently she wrote "When I started the purine diet, it was like lifting a glass jar off of me. All the things that I had missed for five years, like the smell of perfume, the sound of a bird and knowing what a smile was."

In addition to the diet, a trial of oral D-ribose has been conducted in a patient with the ASL deficiency form of purine autism (Salerno *et al.* in press). There was progressive reduction of seizures, which increased again each time following two attempts at crossover. Allopurinol can also be tried as an anticonvulsant in patients with purine disorders (Coleman *et al.* 1986) and severe epilepsy (De Marco and Zagnoni 1988). The first trial of iridine therapy for patients with 5′-nucleotidase elevation was described as successful (Page *et al.* 1997).

AUTISM/STEATORRHEA SYNDROME

The pathophysiology of autism/steatorrhea has not yet been worked out, making it difficult to design specific treatment approaches for this group of children. Horvath *et al.* (1998) issued a report about three children with autism who underwent upper gastrointestinal endoscopy and intravenous administration of secretin to stimulate pancreaticobiliary secretory response; all three had an increased pancreaticobiliary secretory response when compared with non-autistic patients (7.5 to 10 mL/min vs. 1 to 2 mL/min.) The authors reported that, within five weeks of the secretin administration, a significant amelioration of the children's gastrointestinal symptoms was observed. The authors also reported improved eye contact, alertness and expansion of expressive language in the three children. A total reversal of all autistic symptoms was not claimed. Reports not yet published also note that elevated blood levels of serotonin in at least one of the children were lowered into the normal range by the secretin treatment. However, a more recent, large-scale controlled study failed to demonstrate significant positive effects of secretin treatment in autism (Sandler *et al.* 1999).

Secretin is a drug developed originally for use in gastrointestinal testing, a gastrointestinal peptide hormone whose primary action is to increase the volume and bicarbonate content of secreted pancreatic juices. A secretin challenge test is used to identify pancreatic disease. It should also be noted that secretin and secretin receptors have been identified in the brain of a mammal (the rat). It has been suggested that one possible explanation for the improvement noted by some parents may be a diminution of chronic gastrointestinal pain and diarrhea, which allows a child to be more externally focused (Horvath *et al.* 1999).

For good historical reasons, the medical community insists on a double-blind, cross-over study before any therapy can be recommended. A few such studies of secretin have been published (Chez *et al.* 1999, Owley *et al.* 1999, Sandler *et al.* 1999). To date these studies generally have overall negative results; all studied children with autism in general and did not limit the studies to a selected subgroup with steatorrhea. One double-blind, placebo-controlled study on 60 children with autism who have not yet received a specific diagnosis showed no evidence of effectiveness and a significant placebo effect (Sandler *et al.* 1999). Also, in developing a therapy, it is best to understand the mechanism of how secretin, or a peptide similar to it, works. It is important to note that, if this therapy turns out of be of value for a subgroup of patients with one type of autism, there are sure to be side effects (as is true in all effective therapies). These side-effects will be more likely to show up if the therapy is given to a child with a different diagnosis – that is, a child with a subgroup of autism which is not autism/steatorrhea. At present, professionals are divided on the value of secretin as a therapy, calling it "snake oil" (Herlihy 2000) or urging caution regarding early negative results (Gordon 2000).

There is a medical hypothesis that another drug related to the gastrointestinal tract – a histamine-2-receptor blocker called famotidine, which has been reported to possibly be helpful with the deficit (withdrawal) symptoms of schizophrenia – might be useful for the treatment of autism (Linday 1997).

DIET RESPONSIVE AUTISM?
Finally, under the topic of specific therapies, this chapter would not be complete without addressing the question of whether such a thing as *diet responsive autism* exists. The question stays alive, in spite of skepticism, because of studies such as the one by D'Eufemia *et al.* (1996) showing abnormal intestinal permeability in a subgroup of children with autism. These authors reported altered intestinal permeability in 9 out of 21 (43 per cent) patients with autism but none in 40 controls.

Most of the work regarding possible diet responsive autism has focused on two types of foods: milk and wheat products. In 1987, a nurse wrote a popular book telling the story of her son whose autism responded to the removal of milk from his diet (Callahan 1987). This was followed by another testimonial (Braffet 1994). There is evidence of elevated levels of antibodies to some components of milk, particularly casein, in some children with autism, and unusual immunoreactivity in brain areas in rats (Sun *et al.* 1999). Lucarelli *et al.* (1995) have reported higher levels of IgA-specific antibodies for casein, lactalbumin, and beta-lactoglobulin, IgG and IgM-specific for casein in autistic patients compared to findings in controls. These findings led to an open trial of a diet eliminating milk at the University of Rome; that study reported a marked improvement in behavioral symptoms of some patients with infantile autism after a period of 8 weeks (Lucarelli *et al.* 1995). All this raises more questions than it answers. It is necessary to perform crossover studies on such children. Of course, it is extremely challenging to design actual blind studies regarding changes in diet in the exquisitely taste-sensitive children with autism.

As a result of the Callahan book, a number of parents, perhaps understandably, have withheld dairy products (a major source of calcium) from their child, feeling that this is something within their own control that they could do that might help their child. This is happening even though physicians generally have advised parents that the concept of diet responsive autism remains unproven at this time. This development is worrisome because a significant portion of children with autism have abnormally low levels of calcium in their urine, sometimes idiopathically (see Chapter 13) and sometimes secondary to anti-convulsants (see Chapter 12). These low levels of calcium in children with autism may be associated with abnormal BAERs in the electroencephalogram (Thivierge *et al.* 1990) as well as seizures and ocular self-mutilation (Coleman 1989).

Currently there is interest in another possible type of diet responsive autism, based on the elimination of wheat products from the diet. Known as *celiac disease*, it was first reported by Asperger in 1961 in patients with his syndrome (Asperger 1961). In the Kanner type of autism, the first report was by Goodwin and Goodwin (1969), who des-cribed improvement in both behavior and physical condition in a 6-year-old boy on a wheat-free diet, who then had a relapse when placed on a normal diet (Goodwin *et al.* 1971). Since then, there have been other case reports of children reported to have both autism and celiac disease (Rimland 1972, Sullivan 1975, Reichelt *et al.* 1986, Shattock 1988, Braffet 1994). It has long been known that there is a subgroup of autistic children with gastrointestinal problems presenting with diarrhea and steatorrhea; today they are called the autism/steatorrhea syndrome (see Chapter 10). Because of case reports and information obtained from parents and pediatricians about autistic symptoms worsening on foods containing gluten and gliadin, researchers have undertaken studies to determine if celiac disease might underlie the symptoms of steatorrhea in such children. However, a number of studies – both surveys of children with celiac disease and studies of children with autism, including studies in which the children ingested 20 grams of gluten daily for a month prior to testing – have failed to connect these two syndromes in the same individual (Walker-Smith 1973, McCarthy and Coleman 1979, Pavone *et al.* 1997). Fortunately, gastrointestinal biopsies are no longer needed to make the diagnosis of celiac disease in a child; it can be done by blood tests (IgA and IgG antigliadin antibodies; endomysium-specific antibodies (Pavone *et al.* 1997)).

Therapy of symptom complexes within autism
In patients who meet the criteria of an autistic syndrome, often there are symptom complexes that are also seen in other disorders of the central nervous system of children. Although these behaviors are not unique to autism, some of them may often be a troubling part of the clinical management of the person with autism. Discussion of therapeutic management of these problems, where not previously discussed in Chapter 7, is included here.

Hyperactivity/Attention Deficit Disorder

Children with an autistic syndrome have been described with both hypoactivity and hyperactivity. The hyperactivity seen in children with autism may be part of a pattern of hyperarousal behaviors, such as hyperactivity, hyperviligance, stereotyped body movements and even self-stimulation. The distractibility and poor attention span of some of these children often compound their already serious educational problems. Methylphenidate, a commonly-used drug to improve attention span, has been used in autism. In children with autism, other choices include clonidine and naltrexone.

Clonidine, an alpha2 adrenergic receptor partial agonist, is increasingly being used to treat attention deficit/hyperactivity disorders in a variety of patient groups. There are several studies of clonidine performed in patients with autism. Using a transdermal patch, Fankhauser *et al.* (1992) performed a double-blind placebo crossover study in nine males with autism aged 5 to 33 years. They reported that clonidine was effective in reducing hyperactivity and hypervigilance as well as in improving social relationships. Another double-blind placebo crossover study of clonidine in eight male children, performed by Jaselskis *et al.* (1992), demonstrated only modest improvements in irritability and hyperactivity. Side-effects limiting the use of this drug (McCracken and Martin 1997) include drowsiness and sedation, with bradycardia a danger in the event of overdosage. Another dopamine agonist that, in one study, is reported to help hyperactivity in autism is the old-fashioned drug, bromocriptine (Dollfus *et al.* 1992).

Sleep Disorders

A chronic sleep disorder is often a major problem both for the child with autism and the sleep-deprived parents. Traditional approaches include behavioral therapies and sedatives. Also the histamine H1-receptor antagonist niaprazine is reported to help both the sleep disorder and behavior problems in some subjects with autism (Rossi *et al.* 1999). Abnormalities in circadian rhythm have been demonstrated in children with autism (see Chapter 13). After a child has had a complete medical work-up, which has ruled out any autoimmune disorder, melatonin is another option to consider for a child with a disturbance of the chronic sleep–wake cycle (Lord 1998). An oral dose of fast-release melatonin taken at bedtime may be helpful; side-effects or the development of tolerance are rare (Jan and O'Donnell 1996).

Aggression

One of the most disruptive problems of individuals with autism is aggressive behavior, historically treated by behavioral management combined with neuroleptics, anti-depressants and sedating agents. Beta-blockers, such as propranolol, have been used with success for aggression in some patients with autism; there is a good discussion of their mechanism of action and clinical use in a paper by Haspel (1995). Koshes and Rock (1994) have suggested the use of clonidine in an adult with an intermittent explosive disorder. Hillbrand and Scott (1995) report on the value of buspirone with aggressive behavior.

A newer approach to controlling aggression is the use of risperidone, an atypical neuroleptic drug. Data from a double-blind, placebo-controlled study of adults with autism found that risperidone produces reductions in aggression, repetitive behavior and affective symptoms (Longhurst *et al.* 1997). An open study of eleven male out-patients with autism also showed improvements in aggression as well as in explosivity, self-injury and poor sleep hygiene (Horrigan and Barnhill 1997). In a study of eight adults with mental retardation, half of whom had an autistic syndrome, reduced aggression occurred with the use of risperidone (Cohen *et al.* 1998). However, the reports of improvement are not unanimous. In a study involving a single individual with autism who was part of a larger clinically heterogeneous group of retarded children and adolescents receiving risperidone, Schreier (1998) reports that the autistic child, who had aggressive behavior, did not respond to risperidone; it was noted that this child lacked the affective symptoms seen in the other retarded children who did respond to the drug.

Non-specific therapy for autistic symptoms in general

Is there a drug which might reverse autism? Could there be a drug which would reverse some of the core symptoms of autism regardless of etiology? As of 1995, Cook and Leventhal reported that there were no well-established medications to treat core symptoms. Regarding new drugs, particularly those in the serotonin reuptake inhibitor class, I. Rapin (1997) writes that the SSRIs are "certainly not curative of autism."

Historically, one drug studied with the hope of reversing core symptoms was haloperidol, classified as a dopamine-receptor blocker. When it was systematically studied in autism, haloperidol was shown to be more effective than placebo in decreasing hyperactivity, temper tantrums, irritability and withdrawal (Anderson *et al.* 1989). However, in about 30 per cent of the children on the drug, withdrawal and tardive dyskinesias occurred (Campbell *et al.* 1988). Drugs with similar pharmacology, such as pimozide, also had unacceptable side-effects, such as dystonia, in some children (Ernst *et al.* 1993).

This experience with the dopamine-receptor blocker drugs led to a search for new pharmaceuticals for autism that would not cause major side-effects. Several new classes of drugs are now under investigation to see if they can more safely influence the core symptoms of autism. One class has been characterized as atypical antipsychotics, another class as drugs that especially affect the serotonin receptors.

ATYPICAL ANTIPSYCHOTICS

The benzisoxazole derivatives are a relatively new chemical class of drugs. They are believed to act through dopamine type 2 and serotonin type 2A receptor antagonism, as well as antagonism at other unspecified receptors (PDR 1999). An example that has been tested in patients with autism is risperidone. This drug has been reported to be superior to placebo in reducing the overall behavioral symptoms of autism, as well as repetitive behavior, aggression, anxiety, depression and irritability, in 8 out of 14 adults with autism who participated in a double-blind study for 12 weeks (McDougle *et al.* 1998). In an open study of risperidone – 8 out of 10 boys with autism for 12 weeks (Nicolson *et al.* 1998); and 6 patients with autism for 8 weeks (Findling *et al.* 1997) – the children were reported to have improved ratings as measured by the Clinical Global Impressions scale. Purdon *et al.* (1994) also reported clinical improvement in two patients diagnosed as PPD. Recently there has been evidence that, if risperidone is effective, it may continue to be so for at least two years (Dartnall *et al.* 1999). Risperidone has been used in children as young as 23 months to improve social relatedness and reduce aggression (Posey *et al.* 1999b).

Regarding side-effects of risperidone, the drug has been reported to cause weight gain (Kelly *et al.* 1998), hepatotoxicity (Benazzi 1998) and, alas, tardive dyskinesias (Demb and Nguyen 1999). However, it has also been reported to diminish the severity of tardive dyskinesia induced by other neuroleptics (Khan 1997). A caution to keep in mind is that the combining of risperidone with valproate – a drug often used for seizure control in autism – can result in edema (Sanders and Lehrer 1998). When risperidone is combined with SSRIs, enuresis has been reported (Took and Buck 1996).

Another atypical antipsychotic is clozapine (Buckley and Schulz 1996). Clozapine is a most complicated new drug. It interferes with the binding at the dopamine D1, D2, D3, and D5 receptors and has a high affinity for the D4 receptor. It also acts as an antagonist at adrenergic, cholinergic, histaminergic and serotonergic receptors (PDR 1999). The studies of clozapine in autism are few but raise the question about whether it might be clinically efficacious (Zuddas *et al.* 1996, Toren *et al.* 1998). Potential side-effects are not yet documented in autism.

DRUGS THAT MAY ESPECIALLY AFFECT THE SEROTONIN PATHWAY

An early study of tryptophan loading tests in patients with autism demonstrated improvement in those loading tests when the amount of the vitamin B6 co-factor involved in the tryptophan metabolic pathways was increased (Heeley and Roberts 1966). The hope that drugs affecting serotonin might possibly be a panacea for some children with autism was enhanced when it was found that tryptophan depletion led to a significant worsening of symptoms in 65 per cent of patients with autism, compared to a sham depletion (McDougle *et al.* 1996a). Since the symptoms of individuals with major depression, obsessive-compulsive disorder and panic disorder did not worsen after tryptophan depletion, the result in autism raised the possibility that serotonergic dysfunction might be more central to the pathophysiology of autism than to that of the other psychiatric disorders – even disorders which generally respond to treatment with inhibitors of serotonin uptake (Longhurst *et al.* 1997). However, since up to 99 per cent of tryptophan in the body does not go down the serotonin pathway, a great deal more work is needed to understand these research results and to evaluate whether serotonin abnormalities are specific or non-specific in patients with autism (see Chapter 13).

At the moment, there is a high level of interest in drugs which selectively and powerfully inhibit serotonin transport reuptake (SSRIs or SRIs) resulting in potentiation of serotonergic neurotransmission. Besides the obvious interest that these drugs might help patients with the specific diagnosis of IABD, the hope has been raised that SSRIs might help any individual with autism improve core symptoms. Despite sharing the same principal mechanism of action, SRIs are structurally diverse, with variations in their pharmokinetic profiles. For example, in the case of sertraline, its relative potency for dopamine uptake inhibition differentiates it pharmacologically from other SRIs.

277

Fluoxetine is a racemic mixture of different chiral forms that possess varying profiles; it has a long-acting and pharmacologically active metabolite.

At first there was considerable interest in clomipramine, a tricyclic anti-depressant with SRI properties; the drug is effective in suppressing obsessional behavior. However, in spite of promising early reports (Gordon *et al.* 1993, Brasic *et al.* 1994), there have been studies showing that the drug made some young autistic children worse (Magen 1993, Sanchez *et al.* 1996, Brasic *et al.* 1997b). In adults with the autistic syndrome, there is a concern about side-effects, which balances the evidence of efficacy in some individuals (McDougle *et al.* 1992, Brodkin *et al.* 1997).

One of the symptoms of autism that is most disabling for family life is a child's intolerance of change in routine and environment. Steingard *et al.* (1997) have reported that the SRI drug, sertraline, helped 8 out of 9 patients cope with transition-induced behavioral deterioration in the initial stages of an open-label study. In 6 patients, the good results persisted past 7 months of follow-up. There were minimal side-effects. Four of the children's families were identified as having mood and/or anxiety disorders. In another study (McDougle *et al.* 1998), 42 adults with the autistic syndrome participated in a 12-week, open-label trial of sertraline. Twenty-four (57 per cent) showed significant improvement, primarily in repetitive and aggressive symptoms. Statistically significant changes in measures of social relatedness did not occur in this study. It needs to be noted that double-blind studies in autism are yet to be completed with this drug. Also, the side-effects of sertraline in long-term use are unknown in patients with the autistic syndrome; this is a drug with relatively potent dopamine reuptake inhibition.

Fluoxetine, the SRI drug being tested in IABD, was subject to an open trial by Cook *et al.* (1992). They reported that it led to a significant improvement in 15 out of 23 subjects with an autistic syndrome, as measured by the Clinical Global Impressions ratings of Clinical Severity, but 6 of the 15 developed side-effects which interfered with their function. Fatemi *et al.* (1998) performed a retrospective chart review of seven adolescents and young adults with autism treated with fluoxetine alone or in combination with other medications. In this group of patients some improvement was reported, as measured by the Aberrant Behavior Checklist rating scale, in stereotypy, inappropriate speech, irritability and lethargy. Side-effects included initial appetite suppression, vivid dreams and minor hyperactivity. Fluoxetine has also been suggested for control of obsessive-compulsive behavior in autism (Koshes 1997).

Another SRI drug, fluvoxamine, has been reported to significantly reduce maladaptive behavior, obsessive-compulsive symptoms, and aggression; it was also reported to have improved certain aspects of social relatedness, most notably language use (McDougle *et al.* 1996b). The study with these promising results was a double-blind, placebo-controlled experiment. Fluvoxamine was also used in a single case history of a 20-year-old woman with autism, where severe repetitive behavior was reported to improve dramatically (Harvey and Cooray 1995). There is also a single case report of paroxetine reducing the preoccupations and other behavioral symptoms of a 7-year-old boy with autism (Posey *et al.* 1999a).

In view of the evidence of immune dysfunction in some children with autism (see Chapter 13), the possibility of some kind of immune therapy in the future has been raised (Singh 1997). Nothing is yet established although there is evidence for infection-triggered tics and OCD in children (Perlmutter *et al.* 1999).

VITAMINS

Vitamins – specifically pyridoxine (vitamin B6) and ascorbic acid – have been tried as therapy in patients with autism. Sankar (1979) studied 125 children admitted to a psychiatric ward and found no evidence of a pyridoxine deficiency, even though, in 1966, Heeley and Roberts had reported that pyridoxine improved a tryptophan loading test in children with autism. An open trial of pyridoxine by Bönisch (1968) noted some marked improvements in the patients. Rimland (1974), using multivitamins in an open study, located, by clinical trial and error, a subgroup of children with autism who appeared to respond to pyridoxine, relapse on withdrawal and improve when the vitamin was started again. Attention span and other symptoms improved but no claims were made of a complete reversal of autism. Callaway (1977) also noted clinical improvements. Rimland and his colleagues (1978) then undertook a double-blind crossover evaluation of effectiveness of pharmacological doses of pyridoxine in the previously identified subgroup. In this study they were able to correctly identify 11 out of 15 periods when the children were on either placebo or pyridoxine, using only the behavioral data. In thinking about the Rimland *et al.* (1978) study, it is relevant to remember that the subjects were not chosen at random but had been previously selected as pyridoxine responders out of a larger group of children with autism. What this means remains unresolved because it is still unknown which, if any, are the pyridoxine-dependent diseases within the autistic syndrome, and it is not known how to test for any such putative diseases.

The Rimland *et al.* (1978) study sparked the interest of other investigators. The Lelord group in France added magnesium to all their protocols, as a result of a study by their group (Barthélémy *et al.* 1981) which found that trials of pyridoxine alone or magnesium alone were ineffective in their patient group, compared to the clinical effect of the combination of the two. Magnesium depletion has been noted in patients with autism (see Chapter 13). Researchers began looking for objective ways to document the effect of pyridoxine/magnesium. It has been reported that, in children with autism, pyridoxine may lower elevated levels of homovanillic acid (HVA) (Martineau *et al.* 1988), increase the amplitude of middle latency evoked potentials (Lelord *et al.* 1979), and improve the ability to form cross-modal associations as demonstrated by evoked potential conditioning (Martineau *et al.* 1988). In the 1990s, two studies of autism failed to find a clinical response to pyridoxine/magnesium in both low-dose (Tolbert *et al.* 1993) and high-dose (Findling *et al.* 1997) research designs. It should be noted that, when given over a long-term period in pharmacological doses, pyridoxine may cause side-effects such as a sensory peripheral neuropathy, sun blisters, sound sensitivity, stomach upset, enuresis and irritability (Schaumberg *et al.* 1983, Coleman *et al.* 1985). The irritability, sound sensitivity and enuresis are less of a problem if magnesium is given with the pyridoxine.

Regarding another vitamin, ascorbic acid, only very preliminary data are available. Sankar (1979) studied ascorbic acid levels in 125 children admitted to a psychiatric ward and did not find abnormal values. In 1993, Dolske *et al.* gave a high dose (8 gm/70 kg/day) of ascorbic acid to children with autism in residential placement in a double-blind, placebo-controlled experiment. Based on behaviors rated weekly using the Ritvo-Freeman scale, they reported improvements in both the total score and the sensory motor scores.

Problems with side-effects of drugs

Tardive dyskinesia, an involuntary abnormal movement disorder, is a serious untoward effect of some drugs used in autism, particularly those classified as dopamine-receptor blockers.

Some patients with autism who receive long-term neuroleptic medicines develop what appears to be Tourette syndrome when withdrawn from neuroleptics. Stahl (1980) coined the term "tardive Tourette syndrome" to describe this group. In such cases, it is hard to be sure exactly what is happening – the re-emergence of pre-existing stereotypies or the emergence of new ones, the appearance of the Tourette syndrome at this age or Tourette-like withdrawal dyskinesias. In one such case, where severe dyskinesias including tics developed in the month following discontinuation after at least two years on a dopamine-receptor blocker, the child was helped by another drug, clomipramine (Brasic *et al.* 1997b). It facilitated the gradual diminution of the dyskinesias induced by withdrawal of the original dopamine-receptor blocker drug.

Often these dyskinesias closely resemble the stereotypies of autism, making it difficult to differentiate between what is a baseline symptom and what is a drug-induced dyskinesia. Shay *et al.* (1993) used the Abnormal Involuntary Movement Scale (AIMS) to have observers rate the movement disorders in patients as recorded on videotape. The blind raters could only differentiate drug-induced dyskinesias from baseline stereotypies 59 per cent of the time. However, a discriminant function limited to four items on the AIMS test – Item 1 (muscles of facial expression), Item 2 (lips and perioral area), Item 6 (lower extremities), and Item 7 (neck, shoulders, hips) – correctly classified all 9 children with drug-induced dyskinesia, and 8 out of 9 children with baseline stereotypies.

Occasionally, pharmaceuticals used in autism can cause a most serious problem – neuroleptic malignant syndrome (NMS). The three major manifestations of NMS are fever, rigidity and elevated CK levels. Additional characteristic symptoms include tachycardia, tachypnea, altered consciousness and leukocytosis. Fatalities have been reported.

Proposed new therapies

When one compares the medical therapies proposed in the second edition of this textbook in 1992, it is of interest that many of the drugs described in this chapter in this third edition (2000) are newly described. The turnover is great in an eight-year period. This is a sign of a struggling field of medicine without final answers. Thus it is vital to remain open to new concepts and theoretical proposals regarding pharmacotherapy in autism. One such proposal by a major researcher (Carlsson 1998) has suggested the use of glutamate agonists. It will be fascinating to see what the future brings.

REFERENCES

Anderson, L.T., Campbell, M., Adams, P., Small, A.M., Perry, R., Shell, J. (1989) 'The effects of haloperidol on discrimination learning and behavioral symptoms in autistic children.' *American Journal of Psychiatry*, **141**, 1195–1202.

Asperger, H. (1961) 'Die Psychopathologie des coeliak-iekranken Kindes.' *Annales Paediatriae*, **197**, 146–151.

Bartels, E.C. (1943) 'Successful treatment of gout.' *Annals of Internal Medicine*, **18**, 21–28.

Barthélémy, C., Garreau, B., Leddet, I., Ernouf, D., Muh, J.P., Lelord, G. (1981) 'Behavioral and biological effects of oral magnesium, vitamin B6 and combined magnesium-vitamin B6 administration in autistic children.' *Magnesium Bulletin*, **3**, 150–153.

Benazzi, F. (1998) 'Risperidone-induced hepatotoxicity.' *Pharmacopsychiatry*, **31**, 241.

Bönisch, E. (1968) 'Erfahrungen met Pyrithioxin bei hirgeschädigten Kindern mit autistischen Syndrom.' *Praxis de Kinderpsychologie*, **8**, 308–310.

Braffet, C. (1994) 'No milk, no bread please.' *Autism Society of Indiana Quarterly*, **1**, 7–9.

Brasic, J.R., Barnett, J.Y., Kaplan, D., Sheitman, B.B., Aisemberg, P., Lafargue, R.T., Kowalik, S., Tsaltas, M.O., Young, J.G. (1994) 'Clomipramine ameliorates adventitious movements and compulsions in prepubertal boys with autistic disorder and severe mental retardation.' *Neurology*, **44**, 1309–1312.

Brasic, J.R., Barnett, J.Y., Aisemberg, P., Ahn, S.C., Nadrich, R.H., Kaplan, D., Ahmad, R., Mendonca, M. de F. (1997a) 'Dyskinesias subside off all medication in a boy with autistic disorder and severe mental retardation.' *Psychological Reports*, **81**, 755–767.

Brasic, J.R., Barnett, J.Y., Sheitman, B.B., Tsaltas, M.O. (1997b) 'Adverse effects of clomipramine.' *Journal of the American Academy of Child and Adolescent Psychiatry*, **36**, 1165–1166.

Brodkin, E.S., McDougle, C.J., Naylor, S.T., Cohen, D.J., Price, L.H. (1997) 'Clomipramine in adults with pervasive developmental disorders: a prospective open-label investigation.' *Journal of Child and Adolescent Psychopharmacology*, **7**, 109–121.

Buckley, P.F., Schulz, S.C. (1996) 'Clozapine and risperidone: refining and extending their use.' *Harvard Review of Psychiatry*, **4**, 184–199.

Callahan, M. (1987) *Fighting for Tony*. New York: Simon & Schuster.

Callaway, E. (1977) 'Response of infantile autism to large doses of B6.' *Psychological Bulletin*, **13**, 57–58.

Campbell, M., Fish, B., Shapiro, T., Floyd, A. (1971) 'Study of molindone in disturbed children.' *Current Therapeutic Research*, **13**, 28–33.

Campbell, M., Adams, P., Perry, R., Spencer, E.K., Overall, J.E. (1988) 'Tardive and withdrawal dyskinesia in autistic children: a prospective study.' *Psychopharmacological Bulletin*, **24**, 251–255.

Carlsson, M.L. (1998) 'Hypothesis: is infantile autism a hypoglutamatergic disorder? Relevance of glutamate-serotonin interactions for pharmacotherapy.' *Journal of Neural Transmission*, **105**, 525–535.

Chez, M.G., Hammer, M.S., Bagan, B.T., Buchanan, C.P., McCarthy, K.S., Ovrutskaya, I., Nowinski, C.V., Cohen, Z.S. (1999) 'Secretin used in the treatment of autism: a double-blind clinical trial in children.' (Abstract) *Annals of Neurology*, **46**, 523.

Cohen, S.A., Ihrig, K., Lott, R.S., Kerrick, J.M. (1998) 'Risperidone for aggression and self-injurious behavior.' *Journal of Autism and Developmental Disorders*, **28**, 229–233.

Coleman, M. (1989) 'Autism: non-drug biological treatments.' *In:* Gillberg, C. (Ed.) *Diagnosis and Treatment of Autism*. New York: Plenum Press, pp. 219–235.

Coleman, M., Sobel, S., Bhagavan, H.N., Coursin, D.B., Marquardt, A., Guay, M., Hunt, C. (1985) 'A double blind study of vitamin B6 in Down's syndrome infants. Part I – Clinical and biochemical results.' *Journal of Mental Deficiency Research*, **29**, 233–240.

Coleman, M., Landgrebe, M., Landgrebe, A. (1986) 'Purine seizure disorders.' *Epilepsia*, **23**, 263–269.

Cook, E.H., Leventhal, B.L. (1995) 'Autistic disorder and other pervasive disorders.' *Child and Adolescent Psychiatric Clinics of North America*, **4**, 381–399.

—— (1996) 'The serotonin system in autism.' *Current Opinion in Pediatrics*, **8**, 348–354.

Cook, E.H. Jr., Rowlett, R., Jaselskis, C., Leventhal, B.L. (1992) 'Fluoxetine treatment of children and adults with autistic disorder and mental retardation.' *Journal of American Academy of Child and Adolescent Psychiatry*, **31**, 739–745.

Dartnall, N.A., Holmes, J.P., Morgan, S.N., McDougle, C.J. (1999) 'Brief report: Two-year control of behavioral symptoms with risperidone in two profoundly retarded adults with autism.' *Journal of Autism and Developmental Disorders*, **29**, 87–91.

DeLong, G.R., Teague, L.A., McSwain Kamran, M. (1998) 'Effects of fluoxetine treatment in young children with idiopathic autism.' *Developmental Medicine and Child Neurology*, **40**, 551–562.

De Marco, P., Zagnoni, P. (1988) 'Allopurinol in severe epilepsy.' *Neuropsychobiology*, **19**, 51–53.

Demb, H.B., Nguyen, K.T. (1999) 'Movement disorders in children with developmental disabilities taking risperidone.' *Journal of the American Academy of Child and Adolescent Psychiatry*, **38**, 5–6.

D'Eufemia, P., Celli, M., Finocchiaro, R., Pacifico, L., Viozzi, L., Zaccagnini, M., Cardi, E., Giardini, O. (1996) 'Abnormal intestinal permeability in children with autism.' *Acta Paediatrica*, **85**, 1076–1079.

Dollfus, S., Petit, M., Menard, J.F., Lesieur, P. (1992) 'Amisulpride versus bromocriptine in infantile autism: a controlled crossover comparative study of two drugs with opposite effects on dopaminergic function.' *Journal of Autism and Developmental Disorders*, **22**, 47–60.

Dolske, M.C., Spollen, J., McKay, S., Lancashire, E., Tolbert, L. (1993) 'A preliminary trial of ascorbic acid as supplemental therapy for autism.' *Progress in Neuropsychopharmacology and Biological Psychiatry*, **17**, 765–774.

Ernst, M., Gonzalez, N.M., Campbell, M. (1993) 'Acute dystonic reaction with low-dose pimozide.' *Journal of the American Academy of Child and Adolescent Psychiatry*, **32**, 640–642.

Fankhauser, M.P., Karumanchi, V.C., German, M.L., Yates, A., Karumanchi, S.D. (1992) 'A double-blind, placebo–controlled study of the efficacy of transdermal clonidine in autism.' *Journal of Clinical Psychiatry*, **53**, 77–82.

Fatemi, S.H., Realmuto, G.M., Khan, L., Thuras, P. (1998) 'Fluoxetine in treatment of adolescent patients with autism: a longitudinal open trial.' *Journal of Autism and Developmental Disorders*, **28**, 303–307.

Findling, R.L., Maxwell, K., Scotese-Wojtila, L., Huang, J., Yamashita, T., Wiznitzer, M. (1993) 'High-dose pyridoxine and magnesium administration in children with autistic disorder: an absence of salutary effects in a double-blind, placebo-controlled study.' *Journal of Autism and Developmental Disorders*, **27**, 467–478.

Findling, R.L., Maxwell, K., Wiznitzer, M. (1997) 'An open clinical trial of risperidone monotherapy in young children with autistic disorder.' *Psychopharmacology Bulletin*, **33**, 155–159.

Goodwin, M.S., Goodwin, T.C. (1969) 'In a dark mirror.' *Mental Hygiene*, **53**, 550.

Goodwin, M.S., Cowen, M.A., Goodwin, T.C. (1971) 'Malabsorption and cerebral dysfunction. A multivariate and comparative study of autistic children.' *Journal of Autism and Childhood Schizophrenia*, **1**, 48.

Gordon, C.T., State, R.C., Nelson, J.E., Hamburger, S.D., Rapoport, J.L. (1993) 'A double-blind comparison of clomipramine, despramine and placebo in the treatment of autistic disorder.' *Archives of General Psychiatry*, **50**, 441–447.

Gordon, D. (2000) 'Early negative results not the last word on secretin/autism story.' *Gastroenterology*, **118**, 250.

Grafton, E.J.F., James, D.H., Lindsey, M.P. (1998) 'Antipsychotic medication, psychiatric diagnosis and children with intellectual disability: a 12-year follow-up study.' *Journal of Intellectual Disability*, **42**, 49–57.

Gram, L.F., Rafaelsen, O.J. (1972) 'Lithium treatment of psychiatric children and adolescents; a controlled clinical trial.' *Acta Psychiatrica Scandinavica*, **48**, 253–260.

Harvey, R.J., Cooray, S.E. (1995) 'The effective treatment of severe repetitive behaviour with fluvoxamine in a 20 year old autistic female.' *International Clinical Psychopharmacology*, **10**, 201–203.

Haspel, T. (1995) 'Beta-blockers and the treatment of aggression.' *Harvard Review of Psychiatry*, **2**, 274–281.

Heeley, A.F., Roberts, G.E. (1966) 'A study of tryptophan metabolism in psychotic children.' *Developmental Medicine and Child Neurology*, **8**, 708–718.

Herlihy, W.C. (2000) 'Secretin: cure or snake oil for autism in the new millennium?' *Journal of Pediatric Gastroenterological Nutrition*, **30**, 112–114.

Hillbrand, M., Scott, K. (1995) 'The use of buspirone with aggressive behavior.' *Journal of Autism and Developmental Disorders*, **25**, 663–664.

Horrigan, J.P., Barnhill, L.J. (1997) 'Risperidone and explosive aggressive autism.' *Journal of Autism and Developmental Disorders*, **27**, 313–323.

Horvath, K., Stefanatos, G., Sololski, K.N., Wachtel, R., Nabors, L., Tildon, J.T. (1998) 'Improved social and language skills after secretin administration in patients with autism spectrum disorders.' *Journal of the Association of the Academic Minority Physicians*, **9**, 9–15.

282

Horvath, K., Papadimitriou, J.C., Rabsztyn, A., Drachenberg, C., Tildon, J.T. (1999) 'Gastrointestinal abnormalities in children with autistic disorder.' *Journal of Pediatrics*, **135**, 559–563.

Jan, J.E., O'Donnell, M.E. (1996) 'Use of melatonin in the treatment of paediatric sleep disorders.' *Journal of Pineal Research*, **21**, 193–199.

Jaselskis, C.A., Cook, E.H. Jr., Fletcher, K.E., Leventhal, B.L. (1992) 'Clonidine treatment of hyperactive and impulsive children with autistic disorder.' *Journal of Clinical Psychopharmacology*, **12**, 322–327.

Kelly, D.L., Conley, R.R., Love, R.C., Horn, D.S., Ushchak, C.M. (1998) 'Weight gain in adolescents treated with risperidone and conventional antipsychotics over six months.' *Journal of Child and Adolescent Psychopharmacology*, **8**, 151–159.

Kerbeshian, J., Burd, L., Fisher, W. (1987) 'Lithium carbonate in the treatment of two patients with infantile autism and atypical bipolar symptomatology.' *Journal of Clinical Psychopharmacology*, **7**, 401–405.

Khan, B.U. (1997) 'Brief report: Risperidone for severely disturbed behavior and tardive dyskinesia in developmentally disabled adults.' *Journal of Autism and Developmental Disorder*, **27**, 479–489.

Koshes, R.J. (1997) 'Use of fluoxetine for obsessive-compulsive behavior in adults with autism.' *American Journal of Psychiatry*, **154**, 578.

Koshes, R.J., Rock, N.L. (1994) 'Use of clonidine for behavioral control in an adult patient with autism.' (Letter) *American Journal of Psychiatry*, **151**, 1714.

Landgrebe, M. (1976) Appendix IV-B 'The restricted purine diet.' *In:* Coleman, M. (Ed.) *The Autistic Syndromes*. New York: American Elsevier, pp. 325–327.

Lelord, G., Callaway, E., Muh, J.P., Arlot, J.C., Sauvage, D., Garreau, B., Domenech, J. (1979) 'Electrophysiological and biochemical studies in autistic children treated with vitamin B6.' *In:* Lehmann, D., Callaway, E. (Eds) *Human Evoked Potentials*. New York: Plenum Press.

Linday, L.A. (1997) 'Oral famotidine: a potential treatment for children with autism.' *Medical Hypothesis*, **48**, 381–386

Longhurst, J.G., Potenza, M.N., McDougle, C.J. (1997) 'Autism.' (Letter) *New England Journal of Medicine*, **337**, 1555–1556.

Lord, C. (1998) 'What is melatonin? Is it a useful treatment for the sleep problems of autism?' *Journal of Autism and Developmental Disorders*, **28**, 345–346.

Lucarelli, S., Frediani, T., Zingoni, A.M., Ferruzzi, F., Giardini, O., Quintiere, F., Barbato, M., D'Eufemia, P., Cardi, E. (1995) 'Food allergy and infantile autism.' *Panminerva Medica*, **37**, 137–141.

McCarthy, D.M., Coleman, M. (1979) 'Response of intestinal mucosa to gluten challenge in autistic subjects.' *The Lancet*, **ii**, 877–878.

McCracken, J.T., Martin, W. (1997) 'Clonidine side effect.' *Journal of the American Academy of Child and Adolescent Psychiatry*, **36**, 160–161.

McDougle, C.J., Price, L.H., Volkmar, F.R., Goodman, W.K., Ward-O'Brien, D., Nielsen, J., Bregman, J., Cohen, D.J. (1992) 'Clomipramine in autism: preliminary evidence of efficacy.' *Journal of the American Academy of Child and Adolescent Psychiatry*, **31**, 746–750.

McDougle, C.J., Naylor, S.T., Cohen, D.J., Aghajanian, G.K., Heninger, G.R., Price, L.H. (1996a) 'Effects of tryptophan depletion in drug-free adults with autistic disorder.' *Archives of General Psychiatry*, **53**, 993–1000.

McDougle, C.J., Naylor, S.T., Cohen, D.J., Volkmar, F.R., Heninger, G.R., Price, L.H. (1996b) 'A double-blind, placebo-controlled study of fluvoxamine in adults with autistic disorder.' *Archives of General Psychiatry*, **53**, 1001–1008.

McDougle, C.J., Holmes, J.P., Carlson, D.C., Pelton, G.H., Cohen, D.J., Price, L.H. (1998) 'A double-blind, placebo-controlled study of risperidone in adults with autistic disorder and other pervasive developmental disorders.' *Archives of General Psychiatry*, **55**, 633–641.

Magen, J. (1993) 'Negative results with clomipramine.' *Journal of the American Academy of Child and Adolescent Psychiatry*, **32**, 1079–1080.

Martineau, J., Cheliakine, C., Lelord, G. (1988) 'Brief report: An open middle-term study of combined vitamin B6-magnesium in a subgroup of autistic children selected for their sensitivity to this treatment.' *Journal of Autism and Developmental Disorders*, **3**, 435–447.

Nicolson, R., Awad, G., Sloman, L. (1998) 'An open trial of risperidone in young autistic children.' *Journal of the American Academy of Child and Adolescent Psychiatry*, **37**, 372–376.

Owley, T., Steele, E., Corsello, C., Risi, S., McKaig, K., Lord, C., Leventhal, B.L., Cook, E.H. (1999) 'A double-blind, placebo-controlled trial of secretin for the treatment of autistic disorder.' Medscape

283

General Medicine, October 6. Available online at: http://www.medscape.com/Medscape/General: Medicine/journal/1999/v01.n10/mgm1006.owle/mgm1006.owle-01.html

Page, T., Yu, A., Fontane, J., Nyhan, W.L. (1997) 'Developmental disorder associated with increased cellular nucleotidase activity.' *Proceedings of the National Academy of Sciences*, **94**, 11601–11606.

Pavone, L., Fiumara, A., Bottaro, G., Mazzone, D., Coleman, M. (1997) 'Autism and celiac disease: failure to validate the hypothesis that a link might exist.' *Biological Psychiatry*, **42**, 72–75.

PDR = *Physicians Desk Reference* (1999) Montvale, NJ: Medical Economics Company, Inc.

Perlmutter, S.J., Leitman, S.F., Garvey, M.A., Hamburger, S., Feldman, E., Leonard, H.L., Swedo, S.E. (1999) 'Therapeutic plasma exchange and intravenous immunoglobulin for obsessive-compulsive disorder and tic disorders in childhood.' *Lancet*, **354**, 1153–1158.

Posey, D.J., Litwiller, M., Koburn, A., McDougle, C.J. (1999a) 'Paroxetine in autism.' *Journal of the American Academy of Child and Adolescent Psychiatry*, **38**, 111–112.

Posey, D.J., Walsh, K.H., Wilson, G.A., McDougle, C.J. (1999b) 'Risperidone in the treatment of two very young children with autism.' *Journal of Child and Adolescent Psychopharmacology*, **9**, 273–276.

Purdon, S.E., Lit, W., Labelle, A., Jones, B.D. (1994) 'Risperidone in the treatment of pervasive developmental disorder.' *Canadian Journal of Psychiatry*, **39**, 400–405.

Rapin, I. (1997) 'Autism.' (Letter) *New England Journal of Medicine*, **337**, 1556–1557.

Reichelt, K.L., Sarlid, G., Lindback, T., Boler, J.B. (1986) 'Childhood autism: a complex disorder.' *Biological Psychiatry*, **21**, 1279–1290.

Rimland, B. (1972) 'Progress in research.' *Proceedings of the Fourth Annual Meeting of the National Society for Autistic Children, Washington D.C.*.

—— (1974) 'An orthomolecular study of psychotic children.' *Journal of Orthomolecular Psychiatry*, **3**, 3371–3377.

Rimland, B., Callaway, E., Dreyfus, P. (1978) 'The effects of high doses of vitamin B6 on autistic children: a double-blind crossover study.' *American Journal of Psychiatry*, **135**, 472–475.

Rossi, P.G., Posar, A., Parmeggiani, A., Pipitone, E., D'Agata, M. (1999) 'Niaprazine in the treatment of autistic disorder.' *Journal of Child Neurology*, **14**, 547–550.

Salerno, C., D'Eufemia, P., Finocchiaro, R., Celli, M., Spalice, P., Iannetti, P., Crifo, C., Giardini, O. (1999) 'Effect of D-ribose on purine synthesis and neurological symptoms in a patient with adenylosuccinase deficiency.' *Biochimica et Biophysica Acta*, **1453**, 135–140.

Sanchez, L.E., Campbell, M., Small, A.M., Cueva, J.E., Armenteros, J.L., Adams, P.B. (1996) 'A pilot study of clomipramine in young autistic children.' *Journal of the American Academy of Child and Adolescent Psychiatry*, **35**, 537–544.

Sanders, R.D., Lehrer, D.S. (1998) 'Edema associated with addition of risperidone to valproate treatment.' *Journal of Clinical Psychiatry*, **59**, 689–690.

Sandler, A.D., Sutton, K.A., DeWeese, J., Girardi, M.A., Sheppard, V., Bodfish, J.W. (1999) 'Lack of benefit of a single dose of synthetic human secretin in the treatment of autism and pervasive developmental disorder.' *New England Journal of Medicine*, **341**, 1801–1806.

Sankar, D.V.S. (1979) 'Plasma levels of folates, riboflavin, vitamin B6 and ascorbate in severely disturbed children.' *Journal of Autism and Developmental Disorders*, **9**, 73–82.

Schaumburg, H., Kapla, J., Windebank, A., Nick, N., Rasmus, S., Pleasure, D., Brown, M.J. (1983) 'Sensory neuropathy from pyridoxine abuse.' *New England Journal of Medicine*, **309**, 445–448.

Schreier, H.A. (1998) 'Risperidone for young children with mood disorders and aggressive behavior.' *Journal of Child and Adolescent Psychopharmacology*, **8**, 49–59.

Shattock, P. (1988) 'Autism: possible clues to the underlying etiology. A parent's view.' *In:* Wing, L. (Ed.) *Aspects of Autism*. London: Gaskell, pp. 1–18.

Shay, J., Sanchez, L.E., Cueva, J.E., Armenteros, J.L., Overall, J.E., Campbell, M. (1993) 'Neuroleptic-related dyskinesias and stereotypies in autistic children: videotaped ratings.' *Psychopharmacological Bulletin*, **29**, 359–363.

Singh, V.K. (1997) 'Immunotherapy for brain diseases and mental illnesses.' *Progress in Drug Research*, **48**, 129–146.

Snead, R.W., Boon, F., Presberg, J. (1994) 'Paroxetine for self-injurious behavior.' (Letter) *Journal of the American Academy of Child and Adolescent Psychiatry*, **33**, 909–910.

Stahl, S.M. (1980) 'Tardive Tourette syndrome in an autistic patient after long-term neuroleptic administration.' *American Journal of Psychiatry*, **137**, 1267–1269.

Steingard, R., Biederman, J. (1987) 'Lithium responsive manic-like symptoms in two individuals with autism and mental retardation: case report.' *Journal of the American Academy of Child and Adolescent Psychiatry*, **26**, 932–935.

Steingard, R.J., Zimnitzky, B., DeMaso, D.R., Bauman, M.L., Bucci, J.P. (1997) 'Sertraline treatment of transition-associated anxiety and agitation in children with autistic disorder.' *Journal of Child and Adolescent Psychopharmacology*, **7**, 9–15.

Sullivan, R. (1975) 'Hunches on some biological factors in autism.' *Journal of Autism and Childhood Schizophrenia*, **5**, 177–184.

Sun, Z., Cade, J.R., Fregley, M.J., Privette, R.M. (1999) 'B-casomorphin induces Fos-like immunoreactivity in discrete brain regions relevant to schizophrenia and autism.' *Autism*, **3**, 67–83.

Thivierge, J., Bedard, D., Cote, R., Maziade, M. (1990) 'Brainstem auditory evoked response and subcortical abnormalities in autism.' *American Journal of Psychiatry*, **47**, 1609–1613.

Tolbert, L., Haigler, T., Waits, M.M., Dennis, T. (1993) 'Brief report: Lack of response in an autistic population to a low dose clinical trial of pyridoxine plus magnesium.' *Journal of Autism and Developmental Disorders*, **23**, 193–199.

Took, K.J., Buck, B.J. (1996) 'Enuresis with combined risperidone and SSRI use.' *Journal of the American Academy of Child and Adolescent Psychiatry*, **35**, 840–841.

Toren, P., Laor, N., Weizman, A. (1998) 'Use of atypical neuroleptics in child and adolescent psychiatry.' *Journal of Clinical Psychiatry*, **59**, 644–656.

Tsai, L.Y. (1999) 'Psychopharmacology in autism.' *Psychosomatic Medicine*, **61**, 651–656.

Walker-Smith, J. (1973) 'Gastrointestinal disease and autism – the result of a survey.' *Symposium on Autism, Sidney, Australia*. Abbott Laboratories

Zappella, M. (1996) *Autismo Infantile. Studi sull'affettività e le emozioni*. Roma: La Nuova Italia Scientifica, p. 209.

Zuddas, A., Ledda, M.G., Fratta, A., Muglia, P., Cianchetti, C. (1996) 'Clinical effects of clozapine on autistic disorder.' *American Journal of Psychiatry*, **153**, 738.

18
OTHER INTERVENTIONS

There are a number of non-biological interventions that are used in autism and related disorders. Most of these have been developed within the fields of education, behavior modification and neuropsychology/cognitive psychology. Given that, in some cases, the various biological treatments available are of no, or only limited, value, such interventions are reviewed briefly here, so as better to reflect the "state-of-the-art," when it comes to the most commonly used treatment approaches in autism at the time of going to press with this book.

Impact of diagnosis and information: the psychoeducational approach

The word intervention is sometimes taken to mean "treatment." This is often not appropriate. Treatment should be aimed at a specific problem/dysfunction/pathology which can be positively affected by the treatment; a cure is intended. The typical example is antibiotic treatment of a bacterial infection; cures are often achieved. Treatment in this sense, more often than not, is not yet available in autism. However, this state of affairs is not unique to autism, and, contrary to popular belief, treatment in this sense is not available in the vast majority of problems in any branch of medicine.

Almost all of the disorders within the autism spectrum are severely disabling chronic conditions. In the majority of cases no cures are available to date, and any intervention should be performed in order to improve the situation of the individual and family rather than to cure the underlying disorder.

Diagnosis and information are often major components of good treatment. They always constitute essential elements of intervention.

In general, information about the diagnosis, work-up and implications should be as open and detailed as possible, taking into account the specifics and needs of the individual and his/her family. Optimally, both parents should be present when the information is shared. Written information to supplement the oral communication is usually helpful. A written summary of the diagnostic evaluation should be provided in most cases. Excellent leaflets, booklets and books are available in several different languages on many topics relating to autism spectrum disorders.

Prognosis should be discussed after a diagnosis has been made. This issue should never be treated lightly or in terms of definitive statements. In the individual case, outcome is always unknown, even though there is good statistical evidence to indicate which types of outcome are more and which are less likely. The information should always be based on the most up-to-date review of the outcome literature. There is huge variation in respect of outcome, and this range should be acknowledged. It is essential to take a realistic view. Striking over-optimistic or over-pessimistic attitudes is inappropriate and usually serves to prolong the phase in which a family is trying unsuccessfully to reorient after a period of shock and confusion.

Models for crisis development and intervention are very often hopelessly off key in autism. Shock is rarely a question of a one-time experience in disorders such as autism, disintegrative disorder, and Asperger syndrome. Rather, a slow re-learning process (cognitive and affective), trying to adjust to the situation of having an abnormal or unusual child, is set in motion before, at, or years after initial diagnosis. There is no simple solution to the various problems faced by a family with a disabled child, and no two crises are the same. Thus, it is often grossly inappropriate to speak of the need for crisis psychotherapy. What most parents need in connection with a diagnosis of an autism spectrum disorder is information, empathic support and practical help in arranging financial matters, day-care and respite care, for example.

Parent associations
Parent associations, when knowledgeable and effectively organized, can be exceptionally helpful to families of individuals suffering from autism spectrum disorders, and also to the professionals catering for them within the health care system. There has been a tradition that parents and professionals work separately from each other, both with the goal of providing the best available help to affected children. Slowly, this tradition is breaking down, and we are beginning to see the coming together of parents and professionals, both in areas such as organizing conferences and writing books, and in everyday clinical practice.

In tailoring services to meet the needs of children and adolescents with autism and their families, it is essential to find out just what families need and not to impose interventions that are felt by those closest to the patient to be irrelevant. Thus, whenever considering major changes, improvements or the implementation of new services, relevant parent associations should be consulted.

Support groups of other kinds
Apart from parent associations, there are other support groups, including some autism "institutions." Siblings associations, and associations of individuals with Asperger syndrome (without the "admixture" of parents or siblings) are just a few examples of the kinds of support groups that can be very helpful, albeit for very different purposes.

Changing societal attitudes
One of the most important intervention aspects in the field of autism and related disorders is the changing of societal attitudes to the disorders. This has to be a continuous process, which has to be informed by updated knowledge accumulated in research, clinical practice and results obtained in investigations of attitudes on the part of those affected, their families and carers, and people in the community not affected by autism.

Behavior modification programs
There is a considerable literature on the effects of behavior modification in autism, almost all of which relates to studies that have demonstrated positive results. However, there has also been a great deal of debate as to the actual level of what can be achieved in autism by

using various behavior modification techniques. Ivar Lovaas and his colleagues represent an extreme standpoint in claiming that a very large minority of young children with autism exposed to very intensive behavior modification can actually be "cured" (Lovaas *et al.* 1989). The program he used required at least 40 hours a week of intensive training and involved several full-time employed trainers. It also seems that he included a disproportionate number of relatively high-functioning children who already had some degree of verbal ability in the pre-school age period. Pat Howlin and her colleagues, on the other hand, feel that, far from being a cure for autism, a behavior modification program, suited to the individual family's needs and possibilities, can achieve a lot of good in autism, particularly with regard to reduction of major behavior problems, but that IQ and "basic" autism dysfunctions remain unchanged or only marginally positively affected (Hadwin *et al.* 1997). Howlin has advocated a program that includes highly-structured, slow and gradual change, which, in our experience, has been very successful. Bryna Siegel is of the opinion that behavior modification can be very useful in autism, but that 10-20 hours a week, by and large, may be a more realistic frame than the extreme intensity of the Lovaas program (Siegel 1996).

Whatever one's opinion about the relative merits of behavior modification in autism, almost all authorities agree that all intervention programs do and should include measures involving positive behavioral reinforcement. We use such measures in our clinical care of patients with autism and related disorders and find them generally helpful. However, we do not accept the use of punishment in behavior modification programs. We believe that it is unethical to punish individuals who are already suffering under the burden of the severe functional impairment that we call autism.

Special education interventions

The majority of individuals with classic autism and disintegrative disorder also suffer from mental retardation. It should therefore come as no surprise that they require special approaches and measures in the various fields of education. The social, communicative and imaginative impairments associated with autism call for more specific approaches than those that may be sufficient for children and adolescents with mental retardation without autism.

The majority of individuals with Asperger syndrome are not mentally retarded. Indeed, quite a large proportion are of good or superior overall intelligence. Nevertheless, there are cognitive peculiarities and neuropsychological deficits, particularly in the fields of communication and executive functions, and special education interventions are therefore very often required in this group as well.

A model – or rather "philosophy" – for educational interventions in autism spectrum disorders has been developed by Eric Schopler, Margaret Lansing, Gary Mesibov and their group at Chapel Hill, North Carolina. Generally referred to as TEACCH (Treatment and Education of Autistic and other Communication-handicapped Children), the program includes several elements that, by and large, have now become generally accepted as necessary cornerstones in most intervention recommendations for individuals on the autism spectrum (Schopler 1989). These include:

1   A high degree of structure, including a fairly rigorous curriculum for daily-life activities, school subjects, areas that need particular training and leisure activities.
2   A high degree of continuity over time, with regard to people involved in training, physical environment for training, and time of day set aside for training.
3   A highly individualized approach acknowledging the wide degree of variability encountered in autism in terms of intellectual level, degree of autism impairments, and level of general skills.
4   An emphasis on concrete – often, and if possible, visual – ways of teaching subjects and skills.
5   A long-term perspective with regular developmental and educational "check-ups."
6   Acceptance of underlying developmental disorder and a respectful attitude to the individual with autism and his/her family, who need to be informed about and involved in all aspects of intervention.

The North Carolina group has been able to demonstrate that, when the above elements are included in the education program, important gains for the affected individual can be made in most areas (possibly excepting IQ), and that psychosocial adjustment and quality of life for individual and family can be improved.

It has been our experience over several decades that, particularly with regard to middle- and low-functioning individuals with autism, the TEACCH philosophy has a lot to offer affected individuals, and that families, teachers and other professionals are much better able to cope if education/intervention is planned along TEACCH guidelines. It can be very helpful in Asperger syndrome also, but it has to be applied in a very flexible way in these high-functioning individuals within the autism spectrum.

A few studies have been published looking at the effects of trying to educate young children with autism in the field of theory of mind (Ozonoff and Miller 1995, Hadwin *et al.* 1997). Even though children receiving intensive training improve their capacity to solve theory-of-mind tasks in a laboratory setting, so far, it seems that such improvement may not be accompanied by corresponding gains in a real-life setting. However, it does seem reasonable, based on the experience from other interventions in autism, that further training in real-life settings might improve real-life skills. Further studies are needed before generalized recommendations can be issued to the effect that young children with autism should receive specific theory-of-mind training.

Other interventions
Over the years, a plethora of therapies has been suggested to be useful in the treatment of individuals affected by autism. These include dance therapy, pony therapy, dolphin therapy, art therapy, holding therapy, facilitated communication, and auditory integration training. So far, these "alternative" interventions share the common feature of either never having been put under rigorous scientific scrutiny, or having been shown to be of no specific positive value in autism. This is not to say that there may not be any positive effects from these therapies, only that they cannot be recommended for the treatment of the basic impairments characteristic of autism.

Summary

Behavioral and educational modes of intervention have been demonstrated to have positive effects in autism, even though it is too early as yet to say whether they affect the basic impairments in autism in a long-lasting way. All current intervention programs for autism should include an individualized special education curriculum tailored to meet the developmental and educational needs of the child or adolescent (or adult) with the autism spectrum disorder. An element of positive behavior modification should be part of every long-term management plan. There is a need for intensified behavioral intervention research in the whole field of autism and Asperger syndrome. Until more such research is carried out, there is no basis for extravagant claims for miracle cures or extreme improvements.

REFERENCES

Hadwin, J., Baron-Cohen, S., Howlin, P., Hill, K. (1997) 'Does teaching theory of mind have an effect on the ability to develop conversation in children with autism?' *Journal of Autism and Developmental Disorders*, **27**, 519–537.

Lovaas, I., Calouri, K., Jada, J. (1989) 'The nature of behavioural treatment and research with young autistic persons.' *In:* Gillberg, C. (Ed.) *The Nature of Behavioural Treatment and Research with Young Autistic Persons.* New York: Plenum Press, pp. 285–305.

Ozonoff, S., Miller, J.N. (1995) 'Teaching theory of mind: a new approach to social skills training for individuals with autism.' *Journal of Autism and Developmental Disorders*, **25**, 415–433.

Schopler, E. (1989) 'Diagnosis and treatment of autism.' *In:* Gillberg, C. (Ed.) *Diagnosis and Treatment of Autism.* New York: Plenum Press, pp. 167–183.

Siegel, B. (1996) *The World of the Autistic Child: Understanding and Treating Autistic Spectrum Disorders.* New York: Oxford University Press.

19
THE NEUROLOGY OF AUTISM

Children with autism struggle through their developmental sequences as best they can, often in quite unusual ways. An investigation of an 8-year-old boy with autism showed that he was acquiring his phonological system in at least a partly unique way, showing some typical patterns as well as some patterns that rarely appear in normally developing children (Wolk and Edwards 1993). Males are more affected with autism than females, particularly in the apparently higher IQ levels (Volkmar *et al.* 1993). In this higher-functioning group, males are rated to be more severely autistic than females on several measures of early social development but not in other areas (McLennan *et al.* 1993).

These children with autism challenge many previous concepts of developmental brain function and present us with major riddles. In this final chapter, we shall attempt to integrate what is known about autism and to delineate what is not known. The task is not easy. Individuals with an autistic syndrome present in different ways and follow different courses throughout life. Some have marked regressions; others do not. Some develop speech; others do not. Some improve at the end of early childhood; others do not. Some develop seizures; others do not. Some are low-functioning, while others are so high-functioning it is hard to believe that they have the syndrome.

The autistic syndrome comprises a number of disease processes that begin in the fetal and infant brain. We view trying to understand the neurology of autism (the behavioral syndrome) as a task not dissimilar to trying to decipher the neurology of mental retardation (the more cognitively defined syndrome). These are very, very complex questions that make it inappropriate to bemoan the fact that no coherent theory of autism has emerged at this time of medical history.

Human infants are dependent upon the physical and emotional environmental climate provided by their caregivers, yet we do not blame their parents when they develop mental retardation, even though we know that intensive stimulation of a baby can improve the cognitive profile. In the same spirit, we must accurately diagnose each child with an autistic syndrome regarding their underlying disease entity, if that is possible, and give the parents the kind of knowledge and support services that they need to raise a child whose brain is functioning poorly with resulting major behavioral problems.

The question that has been asked by each generation of investigators studying the autistic syndrome is: what information do we have that identifies underlying lesions in a young brain that could lead to such a major dysfunction of the central nervous system? An attempt to present working hypotheses to that question is presented here.

In neurology, the classic questions to answer regarding a patient's lesion are *where* is it? – followed by *what* is it? In pediatric neurology, an additional question is often highly relevant, particularly in young children; that question is *when* did it happen? In this chapter, we shall set up a series of working hypotheses trying to answer these questions, based on current knowledge in the field of autism.

Where?

Question: Which side of the brain is involved in autism, left or right?

Working hypothesis: Both or either.

When neuroscientists first began thinking about where a lesion in the brain might result in autistic symptoms, both the left and right sides of the brain came under careful consideration (Geschwind and Behan 1982, Geschwind and Galaburda 1985). The left side of the brain was of interest because up to half of all individuals with the diagnosis of autism remained mute. Speech processing is not bilateral by the time adulthood is reached; in approximately 98 per cent of adults who are right-handed, linguistic analysis is performed in left brain structures. The possibility of left brain damage was also of interest because of the research flowing from studies of split brain studies, which showed that, when the left brain is not working, the brain tends to think quite literally, a phenomenon documented in some children with autism.

The alternative possibility of right brain dysfunction *also* was of interest for a number of reasons (Sabbagh 1999). One was that children with autism appear to be less lateralized than normal controls of the same age, based on handedness studies. Language processing may be exclusively based in the right hemisphere in up to a third of adults who are ambidextrous or left-handed (Caplan 1995). (However, there is some evidence of involvement of bilateral processing in humans in using the language system (Howard *et al.* 1992), so caution is indicated regarding generalizations.) In a study by Ozonoff and Miller (1996), pragmatic language measures sensitive to right-hemisphere damage were administered to non-retarded adults with autism and to controls matched on age and intellectual ability; subjects with autism performed significantly less well than controls on all measures. This study was similar to a study of right-hemisphere stroke patients (Molloy *et al.* 1990). It should be noted that the statistically significant increase in left-handedness and ambiguous-handedness found in patients with autism, with all that it implies, is not unique. Non-right-handedness in autism is no greater than that found in children with learning disabilities (Cornish and McManus 1996), Down syndrome or epilepsy (Lewin *et al.* 1993). Also, regarding the comparison with stroke patients, caution is needed when comparing developmental with acquired lesions.

However, the right brain was also of interest because this appears to be the site of non-verbal communication – such as gestures and patterns of emphasis that express emotion – which is an area of major difficulty in children with autism. In speaking children with autism, there is difficulty in using language appropriately in social contexts, and in using and interpreting conversational gestures and the emotional tones of speech of other people; this type of language disability is also thought to involve the communicative centers of the right hemisphere (Brumback *et al.* 1996). It is interesting that problems in non-verbal communication, in the presence of apparently normal verbal ability, raise the question of whether Asperger syndrome may be primarily a right-brain disease entity.

Perhaps the most puzzling finding about right/left brain differences in autism is from a study of brain enlargement in autism that showed predominant right-sided enlargement (Piven *et al.* 1996).

Small first suggested in 1976 that there might be unusual cerebral lateralization in autism. Her studies found that children with autism failed to have the higher EEG voltages over the left hemisphere that are found in healthy children, and she raised the question of whether there actually might be a partial or full failure of cerebral lateralization in autism. Indirect backing of the failure of cerebral lateralization hypothesis is found in studies using a non-invasive imaging technique called transcranial ultrasonic Doppler method, which measures the flow dynamics of the middle cerebral arteries. Using auditory stimulation to evoke responses, Bruneau *et al.* (1992) have shown that children with autism display a symmetrical pattern of flow responses – in marked contrast to the lateralized patterns in normal children, and even to the less symmetrical but also still lateralized responses in mentally retarded children. The lack of the usual hemisphere specialization has also been documented by SPECT imaging, comparing children with autism to age-matched normal controls who had greater regional cerebral blood flow to the left side (Chiron *et al.* 1995). The pattern of equal regional cerebral blood flow to both hemispheres seen in the children with autism was independent of handedness, sex and age. This disruption of normal cerebral asymmetries is not unique to autism; it can also be found in patients with dyslexia, attention deficit disorder, Tourette's syndrome and schizophrenia (Peterson 1995).

Reversal of the usual asymmetry of the brain has also been demonstrated. A recent PET study of high-functioning adults with autism showed reverse hemisphere dominance during verbal auditory stimulation (Müller *et al.* 1999). Siegel *et al.* (1992) used PET studies to show that the anterior rectal gyrus region of the brain in autism had left>right asymmetry instead of the usual right>left asymmetry.

Plasticity is a documented characteristic of infant brains, although there is some evidence that the extent of plasticity of the brain of a young child may not be as great as originally thought (Vargha-Kadem *et al.* 1985). A question has been raised about whether plasticity will occur in an infant brain if there is not a specific traumatic event which triggers it, leading to questions regarding the differential effect of prenatal developmental lesions versus postnatal traumatic lesions, which are the basis of much of the documentation regarding brain plasticity. However, in spite of many unresolved issues regarding plasticity of the infant brain, the success that has sometimes been demonstrated in autism by types of behavior modification therapy could be interpreted as modifications of still-plastic neural circuitry of the infant brain (Perry *et al.* 1995), and the very rare spontaneous recovery of a young child from the symptoms of autism must be attributed to change in at least one of the brain systems underlying what is called plasticity. One of the most dramatic examples of the plasticity of the infant brain is a neurosurgical hemispherectomy to remove an epileptic focus in a young child; these children grow up with essentially normal cognition and behavior, with only half of the brain that most children have. It can be argued that the demonstrated success of hemispherectomy operations raises profound questions about the likelihood of functional bilaterality of disease entities of very young children when they do not overcome major handicaps of the central nervous system, either cognitively or in the realms of behavior, as they grow up.

Bilaterality of dysfunction of the cerebral cortex has been demonstrated in both children and adults with autism, using the newest imaging techniques, in several studies. One example is the study of regional cerebral blood flow in six young, severely autistic children, where the temporal and parietal lobes were shown to be bilaterally abnormal, with the lower values in the left hemisphere (Mountz *et al.* 1995). However, other studies using slightly different techniques and a different patient group found little or no difference in cerebral blood flow (see Chapter 14 for a review of all studies).

A more certain way of identifying lesions can be found in patients with tuberous sclerosis who have brain tubers visible on MRI. Although presence of bilateral tubers can be demonstrated in patients with tuberous sclerosis who are not autistic, the converse (unilateral tubers in patients who are autistic) does not seem to be the case (Jambaqué *et al.* 1991). Bilateral lesions (hypodense areas in the temporal regions on both sides by CT) can also be demonstrated in patients with autism and a history of herpes simplex encephalitis (Ghaziuddin *et al.* 1992). Even children with unusual forms of autism appear to have bilateral lesions; children with autism and documented visual agnosia display bilateral lesions. One child, with a right temporo-occipital cortical dysplasia surgically removed at the age of 7 years, was shown to have a left frontal hypometabolism together with the right occipital defect (Jambaqué *et al.* 1998). A 2-year-old, with a visual agnosia characterized by aspects of associative and apperceptive agnosia, was found by MRI to have bilateral temporo-occipital and right temporal encephalomalacia (Mottron *et al.* 1997).

It should be noted that autistic patients with one-sided lesions pose an apparent problem to any bilaterality hypothesis. There are clear-cut examples of one-sided lesions, such as the case of autistic regression reported by Neville *et al.* (1997), where the patient had a right-sided temporal lobe tumor. In this tumor patient, however, there was prior evidence of subclinical seizure activity in both temporal lobes by EEG. Another example is infants with infantile spasms who have seizure-free outcomes after resection of a focal one-sided epileptogenic lesion (H.T. Chugani *et al.* 1993, Wyllie *et al.* 1998). However, these patients all had bilateral hypsarrhythmia on EEG prior to the surgery. This phenomenon, of bilateral functional disability accompanying a one-sided structural lesion, is well documented in many examples of unilateral lesions of the brain in neurology.

For a hypothesis to be valid in science, it should have predictive value. In 1996, a paper was published indicating a laboratory test that could predict DSM-IV autism in a great majority of the patient group under study (H.T. Chugani *et al.* 1996). Out of more than 100 babies with the infantile spasm syndrome, these authors were able to follow 14 out of the 18 babies who had a special pattern by PET study of brain glucose utilization. What these infants demonstrated was a bilateral hypometabolism limited to the temporal lobes on PET studies. In the prospective study of long-term outcome of the 14 children who were able to be followed-up, 10 (71 per cent) met DSM-IV criteria for autism. They all also had severe developmental delay and minimal or absent language development.

The authors state that patients with infantile spasms and bitemporal glucose hypo-metabolism on PET comprise a relatively homogeneous group – whose likely outcome can be predicted. It is possible that some of them may have had tuberous sclerosis, as in the Calderon Gonzalez *et al.* tuberous sclerosis series (1994), where 5 out of 7 of the children with autism had infantile spasms. This paper also states that the difference between the children who did or did not have autism appears to be related, to a great extent, to the anatomical location of tubers.

EXACTLY WHERE?

Exactly where in the brain are the lesions that result in autistic symptoms? Are they lesions in specific anatomical locations, or are they dysfunctions of certain metabolic pathways in the brain, or exactly what are we talking about?

To start with neuroanatomy, in 1998 Kates *et al.* used an imaging study to define neuroanatomical differences in a pair of monozygotic male twins discordant for strictly defined autism. The unaffected twin, while not fulfilling the full range of autism, did have constrictions in social interaction and play. On MRI, the affected twin had smaller caudate, amygdaloid and hippocampal volumes and smaller cerebellar vermis lobules VI and VII, in comparison with his brother. However, both twins evidenced disproportion-ately reduced volumes of the superior temporal gyrus and the frontal lobe, relative to unaffected peers. A look at these six anatomical areas of the brain in individuals with autism, plus other anatomical areas suggested by the research literature, will now be undertaken.

PREFRONTAL AND FRONTAL LOBE

Problems with the medial prefrontal cortex have been demonstrated by modern imaging techniques in Asperger's syndrome, in high-functioning patients with autism, and in 13-year-olds with autism (see Chapter 14). Recently, dysfunction of the circuitry of the prefrontal cortex (and its connections with the parietal cortex) has been shown by tasks involving visual saccades (Minshew *et al.* 1999). In autistic patients with macrocephaly, the frontal lobes are not enlarged in the presence of enlargement of the temporal, parietal and occipital lobes by MRI (Piven *et al.* 1996); this could be interpreted either positively or negatively. Focal regions of decreased uptake of alpha[^{11}C]methyl L-tryptophan, inter-preted as serotonin, have been shown in the frontal cortex of boys with autism (D.C. Chugani *et al.* 1999).

THE PARIETAL LOBE

A retrospective review of SPET techniques found focal areas of decreased perfusion in posterior parietal area in 10 out of 23 young children with autism (Ryu *et al.* 1999). It is of interest that the area of thinning of the corpus callosum, discussed below, has fibers primarily from the posterior parietal area. In groups of tests that reflect parietal lobe func-tion, the neurological abnormalities detectable by clinical examination were significantly greater for autistic subjects than for normal controls (Haas *et al.* 1996).

THE OCCIPITAL LOBE

Several electrophysiological studies have shown that there is a subgroup of children with autism with significantly smaller visual event-related potential P3 waves (Verbaten *et al.* 1991). It has been suggested that this means that there is understimulation of the occipital lobe by visual stimuli in autistic children (Kemner *et al.* 1995). Although there are cases of visual agnosia and autism in the literature (Mottron *et al.* 1997, Jambaqué *et al.* 1998), the cases involve other lobes such as the temporal lobe.

THALAMUS

The thalamus has been proposed as a dysfunctional nucleus in autism because "the thalamus is a grey matter substation serving auditory, visual and tactile pathways. The only sensory system not processed through the thalamus – the olfactory pathway – is also the only system which appears to be quite intact in many young autistic children" (Coleman 1978, see also Coleman 1979). There is evidence from electrophysiological, autonomic, occupational therapy (Ermer and Dunn 1998) and behavioral studies, indicating that some young children with autism may have impairments in the registration, processing and response to those external stimuli that transverse the thalamus. On the other hand, besides clinical observations (where children with autism identify newcomers by smelling them), there is evidence that olfaction is intact in autism. A research study of unpleasant odors, rated by facial responses, found them more accurately classified in 10 mute children classified as PPD than in matched normal controls (Soussignan *et al.* 1995). A retrospective review of SPET studies in young children with autism found focal areas of decreased perfusion of the thalamus in 19 out of 23 of these children (Ryu *et al.* 1999). Focal regions of decreased uptake of alpha[^{11}C]methyl-L-tryptophan in the thalamus have been reported in boys with autism (Chugani *et al.* 1999) and it is known that a disruption of synaptic connection in sensory cortical regions can result from experimental increase or decrease of brain serotonin before puberty.

THE BASAL GANGLIA

The adventitious movements seen in some children with autism have raised concerns about basal ganglia function in such patients. These adventitious movements include hand-flapping, patting, clasping and posturing, facial grimacing, choreic and athetotic postures, jumping and rocking (Walker and Coleman 1976). There is a CT study showing evidence of bilateral caudate atrophy in nine adults with autism (Jacobson *et al.* 1988); in contrast, MRI scans of 35 relatively high-functioning persons with autism (Sears *et al.* 1999), as well as studies of the fragile X syndrome, show evidence of increased volume in the caudate (see Chapter 11). A retrospective review of SPET studies in young children with autism found focal areas of decreased perfusion of the basal ganglia in 5 out of 23 of these children (Ryu *et al.* 1999).

THE CORPUS CALLOSUM

Megaloencephaly is now well documented in the brains of some individuals with autism (see Chapter 14). In view of this finding, it appeared puzzling when reports were published of a corpus callosum diminished in size, even including an MRI study where enlarged cortical lobes were reported (Piven et al. 1996). It was in 1992 that Filipek et al. noted that the corpus callosum was significantly smaller in individuals with autism in their study. In 1993, Courchesne et al. noted thinning of the corpus callosum, especially along the posterior body, in 2 out of 21 patients with autism. In 1994, Berthier observed posterior thinning of the corpus callosum in subjects with Asperger syndrome. Egaas et al. (1995) and Saitoh et al. (1995) reported smaller areas of the posterior subregions of the corpus callosum of autistic persons. To check whether it might be a decrease of myelin rather than a decrease of axons, this group performed an NMR study on the corpus callosum and interpreted their results to mean that callosal narrowing was due to diminution in the number of axons (Belmonte et al. 1995). An MRI study of 35 subjects with autism compared them to age- and IQ-matched healthy controls and adjusted all results for total brain size; again a decrease was reported in the body and posterior subregions of the corpus callosum (Piven et al. 1997a). The same group of patients had previously been shown to have regional brain enlargement (Piven et al. 1996). The posterior subregions of the corpus callosum, described as thin in so many of these studies, are where parietal cortical fibers are concentrated. It is of note that one set of developmental studies that shows thinning or abnormal development of the corpus callosum is the set of studies in patients with subcortical heterotopia (Barkovich 1996). A recent careful study by MRI of the seven subregions of the corpus callosum in 27 low-IQ individuals with autism found significantly smaller corpus callosum, most marked in the body (Manes et al. 1999).

Postmortem studies are in their infancy; however, brains of two autistic individuals have shown thinning (Guerin et al. 1996) and abnormal development (Bailey et al. 1998) of the corpus callosum.

THE TEMPORAL LOBE
There is both clinical and experimental evidence from animals suggesting that the medial temporal lobe, more specifically the amygdaloid complex, may be involved in autistic behaviors (Bachevalier 1994). Human studies of bilateral amygdala damage, either due to stereotaxic operation (Scott et al. 1997) or Urbach-Wiethe disease (Adolphs et al. 1995), show impairment of interpreting the facial expression of emotion in the presence of normal perception of faces, and impairment of perception of the intonation patterns essential to the perception of vocal affect, despite otherwise normal hearing. Functional MRI studies also point to the temporal lobes (Baron-Cohen et al. 1999). Tumors have been reported in autistic patients in both temporal lobes, and SPECT and SPET studies have demonstrated hypoperfusion of the temporal lobes in some patients (see Chapter 14). In fact, bilateral hypometabolism of the temporal lobes in early infancy has been used to predict DSM-IV autism (H.T. Chugani et al. 1996). Patients with early-life bilateral hippocampal sclerosis, who have isolated bilateral anterior temporal lobe hypometablism by PET, have deficits similar to those of severe infantile autism (DeLong and Heinz 1997). Neuropsychological findings in young children with autism have also suggested functional abnormality of the medial temporal lobe (Dawson 1996, Dawson et al. 1998). (See also the limbic system, discussed next.)

The Limbic System

The limbic system consists of the olfactory nerves, tract, nucleus and gyri, the pyriform lobe, the amygdaloid complex of nuclei, the fornix, hippocampal formation, including the dentate gyrus and subiculum, the cingulate and parahippocampal gyrus and septal areas. Intimately related to the limbic system are other important brain structures such as the hypothalamus, medial part of the thalamus, the prefrontal cortex and anterior commissure.

In neuropathological studies of autism, Kemper and Bauman (1998) found small, densely distributed neurons in the amygdala, the entorhinal cortex, the septal nuclei, and the hippocampus, especially in fields CA1 and CA4. They interpreted their results as evidence of maturational delay in autism which is confined to the limbic system. Dopamine selectively inhibits the direct cortical pathway to the CA1 hippocampal region (Otmakhova and Lisman 1999). It should be noted that the UBE3A gene of chromosome 15, whose silencing results in one of the double syndromes (Angelman syndrome), is expressed solely from the murine maternal chromosome in the hippocampus and cerebellar Purkinje cells (see Chapter 15). A theory that autism may be a developmental syndrome of hippocampal dysfunction has been proposed (DeLong 1992). An MRI study of part of the limbic system (the hippocampus proper including the subiculum and the dentate gyrus) was performed by Saitoh *et al.* (1995) on 33 autistic patients, aged 6 to 42 years, comparing them to 23 age-matched normal healthy volunteers. No significant difference was demonstrated; while another study found the hippocampus and amygdala reduced in volume, particularly in relation to total brain volume (Aylward *et al.* 1999). Hippocampal volume can be reduced by seizure activity.

Because of the clinical presentation of autism, the limbic system seems an obvious place to look for lesions; the hippocampal area has particularly strong representation in studies. Yet some are disappointed that not more data has turned up for the limbic system as a whole. However, if one turns from areas of deficit to areas of strength in autism, at least part of the limbic system may be performing well or even at a compensatory superior level. The most functional sensory system of many children with autism is the olfactory system, which is part of the limbic pathways. Also, there is increasing evidence that some aspects of memory, whose pathways include the amygdala and the hippocampus, may be intact and working in some dimensions, at least in savants. There is even evidence that the ability to process affect in musical stimuli is not beyond the reach of some children with autism or Asperger syndrome (Heaton *et al.* 1999).

Brainstem

As early as 1964, Rimland raised the question of whether the brainstem, in particular the reticular formation, might be involved in the cognitive dysfunction of autism. There have been several studies which found the pons to be anatomically altered (smaller or shortened) in patients with autism (see the Rodier study discussed below, and the studies discussed in Chapter 14). In 1986, a short-latency somatosensory evoked potential study performed by Hashimoto *et al.* described a larger brainstem latency in autism. However, since then, at least 11 auditory brainstem response studies in autism, designed to test the integrity of auditory brainstem pathways, have produced contradictory results to date

(Klin 1993). These studies are said to be suggestive, rather than supportive, of brainstem involvement in autism.

CEREBELLUM

The cerebellum, mostly studied regarding its role in movement and motor control, is now understood to be involved in cognition (Schmahmann 1997). At one point, it was hoped that hypoplasia of cerebellar vermal lobules VI and VII might be a marker for autism. But this finding was found to be neither consistent nor unique for autism (Schaefer *et al.* 1996). It is not that cerebellar abnormalities in autism have not been found in the 15 autopsy and quantitative MRI reports from nine laboratories involving a total of 226 cases of autism (Courchesne *et al.* 1994). Both hypoplasia and hyperplasia of the posterior vermis and hemispheres have been reported. Posterior vermal lobules VI and VII were originally singled out as the most hypoplasic. But they are not specific to autism; they are seen in other neurogenetic syndromes in children without autism and even in leukemia patients who have had radiation to the brain (see Chapter 14). In a careful MRI study of 35 autistic subjects and 36 controls, Piven *et al.* (1997b) found no abnormalities in the size of cerebellar lobules VI and VII, but did find that the volume of the total cerebellum was significantly increased. On the other hand, postmortem studies from the major neuropathological centers to date agree on little else, but mostly are consistent in reporting Purkinje neuron loss in the cerebellar cortex (see Chapter 14). The UBE3A gene, whose silencing causes a double syndrome (Angelman syndrome), is expressed from the murine maternal chromosome in the hippocampus and cerebellar Purkinje cells. A retrospective review of SPET with correlative MRI found that focal areas of decreased perfusion occurred in the cerebellar hemispheres in 20 out of 23 young children who met DSM-IV criteria for autism (Ryu *et al.* 1999); this was the highest percentage of this study. A study of alpha [11C]methyl-L-tryptophan with PET found an increased uptake in the dentate nucleus of the cerebellum, where Purkinje cells project (Chugani *et al.* 1997). In groups of tests that reflect cerebellar function, the neurological abnormalities detectable by clinical examination were significantly greater for autistic subjects than for normal controls (Haas *et al.* 1996). It should be noted that cerebellar mutism and personality changes have followed surgical removal of medulloblastoma of the cerebellum in children.

A finding of marked cerebellar dysplasia on MRI can be of value in the differential diagnosis of autism; within the autistic syndrome, certain disease entities are much more likely to have cerebellar dysplasia (see Chapter 16).

Extra question: Approximately half of all children with autism do not speak. Is their brain affected differently compared to children with autism who do speak?

Working hypothesis: Although there undoubtedly are neurodevelopmental difficulties elsewhere in the central nervous system in mute patients, it has been suggested that some of the children do not speak because they may have a selective loss of neurons in the motor nuclei of cranial nerves which control human speech.

Lack of spoken words is a part of the overall lack of communication that so characterizes many children with autism. Lack of spoken and gestural utterance are most likely related, and it can be argued that the same neural system may be responsible for the control of both voice and hands at the level of initiation of motor activity (Hammond (Ed.) 1990). In the case of autistic children who are able to communicate by typing, even though they remain virtually mute, the question arises as to whether there is any possible additional factor that might prevent vocal communication.

One putative answer to that question has arisen from careful study of some of the double syndromes. Thalidomide can lead to autism when exposure occurs during the period between the 20th and 24th day of gestation, around the time of closure of the neural tube (see Chapter 11). The neurological deficits of the thalidomide children with autism indicate that they have sustained injuries to the cranial nerve motor nuclei. Moebius syndrome (see Chapter 11) is a syndrome of cranial nerve damage; it has a higher percentage of cases with autism than most of the other double syndromes. In 1996, Rodier *et al.* autopsied the brainstem of a non-thalidomide case of autism and compared it with a control brain. The brainstem of the autopsy case showed abnormalities predicted by thalidomide cases; it also showed shortening of the brainstem between the trapezoid body and the inferior olive. Other neuropathological cases have also shown evidence of shortened brainstems and problems with the inferior olive (see Chapter 14). A possible rat model of the developmental injury that might cause autism has been developed by Rodier *et al.* (1997). Rodier bombarded mother rats with 350 mg/kg of valproic acid (a teratogen which can cause autism (see Chapter 11)) during the time of gestational neural tube closure in rats. Neuron counts showed reductions of cell numbers in the cranial nerve motor nuclei, particularly the earliest-forming motor nuclei (V and XII). Rodier *et al.* (1996) concluded that the autopsy data, combined with the experimental data from rats, led to the hypothesis that injuries occurring during or just after neural plate closure can lead to a selective loss of neurons derived from the basal plate of the rhombencephalon. This adds two new lines of evidence that place the initiating injury for some forms of autism around the time of neural tube closure. An MRI study in 1992, which found the midbrain and pons to be significantly smaller compared to the size of the cranium in patients with autism, reported that the reduction in brainstem tended to be greater in the low DQ/IQ group – who were presumably more likely to be mute – compared to the higher-functioning children (Hashimoto *et al.* 1992).

There must, however, be a caveat to this interesting work. Widespread indirect effects are common, particularly regarding exact timing of neuropathological factors in the developing central nervous system. The role of the cerebellum in language development is not yet understood. Further neuropathological data from a series of mute cases are needed.

SUMMARY OF WHERE?

Since there is evidence from all over the central nervous system regarding a possible lesion in autism, no focal defect has been consistently demonstrated. Structural abnormalities do not necessarily indicate the site of the pathogenic process, although they are often helpful in diseases of the central nervous system. Also, methodological problems make comparisons between studies difficult. Functional neuroimaging has emphasized the unusual balances between interregional and interhemispheric brain metabolism and blood flow (Deb and Thompson 1998). Abnormalities of the frontal and prefrontal lobes, temporal lobes, corpus callosum and cerebellum stand out among the research findings to date. The combination of two centers – the hippocampus and the cerebellum – has a selectively high expression of FMRI (the fragile X syndrome) and UBE3A (the gene silenced in Angelman syndrome). The recent identification of impairment of thalamic and parietal perfusion awaits further verification. Shortening of the brainstem may turn out to be a relevant finding, especially in mute individuals. However, it should be kept in mind that a single pathogenic process, such as an enzyme abnormality, may result in widespread impairment of multiple areas of the central nervous system. The answer may not lie in neuroanatomy *per se* in many cases. There is simply no substitute for identification of the underlying basic disease process, individual by individual.

What?

Question: What causes autism?

Working hypothesis: Autism is an etiologically heterogeneous entity caused by many different diseases; it is a final common pathway syndrome based on the fact that there are only a finite number of ways for so young a brain to react to injury.

The symptoms of autism are caused by a variety of different etiologies; in reality, there is no such disease as "autism"; there is only the autistic syndrome. Many of the findings discussed throughout this book are based on studies of autistic patients grouped together as one entity, yet these studies reinforce the heterogeneity of the autistic syndrome over and over again. There are now many established subgroups.

There is strong evidence that many of the underlying disease entities have a genetic basis. A number of different genetic patterns have already been demonstrated in disease entities which include patients with autism (see Chapter 15). A genetic hypothesis – the imprinted X-liability threshold – has been suggested to explain the preponderance of males in autism (Skuse 2000). Non-genetic factors may also be relevant, as suggested by the "two hit hypothesis." In such disease entities, a second hit is thought to be needed in addition to the genetic error. The second hit might be a somatic mutation caused by infection, toxins, background radiation or other environmental factors. Based on what has been found so far in molecular biology studies in general, it is likely that most of the monogenetic diseases that present with autistic symptoms will be identified as rare diseases.

The relevance of infectious diseases to autism is poorly understood and is a major area for research. The excess of March birthdays in children with autism is striking (Gillberg 1990, Mouridsen *et al.* 1994) and raises the question of whether some susceptible fetuses were exposed to viral pandemics in those falls/winters prior to the excess of March birthdays. The role of immune and autoimmune abnormalities found in many children with autism will have to be explained on either an infectious or genetic basis.

SUMMARY OF WHAT?

Autism is not one disease; it is not a medical diagnosis. It is many disease entities that occur in the central nervous system at the earliest time periods in the life of a child, pushing that child's development and behavior into abnormal patterns. To find out *what* is wrong with a child, there is no substitute for an individualized work-up to identify that child's particular disease entity.

When?

Question: When, during development, is the central nervous system vulnerable to being damaged so that autistic symptoms result?

Working hypothesis: The autistic syndrome is, in most cases, a neurodevelopmental syndrome beginning during fetal life. In addition, very occasionally, injuries can occur to the brain perinatally or postnatally.

Studies from many different disciplines – neuropathology (see Chapter 14), neurophysiology (McClelland *et al.* 1992), modern imaging studies (see Chapter 14), and evidence from the multiple congenital anomaly (MCA) syndromes which have a subgroup with autism – all point toward an intrauterine maturational defect in autism. Thus, in trying to determine exactly when a brain insult has occurred in a child with autism, there is information available from a number of disciplines. What needs to be determined is the developmental timing of such an insult, with its possible disruption of a critical phase of neurogenesis, in fetuses that survive the insult.

Patients with autistic features can be classified in many ways. One way of classifying them is by the presence or absence of dysmorphic facial and other physical stigmata (see Chapter 16). The brain seems vulnerable to developing future autistic features during both the first and second trimesters. The first trimester time window of vulnerability (seen in thalidomide cases, patients with Moebius syndrome, etc.) would be the period when children with autism who have dysmorphic facial features are most likely to have been damaged. On the other hand, injury during the second trimester time window (as seen in rubella autism, diseases with malformations of cortical development, etc.) would occur at a time after the face is fully formed, so the disease process has no distorting effect on the facial features or the rest of the body (Coleman 1994). (Also, non-stigmatized facial features would also be seen in any etiology of the autistic symptoms that occur in the perinatal or postnatal period.)

Regarding the first trimester time window, thalidomide embryopathy associated with autism appeared to be limited to the period 20–24 days after conception (Stromland *et al.* 1994). Also, autopsy and quantitative magnetic resonance imaging have identified abnormalities in specific areas of the brain in individuals with autism (Courchesne 1997). These are the areas where neurogenesis of certain neuron types occurs during approximately the fifth week of gestation. Specifically what has been found is dysgenesis of the facial nucleus, increased neuron-packing density of the medial, cortical and central nuclei of the amygdala and medium septum, agenesis of the superior olive, hypoplasia of the brainstem and posterior cerebellum, and reduced numbers of Purkinje neurons. There is evidence from Moebius syndrome that uterine contractions, either occurring naturally or brought about by abortifacient drugs, may result in the syndrome during the gestational six- to seven-week time frame. The pattern of malformations in Moebius syndrome and the fetal cocaine syndrome (both of which have subgroups of children with autistic features) suggests that there is a zone of vascular vulnerability or ischemic sensitivity in the paramedian region of the developing brainstem during this period – Leong and Ashwell (1997) found mineralized foci in paramedian wedge-shaped areas of the pontine and medullary tegmentum in the postmortem examination of the brain of an infant with Moebius syndrome.

Regarding the second trimester window, this also appears to be a time of special risk for autism, as, for example, in the cases of infection during a pregnancy that result in a child with autism (Coleman 1994). In the only prospective study ever completed of pre-natal factors, comparing children who developed early childhood psychosis with normal and mentally retarded controls, there was a statistically significant finding of second trimester bleeding limited to the mothers of the psychotic children (Torrey *et al.* 1975). The second trimester is when human malformations of cortical development, formerly known as neuronal migration disorders, occur. The emerging molecular genetics of brain malformation is beginning to unravel the complex signaling mechanisms that regulate cortical assembly. It is already established that genetically inherited disorders of human migration represent important etiologies of epilepsy and mental retardation – will autism be next? In autistic studies (see Chapter 14), it is interesting that the malformations of cortical development (pachygyria, macrogyria, polymicrogyria) in the brain have been reported primarily in high-functioning individuals with autism and Asperger syndrome, if a review is limited to imaging studies. The apparent concentration of these neuronal migration anomalies in the higher-functioning groups adds to the speculation that many children with autism who are little stigmatized and have adequate language may have suffered second, rather than first, trimester insults.

However, the greater detail possible in neuropathological studies indicates that individuals with autism who are characterized as lower-functioning may also have evidence of abnormalities or malformations of cortical development, suggesting that their disease processes were also present during the second trimester. If these children are stigmatized, this could be interpreted to represent a continuation of processes that began earlier in gestation.

Is the perinatal period another period of special risk? This appears to be a rare phenomenon. Several large, case-controlled studies have demonstrated that obstetrical complications at the time of birth do not appear to increase the risk for later autism (Piven *et al.* 1993, Cryan *et al.* 1996). Family studies suggest that obstetric abnormalities in autistic subjects may derive from previous abnormality in the fetus in the first place (Bolton *et al.* 1994). However, there are cases of autism that have a history of neonatal herpes encephalitis (see Chapter 11).

Finally, there is some evidence that disease processes may occur or may continue in some patients with autism well after the perinatal period. Quite rarely, an early childhood illness, such as meningitis, may be implicated. There is also data suggesting that the underlying disease entity might sometimes continue forward from prenatal to postnatal periods. The macrocephaly data (see Chapter 14) suggests that the overgrowth could be related to mistakes in the programming for adequate pruning as the central nervous system grows (Minshew 1996). Neuropathology data raise the possibility of a continuing disease process during childhood in some cases (Kemper and Bauman 1998).

Conclusion

There are a finite number of ways in which the infant brain can respond to injury. Two of them are autism and mental retardation, both syndromes of early life that have many different etiologies. There is overwhelming evidence for organicity in both disorders. The organicity may show itself in diverse ways. Both mental retardation and the autistic syndromes have large numbers of children with abnormal cranial circumferences; however, a microcephalic child is likely to be retarded; a macrocephalic child might possibly have autism.

Of course, it should be noted that the distinctions between the two groups of children, the retarded and the autistic, are often not so clearly defined in any particular patient, perhaps because both suffer damage to the central nervous system during the same time period of early life. Retarded individuals had a prevalence of a strictly defined autistic disorder (DSM-III-R) of 11.7 per cent in one study (Nordin and Gillberg 1996); the figure rises to 20 per cent for autistic symptoms in general. Conversely, large numbers of children who meet the strictest criteria of autism have real or apparent intellectual limitations, although some are normal or gifted.

Autism, in most cases, appears to be due to a neurodevelopmental disease process of the central nervous system – a cascade of neurodevelopmental abnormalities that lead to neural misconnection, which leads, in turn, to impaired behaviors. The disease process usually begins *in utero*, although occasional cases occur postpartum. In most of the diseases involved, genetic factors can be identified; other factors include infectious and toxic insults to the brain.

Is there one medical therapy for autism, or is such a therapy likely to be developed? The answer is "no," just as there is no one medical therapy for mental retardation. There is simply no way of avoiding the painstaking task of diagnosing each child, one by one (see Chapter 16), in a search for an exact diagnosis which might lead to rational family counseling and targeted educational and medical treatment. Research in autism has accelerated in recent years; many of today's puzzling findings are likely to be explained by future studies. A possible animal model of autism – the GS guinea-pig (Castron *et al.* 1998) – has become available. Early diagnosis is an important goal; both infectious and metabolic factors could, theoretically, yield to targeted therapies.

A number of children with autism are now entering regular classrooms, thanks to early educational programs and pharmacotherapy. This is a major move forward in the field, even though the children usually carry with them other problems, such as social or attention-span deficits. We look forward to the day when these beautiful, enigmatic children can be identified in the neonatal period, or very early in life, and receive medical and educational therapies designed for major amelioration or actual reversal of their individual disease processes.

REFERENCES

Adolphs, R., Tranel, D., Damasio, H., Damasio, H.R. (1995) 'Fear and the human amygdala.' *Journal of Neuroscience*, **15**, 5879–5891.

Aylward, E.H., Minshew, N.J., Goldstein, G., Honeycutt, N.A., Augustine, A.M., Yates, K.O., Barta, P.E., Pearlson, G.D. (1999) 'MRI volumes of amygdala and hippocampus in non-mentally retarded autistic adolescents and adults.' *Neurology*, **53**, 2145–2150.

Bachevalier, J. (1994) 'Medial temporal lobe structures and autism: a review of clinical and experimental findings.' *Neuropsychologia*, **32**, 627–648.

Bailey, A., Luthert, P., Dean, A., Harding, B., Janota, I., Montgomery, M., Rutter, M., Lantos, P. (1998) 'A clinicopathological study of autism.' *Brain*, **121**, 889–905.

Barkovich, A.J. (1996) 'Subcortical heterotopia: a distinct clinicoradiologic entity.' *AJNR American Journal of Neuroradiology*, **17**, 1315–1322.

Baron-Cohen, S., Ring, H.A., Wheelwright, S., Bullmore, E.T., Brammer, M.J., Simmons, A., Williams, S.C. (1999) 'Social intelligence in the normal and autistic brain: an fMRI study.' *European Journal of Neuroscience*, **11**, 1891–1898.

Belmonte, M., Egaas, B., Townsend, J., Courchesne, E. (1995) 'NMR intensity of corpus callosum differs with age but not with diagnosis of autism.' *Neuroreport*, **6**, 1253–1256.

Berthier, M.L. (1994) 'Corticocallosal anomalies in Asperger's syndrome.' (Letter) *AJR American Journal of Roentgenology*, **162**, 236–237.

Bolton, P., Macdonald, H., Pickles, A., Rios, P., Goode, S., Crowson, M., Bailey, A., Rutter, M. (1994) 'A case-controlled family history study of autism.' *Journal of Child Psychology and Psychiatry*, **35**, 877–900.

Brumback, R., Harper, C., Weinberg, W. (1996) 'Nonverbal learning disabilities, Asperger's syndrome, pervasive developmental disorder – should we care?' (Editorial) *Journal of Child Neurology*, **11**, 427–429.

Bruneau, N., Dourneau, M.C., Garreau, B., Pourcelot, L., Lelord, G. (1992) 'Blood flow response to auditory stimulations in normal, mentally retarded, and autistic children: a preliminary transcranial Doppler ultrasonographic study of the middle cerebral arteries.' *Biological Psychiatry*, **32**, 691–696.

Calderon Gonzalez, R., Trevino Welsch, J., Calderon Sepulveda, A. (1994) 'Autism in tuberous sclerosis.' (In Spanish) *Gaceta Medica de Mexico*, **130**, 374–379.

Caplan, D. (1995) 'The cognitive neuroscience of syntactic processing.' *In:* Gazzaniga, M.S. (Ed.) *The Cognitive Neurosciences.*, Cambridge, Mass.: MIT Press.

Castron, J., Yon, E., Mellier, D., Godfrey, H.P., Delhaye-Bouchard, N., Mariani, J. (1998) *Supplement . . . to the European Journal of Neuroscience*, **10**, 2677–2684.

Chiron, C., Leboyer, M., Leon, F., Jambaqué, I., Nuttin, C., Syrota, A. (1995) 'SPECT of the brain in childhood autism: evidence for a lack of normal hemisphere asymmetry.' *Developmental Medicine and Child Neurology*, **37**, 849–860.

Chugani, D.C., Muzik, O., Rothermel, R., Behen, M., Chakraborry, P., Manger, T., de Silva, E.A., Chugani, H.T. (1997) 'Altered serotonin synthesis in the dentatothalamocortical pathway in autistic boys.' *Annals of Neurology*, **14**, 666–669.

Chugani, D.C., Muzik, O., Behen, M., Rothermel, R., Janisse, J.J., Lee, J., Chugani, H.T. (1999) 'Developmental changes in brain serotonin synthesis capacity in autistic and nonautistic children.' *Annals of Neurology*, **45**, 287–295.

Chugani, H.T., Shewmon, D.A., Shields, W.D., Sankar, R., Comair, Y., Vintero, H.V., Peacock, W.J. (1993) 'Surgery for intractable infantile spasms: neuroimaging perspectives.' *Epilepsia*, **34**, 764–771.

Chugani, H.T., Da Silva, E., Chugani, D.C. (1996) 'Infantile spasms: III. Prognostic implications of bitemporal hypometabolism on positron emission tomography.' *Annals of Neurology*, **39**, 643–649.

Coleman, M. (1978) 'The autistic syndromes.' *In:* Wortis, J. (Ed.) *Mental Retardation and Developmental Disabilities. Volume X.* New York: Brunner/Mazel Inc., pp. 65–76.

—— (1979) 'Studies of the autistic syndromes.' *In:* Katzman, R. (Ed.) *Congenital and Acquired Cognitive Disorders.* New York: Raven Press, pp. 265–275.

—— (1994) 'Second trimester of gestation: a time of risk for classical autism?' *Developmental Brain Dysfunction*, **7**, 104–109.

Cornish, K.M., McManus, I.C. (1996) 'Hand preference and hand skill in children with autism.' *Journal of Autism and Developmental Disorders*, **26**, 597–609.

Courchesne, E. (1997) 'Brainstem, cerebellar and limbic neuroanatomical abnormalities in autism.' *Current Opinion in Neurobiology*, **7**, 568.

Courchesne, E., Press, G.A., Yeung-Courchesne, R. (1993) 'Parietal lobe abnormalities detected by MR in patients with infantile autism.' *AJR American Journal of Roentgenology*, **160**, 387–393.

Courchesne, E., Townsend, J., Saitoh, O. (1994) 'The brain in infantile autism: posterior fossa structures are abnormal.' *Neurology*, **44**, 214–223.

Cryan, E., Byrne, M., O'Donovan, A., O'Callaghan, E. (1996) 'Brief report: A case–control study of obstetric complications and later autistic disorder.' *Journal of Autism and Developmental Disorders*, **26**, 453–460.

Dawson, G. (1996) 'Neuropsychology of autism: a report on the state of the science.' *Journal of Autism and Developmental Disorders*, **26**, 179–184.

Dawson, G., Meltzoff, A.N., Osterling, J., Rinaldi, J. (1998) 'Neuropsychological correlates of early symptoms of autism.' *Child Development*, **69**, 1276–1285.

Deb, S., Thompson, B. (1998) 'Neuroimaging in autism.' *British Journal of Psychiatry*, **173**, 299–302.

DeLong, G.R. (1992) 'Autism, amnesia, hippocampus, and learning.' *Neuroscience and Biobehavioral Review* , **16**, 63–70.

DeLong, G.R., Heinz, E.R. (1997) 'The clinical syndrome of early-life bilateral hippocampal sclerosis.' *Annals of Neurology*, **42**, 11–17.

Egaas, B., Courchesne, E., Saitoh, O. (1995) 'Relative size of the corpus callosum in autism.' *Archives of Neurology*, **52**, 794–801.

Ermer, J., Dunn, W. (1998) 'The Sensory Profile: A discriminant analysis of children with and children without disabilities.' *The American Journal of Occupational Therapy*, **52**, 283–290.

Filipek, P.A., Richelme, C., Kennedy, C.N., Rademacher, J., Pitcher, D.A., Zidel, S., Caviness, V.S. (1992) 'Morphometric analysis of the brain in developmental language disorders and autism.' (Abstract) *Annals of Neurology*, **32**, 475.

Furtado, S., Suchowersky, O., Rewcastle, B., Graham, L., Klimek, M.L., Garber, A. (1996) 'Relationship between trinucleotide repeats and neuropathological changes in Huntington's disease.' *Annals of Neurology*, **39**, 132–136.

Geschwind, N., Behan, P. (1982) 'Left-handedness: association with immune disease, migraine and developmental learning disorders.' *Proceedings of the National Academy of Sciences USA*, **79**, 5097–5100.

Geschwind, N., Galaburda, A.M. (1985) 'Cerebral lateralization: biological mechanism, associations and pathology.' *Archives of Neurology*, **42**, 428–454.

Ghaziuddin, M., Tsai, L.Y., Eilers, L., Ghaziuddin, N. (1992) 'Brief report: Autism and herpes simplex encephalitis.' *Journal of Autism and Developmental Disorders*, **22**, 107–113.

Gillberg, C. (1990) 'Do children with autism have March birthdays?' *Acta Psychiatrica Scandinavica*, **82**, 152–156.

Guerin, P., Lyon, G., Barthélémy, C., Sostak, E., Chevrollier, V., Garreau, B., Lelord, G. (1996) 'Neuropathological study of a case of autistic syndrome with severe mental retardation.' *Developmental Medicine and Child Neurology*, **38**, 203–211.

Haas, R.H., Townsend, J., Courchesne, E., Lincoln, A.J., Schreibman, L., Yeung-Courchesne, R. (1996) 'Neurologic abnormalities in infantile autism.' *Journal of Child Neurology*, **11**, 84–92.

Hammond, G.R. (Ed.) (1990) *Cerebral Control of Speech and Limb Movements*. Amsterdam: North-Holland.

Hashimoto, T., Tayama, M., Miyao, M. (1986) 'Short latency somatosensory evoked potentials in children with autism.' *Brain and Development*, **8**, 428–432.

Hashimoto, T., Tayama, M., Miyazaki, M., Sakurama, N., Yoshimoto, T., Murakawa, K., Kuroda, Y. (1992) 'Reduced brainstem size in children with autism.' *Brain Development*, **14**, 94–97.

Heaton, P., Hermelin, B., Pring, L. (1999) 'Can children with autistic spectrum disorders perceive affect in music? An experimental investigation.' *Psychological Medicine*, **29**, 1405–1410.

Howard, D., Patterson, K., Wise, R., Brown, W.D., Friston, K., Weiler, C., Frackowiak, R.S.J. (1992) 'The cortical locations in language and language-impaired children.' *Brain*, **115**, 1769–1782.

Jacobson, R., Le Couteur, A., Howlin, P., Rutter, M. (1988) 'Selective subcortical abnormalities in autism.' *Psychological Medicine*, **18**, 39–48.

Jambaqué, I., Cusmai, R., Curatolo, P., Cortesi, F., Perrot, C., Dulac, O. (1991) 'Neuropsychological aspects of tuberous sclerosis in relation to epilepsy and MRI findings.' *Developmental Medicine and Child Neurology*, **33**, 698–705.

Jambaqué, I., Mottron, L., Ponsot, G., Chiron, C. (1998) 'Autism and visual agnosia in a child with right occipital lobectomy.' *Journal of Neurology, Neurosurgery and Psychiatry*, **65**, 555–560.

Kates, W.R., Mostofsky, S.H., Zimmerman, A.W., Mazzocco, M.M., Landa, R., Warsofsky, I.S., Kaufmann, W.E., Reiss, A.L. (1998) 'Neuroanatomical and neurocognitive differences in a pair of monozygous twins discordant for strictly defined autism.' *Annals of Neurology*, **43**, 782–791.

Kemner, C., Verbaten, M.N., Cuperus, J.M., Camfferman, G., van Engeland, H. (1995) 'Auditory event-related brain potentials in autistic children and three different control groups.' *Biological Psychiatry*, **38**, 150–165.

Kemper, T.L., Bauman, M. (1998) 'Neuropathology of infantile autism.' *Journal of Neuropathology and Experimental Neurology*, **57**, 645–652.

Klin, A. (1993) 'Auditory brainstem responses in autism: brainstem dysfunction or peripheral hearing loss?' *Journal of Autism and Developmental Disorders*, **23**, 15–23.

Leong, S., Ashwell, K.W. (1997) 'Is there a zone of vascular vulnerability in the fetal brain stem?' *Neurotoxicology and Teratology*, **19**, 265–275.

Lewin, J., Kohen, D., Mathew, G. (1993) 'Handedness in mental handicap: investigation into populations of Down's syndrome, epilepsy and autism.' *British Journal of Psychiatry*, **163**, 674–676.

McClelland, R.J., Eyre, D.G., Watson, D., Calvert, G.J., Sherrard, E. (1992) 'Central conduction time in childhood autism.' *British Journal of Psychiatry*, **160**, 659–663.

McLennan, J.D., Lord, C., Schopler, E. (1993) 'Sex differences in higher functioning people with autism.' *Journal of Autism and Developmental Differences*, **23**, 217–227.

McManus, I.C., Murray, B., Doyle, K., Baron-Cohen, S. (1992) 'Handedness in childhood autism shows a dissociation of skill and handedness.' *Cortex*, **28**, 373–381.

Manes, F., Piven, J., Vrancic, D., Nanclares, V., Plebst, C., Starkstein, S.E. (1999) 'An MRI study of the corpus callosum and cerebellum in mentally retarded autistic individuals.' *Journal of Neuropsychiatry and Clinical Neuroscience*, **11**, 470–474.

Minshew, N.J. (1996) 'Brief report: Brain mechanisms in autism: functional and structural abnormalities.' *Journal of Autism and Developmental Disorders*, **26**, 205–209.

Minshew, N.J., Luna, B., Sweeney, J.A. (1999) 'Oculomotor evidence for neocortical systems but not cerebellar dysfunction in autism.' *Neurology*, **52**, 917–922.

Molloy, A.M., Brownell, H.M., Gardner. *In:* Joanette, Y., Brownell, H.M. (Eds) (1990) *Discourse Ability and Brain Damage: Theoretical and Empirical Perspectives.* New York: Springer-Verlag, pp. 113–130.

Mottron, L., Mineau, S., Decarie, J.C., Jambaqué, I., Labrecque, R., Pepin, J.P., Aroichane, M. (1997) 'Visual agnosia with bilateral temporo-occipital brain lesions in a child with autistic disorder: a case study.' *Developmental Medicine and Child Neurology*, **39**, 699–705.

Mountz, J.M., Tolbert, L.C., Lill, D.W., Katholi, C.R., Liu, H.G. (1995) 'Functional deficits in autistic disorder: characterization by technetium-99m-HMPAO and SPECT.' *Journal of Nuclear Medicine*, **36**, 1156–1162.

Mouridsen, S.E., Nielsen, S., Rich, B., Isager, T. (1994) 'Season of birth in infantile autism and other types of childhood psychoses.' *Child Psychiatry and Human Development*, **25**, 31–43.

Müller, R.-A., Behen, M.E., Rothermel, R.D., Chugani, D.C., Muzik, O., Manger, T.J., Chugani, H.T. (1999) 'Brain mapping of language and auditory perception in high functioning autistic adults: a PET study.' *Journal of Autism and Developmental Disabilities*, **29**, 19–30.

Neville, B.G., Harkness, W.F., Cross, J.H., Cass, H.C., Burch, V.C., Lees, J.A., Taylor, D.C. (1997) 'Surgical treatment of severe autistic regression in childhood epilepsy.' *Pediatric Neurology*, **16**, 137–140.

Nordin, V., Gillberg, C. (1996) 'Autism spectrum disorders in children with physical or mental disability or both. I: Clinical and epidemiological aspects.' *Developmental Medicine and Child Neurology*, **38**, 297–313.

Onodero, O., Idezuko, J., Igarashi, S., Takiyama, Y., Endo, K., Takano, H., Oyake, M., Tanaka, H., Inuzuka, T., Hayashi, T., Yuasa, T., Ito, J., Miyatake, T., Tsuji, S. (1998) 'Progressive atrophy of cerebellum and brainstem as a function of age and the size of the expanded CAG repeats in the *MJD1* gene in Machado-Joseph disease.' *Annals of Neurology*, **43**, 288–296.

Otmakhova, N.A., Lisman, J.E. (1999) 'Dopamine selectively inhibits the direct cortical pathway to the CA1 hippocampal region.' *Journal of Neuroscience*, **19**, 1437–1445.

Ozonoff, S., Miller, J.N. (1996) 'An exploration of right-brain hemisphere contributions to the pragmatic impairments of autism.' *Brain and Language*, **52**, 411–434.

Perry, R., Cohen, I., DeCarlo, R. (1995) 'Case study: deterioration, autism and recovery in two siblings.' *Journal of the American Academy of Child and Adolescent Psychiatry*, **34**, 232–237.

Peterson, B.S. (1995) 'Neuroimaging in child and adolescent neuropsychiatric disorders.' *Journal of the American Academy of Child and Adolescent Psychiatry*, **34**, 1560–1576.

Piven, J., Simon, J., Chase, G.A., Wzorek, M., Landa, R., Gayle, J., Folstein, S. (1993) 'The etiology of autism: pre-, peri- and neonatal factors. *Journal of the American Academy of Child and Adolescent Psychiatry*, **32**, 1256–1263.

Piven, J., Arndt, S., Bailey, J., Andreasen, N. (1996) 'Regional brain enlargement in autism: magnetic resonance imaging study.' *Journal of the American Academy of Child and Adolescent Psychiatry*, **35**, 530–536.

Piven, J., Bailey, J., Ranson, B.J., Arndt, S. (1997a) 'An MRI study of the corpus callosum in autism.' *American Journal of Psychiatry*, **154**, 1051–1056.

Piven, J., Saliba, K., Bailey, J., Arndt, S. (1997b) 'An MRI study of autism: the cerebellum revisited.' *Neurology*, **49**, 546–551.

Rimland, B. (1964) *Infantile Autism: The Syndrome and its Implications for a Neural Theory of Behavior.* Englewood Cliffs, NJ: Prentice-Hall.

Rodier, P.M., Ingram, J.L., Tisdale, B., Nelson, S., Romano, J. (1996) 'Embryological origin for autism: developmental anomalies of the cranial nerve nuclei.' *Journal of Comparative Neurology*, **370**, 247–261.

Rodier, P.M., Ingram, J.L., Tisdale, B., Croog, V.J. (1997) 'Linking etiologies in humans and animal models: studies of autism.' *Reproductive Toxicology*, **11**, 417–422.

Ryu, Y.H., Lee, J.D., Yoon, P.H., Kim, D.I., Lee, H.B., Shin, Y.J. (1999) 'Perfusion impairments in infantile autism on technetium-99m ethyl cysteinate dimer brain single-photon emission tomography: comparison with findings on magnetic resonance imaging.' *European Journal of Nuclear Medicine*, **26**, 253–259.

Sabbagh, M.A. (1999) 'Communicative intentions and language: evidence from right-hemisphere damage and autism.' *Brain Language*, **70**, 29–69.

Saitoh, O., Courchesne, E., Egaas, B., Lincoln, A.J., Schreibman, L. (1995) 'Cross-sectional area of the posterior hippocampus in autistic patients with cerebellar and corpus callosum abnormalities.' *Neurology*, **45**, 317–324.

Schaefer, G.B., Thompson, J.N. Jr., Bodensteiner J.B., McConnell, J.M., Kimberling, W.J., Gay, C.T., Dutton, W.D., Hutchings, D.C., Gray, S.B. (1996) 'Hypoplasia of the cerebellar vermis in neurogenetic syndromes.' *Annals of Neurology*, **39**, 382–385.

Schmahmann, J.D. (1997) 'Rediscovery of an early concept.' *International Review of Neurobiology*, **41**, 3–21.

Scott, S.K., Young, A.W., Calder, A.J., Hellawell, D.J., Aggleton, J.P., Johnson, M. (1997) 'Impaired auditory recognition of fear and anger following bilateral amygdala lesions.' *Nature*, **385**, 254–257.

Sears, L.L., Vest, C., Mohamed, S., Bailey, J., Ranson, B.J., Piven, J. (1999) 'An MRI study of the basal ganglia in autism.' *Progress in Neuropsychopharmacology and Biological Psychiatry*, **23**, 613–624.

Siegel, B.V. Jr., Asarnow, R., Tanguay, P., Call, J.D., Abel, L., Ho, A., Lott, I., Buchsbaum, M.S. (1992) 'Regional cerebral glucose metabolism and attention in adults with a history of childhood autism.' *Journal of Neuropsychiatry and Clinical Neuroscience*, **4**, 406–414.

Skuse, D.H. (2000) 'Imprinting, the X-chromosome, and the male brain: explaining sex differences in the liability to autism.' *Pediatric Research*, **47**, 9–16.

Small, J.G. (1976) 'EEG and neurophysiological studies of early infantile autism.' *Biological Psychiatry*, **10**, 385–397.

Soussignan, R., Schaal, B., Schmidt, G., Nadel, J. (1995) 'Facial responsiveness to odours in normal and pervasively developmental disordered children.' *Chemical Senses*, **20**, 47–59.

Stromland, K., Nordin, V., Miller, M., Akerstrom, B., Gillberg, C. (1994) 'Autism in thalidomide embryopathy: a population study.' *Developmental Medicine and Child Neurology*, **36**, 351–356.

Torrey, E.F., Hersh, S.P., McCabe, K.D. (1975) 'Early childhood psychosis and bleeding during pregnancy: a prospective study of gravid children and their offspring.' *Journal of Autism and Childhood Schizophrenia*, **5**, 287–297.

Vargha-Kadem, F., O'Gorman, A.M., Watters, G.V. (1985) 'Aphasia and handedness in relation to hemispheric side, age of injury and severity of cerebral lesion during childhood.' *Brain*, **108**, 677–696.

Verbaten, M.N., Roelofs, J.W, van Engeland, H., Kenemans, J.K., Slangen, J.L. (1991) 'Abnormal visual event-related potentials of autistic children.' *Journal of Autism and Developmental Disorders*, **21**, 449–470.

Volkmar, F.R., Szatmari, P., Sparrow, S.S. (1993) 'Sex differences in pervasive developmental disorders.' *Journal of Autism and Developmental Disorders*, **23**, 579–591.

Walker, H.A., Coleman, M. (1976) 'Characteristics of adventitious movements in autistic children.' *In:* Coleman, M. (Ed.) *The Autistic Syndromes*. Amsterdam: North-Holland.

Wolk, L., Edwards, M.L. (1993) 'The emerging phonological system of an autistic child.' *Journal of Communication Disorders*, **26**, 161–177.

Wyllie, E., Comair, Y.G., Kotagal, P., Bulacio, J., Bingaman, W., Ruggieri, P. (1998) 'Seizure outcome and epilepsy surgery in children and adolescents.' *Annals of Neurology*, **44**, 740–748.

APPENDIX 1
GLOSSARY OF GENETIC TERMS

Although medical vocabulary used in this book will be obvious to most professional readers, there has been such rapid recent development of molecular genetics that a glossary might be of value for some busy clinicians. Also, for the student and educated lay reader, a number of standard terms in genetics and a few less familiar medical terms are defined.

Alleles (allelomorphic genes).   Alleles are genes that are located at the same locus on the same chromosome and that are concerned about the same category of information, with a very slight variation from each other. For example, the genes of blood groups A, B and O are alleles. A null allele fails to produce the gene product – a protein.

Aneuoploid/aneuoploidy.   Any number of chromosomes other than the diploid number of 46 chromosomes or, in the gametes, the haploid number of 23.

Anticipation/genetic anticipation (in a family history).   This is the phenomenon of the worsening of the disease phenotype over successive generations. In family histories with anticipation, a grandparent may have the disease in the first generation, the parent in the second generation and an infant in the third generation. Naturally, the clinical presentation of the disease looks somewhat different in different generations because the age of the patient at time of onset determines how the body and brain react to the genetic insult. (For the mechanism causing anticipation, see *Trinucleotide repeat expansion.*)

Autosomes.   Autosomal chromosomes, in pairs, are chromosome numbers 1 to 22 (in contrast to the gonosomes).

Chromatin.   The DNA-protein complex which forms chromosomes is termed chromatin during the interphase of the cell.

Chromosomes.   By microscope, chromosomes appear as threadlike concentrations of nuclear chromatin visible during meiosis and mitosis. In actuality, they are single linear duplex DNA molecules complexed with numerous proteins. The parts of a chromosome are:

- the *centromere*, which is the constricted middle section of the chromosome which divides it into long and short arms.
- the *long arm*, which is called 'q'.
- the *short arm*, which is called 'p' (from the French 'petit', meaning small).
- the *telomeres* (at the ends of the arms).

The aberrations of chromosomes include:

isodidentric chromosome
monosomy
ring chromosome
tetrasomy
trisomy.

Codon. In the coding sequence of a gene, each set of three DNA bases forms a codon, the genetic code for the incorporation of one of the 20 amino acids found in proteins. A codon is a triplet of bases in a DNA molecule that codes for one amino acid.

Continuous gene syndrome. Recognizable pattern of malformation associated with the loss of several genes that are physically adjacent to each other on a critical chromosome segment. Example: velocardiofacial/DiGeorge syndrome (deletion 22q11.21).

Deletion. A part of the chromosomal arm is missing.

Diploid. Two haploid sets of 23 chromosomes each = 46 chromosomes.

DNA (deoxyribonucleic acid). A sequence of nucleotides, usually double-stranded. Each DNA molecule is a long chain made up of four basic chemical building blocks called nucleotides. A nucleotide can have any of the four bases: adenine (A), thymine (T), guanine (G), or cytosine (C). These nucleotides, in sets of three called trinucleotides or DNA triplets, are the alphabet of inheritance.

Dominant trait. A trait that is expressed in the phenotype in the heterozygous state.

Duplication. The presence of a segment of a chromosome in a double amount on the same chromosome.

Exons. Coding parts of genes for structural proteins (non-coding parts are called *introns*).

Gamete. Mature germ-cell of either sex (ovum or sperm) with a haploid set of 23 chromosomes in normal circumstances.

Genes. Units of genetic information consisting of DNA. The double-stranded macromolecule DNA consists of two complementary strands that wrap around one another to form a double helix. Each strand is a linear arrangement of nucleotides with four different bases: adenine (A), thymine (T), cytosine (C) and guanine (G). The two DNA strands are held together by hydrogen bonds formed between the complementary bases G and C, or between A and T. The genes are divided into regions, such as:

promoter region
extron
intron.

Genomic imprinting. A phenomenon seen in autosomes where there is inactivation of genes or chromosomal regions on one of two matched chromosomes. This leads to preferential expression of an allele depending upon its parental origin. This results in transmission of a disease in a manner that is dependent upon the sex of the transmitting parent (see *Imprinting* below).

Gonosomes. The chromosomes that determine the sex of the individual, called X and Y, also called the 23rd pair of chromosomes. XX = female; XY = male.

Haploid/haplotype/haploidy. One set of 23 chromosomes, as found in the gametes.

Holoprosencephaly. A brain malformation where the forebrain is not divided into two hemispheres but consists of a single sac enclosing an undivided ventricle (holosphere). The corpus callosum, septum pellucidum and falxum cerebri are absent. The diencephalon and thalmi are fused and the rhinencephalon may be single or totally absent.

Imprinting. The expression of a gene sequence is dependent on parent of origin; the process operates at the transcriptional level and usually involves differential DNA methylation. (Methylation, a very complex process, has some function in silencing the expression of a gene.) Example: Angelman syndrome (deletion of maternal allele).

Inversion. A fragment of a chromosome may break off, become inverted, and fuse again with the same chromosome so that a distorted sequence of genes results.

Isochromosome. Chromosome with two identical halves (sometimes two identical short arms, sometimes two identical long arms).

Isodicentric. Chromosome complexes with two centromeres.

Messenger RNA (mRNA). The protein-coding instructions found in the DNA sequence of a gene are first transcribed into mRNA. The mRNA is translocated from the nucleus of a cell into its cytoplasm, where it is translated by ribosomes into a string of amino acids (protein synthesis).

Microsatellite markers. Throughout the human genome, there are tandem repeats of simple sequence (di-, tri-, tetranucleotide repeats) that occur frequently and randomly. These microsatellite markers are highly polymorphic due to the variation in the number of repeat units, and the rate of mutation is low enough to allow their use in genetic analysis. Because they are short (<100bp) and surrounded by unique sequence DNA, they can easily be detected by the Polymerase Chain Reaction (PRC).

Mitochondria and their DNA. The mitochondria are organelles in the cytoplasm of the cell that generate energy for cellular processes. They have their own unique extra-chromosomal DNA which is distinct from the DNA in the nucleus and is either sporadic (usually deletions) or inherited maternally (usually point mutations). Each mitochondrion contains 2 to 10 DNA molecules, and each cell contains multiple mitochondria. Thus, normal and mutant mitochondrial DNA can coexist within the same cell. This condition, known as *heteroplasmy*, allows an otherwise lethal mutation to persist. *Homoplasmy* is the presence of either consistently normal or consistently mutant mitochondrial DNA. Complexes I, II, III and V may be encoded by either mtDNA or nuclear DNA; Complex IV is encoded only by nuclear DNA.

312

Mosaicism (mixoploidy). Two or more cell populations (clones), each with a different karyotype, in the same individual.

Mutation. A mutation can be defined as any change in the primary nucleotide sequence of DNA. Mutations involving single nucleotides are known as point mutations. Mutations referred to in this book include:

> *Base substitutions*
> *Deletions*
> *Insertions*
> *Missense point mutation* – a substitution of the exact order of nucleotides in the coding region of a gene
> *Splicing or splice site mutation* – mutations in the intronic sequences may create splice donor or splice acceptor sites, resulting in an abnormally spliced mRNA from the mutated gene.

Pseudoautosomal region (PAR). The sections on the X and Y chromosomes that share homology.

Recessive trait. A trait which is only expressed in the phenotype if it is in the homozygous state.

RFLPs. Restricted fragment length polymorphisms, or suite of DNA markers; they are inherited.

Ring chromosome. A chromosome in the form of a ring. There is deletion in the long and short arms and fusion of the two breakpoints, forming a ring.

RNA (Ribonucleic acid). A sequence of nucleotides, usually single-stranded.

Transgenes. Foreign genes introduced directly into the nucleus of a fertilized egg, integrated into nuclear DNA, and expressed in the phenotype. These are genetic chimera.

Translocation. Transfer of a piece of one chromosome to another chromosome. If two non-homologous chromosomes exchange pieces, the translocation is balanced.

Trinucleotide repeat expansion. The nucleotides in DNA come in sets of three – called trinucleotides or DNA triplets. The trinucleotides often repeat within a gene. The number of repeats can sometimes expand beyond the usual number of repeats. Such expansions (and, rarely, contractions) are associated with malfunction of the gene and a subsequent genetic disease. An example of the abnormal number of repeats is the excessive number of the C(cytosine) G(guanine) G(guanine) sequences in the fragile X syndrome.

Trisomy. Two haploid sets of 23 chromosomes plus one extra chromosome. The total number of chromosomes is 47 (rather than the usual 46).

Uniparental disomy (idiodisomy). The inheritance of two maternal copies of the same chromosome or two paternal copies of the same chromosome.

Zygote. The union of egg and sperm at fertilization.

APPENDIX 2
CHARTER FOR PERSONS WITH AUTISM *

People with autism should share the same rights and privileges enjoyed by all of the European population where such are appropriate and in the best interests of the person with autism.

Those rights should be enhanced, protected and enforced by appropriate legislation in each state.

The United Nations declarations on the Rights of Mentally Retarded Persons (1971) and the Rights of Handicapped Persons (1975) and other relevant declarations on Human rights should be considered and, in particular, for people with autism the following should be included.

1. THE RIGHT of people with autism to live independent and full lives to the limit of their potential.
2. THE RIGHT of people with autism to an accessible, unbiased and accurate clinical diagnosis.
3. THE RIGHT of people with autism to accessible and appropriate education.
4. THE RIGHT of people with autism (and their representatives) to be involved in all decisions affecting their future; the wishes of the individual must be, as far as possible, ascertained and respected.
5. THE RIGHT of people with autism to accessible and suitable housing.
6. THE RIGHT of people with autism to the equipment, assistance and support services necessary to live a fully productive life with dignity and independence.
7. THE RIGHT of people with autism to an income or wage sufficient to provide adequate food, accommodation and the other necessities of life.
8. THE RIGHT of people with autism to participate, as far as possible, in the development and management of services provided for their wellbeing.
9. THE RIGHT of people with autism to appropriate counselling and care for their physical, mental and spiritual health; this includes the provision of appropriate treatment and medication administered in the best interest of the individual with protective measures taken.
10. THE RIGHT of people with autism to meaningful employment and vocational training without discrimination or stereotype; training and employment should have regard to the ability and choice of the individual.

---

* from Europe

11. THE RIGHT of people with autism to accessible transport and freedom of movement.
12. THE RIGHT of people with autism to participate in and benefit from culture, entertainment, recreation and sport.
13. THE RIGHT of people with autism of equal access to and use of all facilities, services and activities in the community.
14. THE RIGHT of people with autism to sexual and other relationships, including marriage, without exploitation or coercion.
15. THE RIGHT of people with autism (and their representatives) to legal representation and assistance and to the full protection of all legal rights.
16. THE RIGHT of people with autism to freedom from fear or threat of unwarranted incarceration in psychiatric hospitals or any other restrictive institution.
17. THE RIGHT of people with autism to freedom from abusive physical treatment or neglect.
18. THE RIGHT of people with autism to freedom from pharmocological abuse or misuse.
19. THE RIGHT of access of people with autism (and their representatives) to all information contained in their personal, medical, psychiatric and educational records.

Presented at the 4th Autism-Europe Congress, Den Haag, May 10th 1992, prepared by the World Autism Organization

The only limits included in the statutes are with regard to the definition of autism, and some basic rights of autistic people which are expressed in the "Autism Europe Charter of Rights":

1 The definition is that of the DSM-IV, stating that autism is a neurological disorder, not a psychogenic disorder;
2 The Charter for Persons with Autism was voted by the general assembly of Autism Europe in 1992 and approved by the European Parliament in 1996 as a basic right for autistic people.

INDEX

Note: page numbers in *italics* refer to figures and tables

321